DATE DUE

DEC 1 0 1990		
NOV 2 6	D U	FEB -8 1984
DEC 1 1990	JAN 2 3 1984	
FEB 1 1 1981	JAN 2 4 1984	
MAR - 4 1981	JAN 2 4 1984	
MAR 2 5 1981	NOV 2 8 1984	
RENEWED APR 2 2 1981		
MAY 2 1981 B R		
MAY - 3 1981	NOV 2 8 1984 B R	
MAR - 3 1982	DEC 3 1984	
MAR 2 4 1982		
MAR 2 3 1982 B R	DEC 5 1986	
MAR 2 2 1982	MAY 1 7 1993	
DEC 1 4 1983		
DEC 5 1983 B R		
DEC 6 1983		

REHABILITATION PRACTICES
WITH THE PHYSICALLY DISABLED

Rehabilitation Practices with the Physically Disabled

EDITED BY

JAMES F. GARRETT AND EDNA S. LEVINE

Columbia University Press

NEW YORK AND LONDON

Library of Congress Cataloging in Publication Data

Garrett, James F.
  Rehabilitation practices with the physically
disabled.
  Includes bibliographies.
  1. Physically handicapped—Rehabilitation—
United States—Addresses, essays, lectures.
  2. Physically handicapped—Rehabilitation—Addresses,
essays, lectures.   I. Levine, Edna (Simon),
II. Title.
HD7256.U5G28   362.4   72-13875
ISBN 0-231-03523-3

For Mary and Morton,
who are with us in these pages

FOREWORD

THIS FOREWORD WAS WRITTEN while Congressional hearings on rehabilitation legislation were underway. Legislative inquiry into the philosophy of rehabilitation, its scope, and its practices is the most penetrating the writer has observed in his more than twenty years in Washington. It is evident that times have changed, not just in general, but in rehabilitation. With the federal investment in rehabilitation programs approaching one billion dollars per annum, the budget makers and the budget watchers are scrutinizing rehabilitation activity much more closely than they ever have before, and the politician is becoming much more interested.

Although rehabilitation agencies have generally been regarded as "accounting" for what they do and the results they achieve better than other human service agencies, it is evident that more accurate and revealing standards of accountability must be developed. Concern is being expressed not for just how *many* are served but also for just *who* are served. Concern is expressed as to whether those who need services the most, the severely disabled, are being served before others who may not be so severely disabled. Concern is expressed for those who are not served. Who are they? What are their needs? What happens to them?

In this connection, Congress is seriously considering whether federal rehabilitation support should be limited to those who have vocational goals which they may be reasonably expected to achieve. Are there not other legitimate rehabilitation goals toward which rehabilitation services should be directed? Does not every handicapped individual deserve the opportunity to become as independent as possible, live as comfortably as possible, whether or not he may be expected to enter the labor market? Congress appears ready to provide resources for the rehabilitation of such people, and the passage of "independent living" legislation this year seems almost sure.

Questions are being asked, also, about research and training programs. Are those educated to be rehabilitationists doing better than those whose entry to rehabilitation activity is incidental? Is research "paying off" in terms of improved services to those traditionally considered to be handicapped and to others whose needs seem to be amendable to rehabilitation services? The spinal cord injured, the renal disease victim, the epileptic individual—all are examples.

Another group of concerns is in the area of social reform. Such concerns include those involving the right of handicapped people to get a good general education and to develop vocational skills; the right to a job one is capable of performing; the right of access to public buildings, housing, and transportation. Most important of all, there is being articulated more clearly than ever before the rights of handicapped individuals to be involved in a meaningful way in the development of policies and procedures that govern the provision of services handicapped people will receive.

To say that there is great public concern for the scope, quality, and procedures in rehabilitation is not to be interpreted as meaning that rehabilitation is under attack. Actually, Congressional committees, as well as other groups who have occasion to study rehabilitation activity, are generally complimentary to these programs. As the House Committee on Education and Labor expressed it in a recent report, rehabilitation programs are too good to be permitted to go their way without public knowledge of their aims, methods, and accomplishments.

Now, let us speak of the book to which this statement is a foreword. Rehabilitation people are known more for the services they deliver than for their literary skills. Fortunately, however, there are some who realize that the only way we can keep from making the same mistakes over and over is the recording of results or experience. James Garrett and Edna Levine are among those who themselves write and encourage others to write. The result of their latest effort is this book, which contains sixteen articles by as many authors, all recognized as individuals who have "lived" the subjects they address. As the title implies, the emphasis is upon *practice,* not theory, or research, but practice: how to apply the knowledge we have in the rehabilitation of handicapped individuals.

The subject matter of the articles is relevant to the concerns which have been expressed here. They consider and report results of rehabilitation efforts directed toward helping some of our most severely handicapped citizens. The book deserves wide distribution and careful reading.

E. B. WHITTEN
Executive Director
National Rehabilitation Association

PREFACE

THERE IS HARDLY a more ubiquitous word today in our lexicon than rehabilitation. We not only have rehabilitation for people, but also for our cities, ghettos, docks, waterfronts, buildings, even our national spirit. That such widespread use of the term connotes acceptance of a concept may be a truism. However, this may also suggest broad confusion.

The concept of restoring an individual to some prior state of well-being has gradually been accepted in our thinking over the past half-century. From modest beginnings with a few medical practitioners and a small state-federal program of vocational rehabilitation, the movement has taken on national and international significance. Agreements in the United States Congress are directed not to the value of the program but to how great the financial return is on every dollar appropriated.

The delivery of rehabilitation services is a complex process. It is regularly accepted that rehabilitation is the restoration of a handicapped individual to his fullest physical, mental, social, vocational, and economic usefulness. The cornerstone of the process is an integrated service delivery system based upon teamwork by diverse professionals and associated personnel. To achieve the depth and variety of service which the handicapped need is the great challenge.

Most of those involved in this service delivery system have been trained for solo practice. Collocation does not per se make for teamwork. Professional prerogatives and legal responsibilities are not readily set aside. Continuity of service presupposes a system—but much of our society is really a nonsystem. Rehabilitation calls for a fine orchestration of services.

Rehabilitation has been called a state of mind, an attitude, a philosophy, a set of methods and techniques, a discipline. It is all of these and more; it is commitment of faith in one's fellow man. It believes in accepting individuals for what they are, in joint or contractual goal setting, in higher levels of aspiration, and in society's commitment to and responsibility for the disadvantaged. For some it is man's response to his fellow man.

Programs for the disabled have shown growth and development over the years. From a vocational training process around a disability, the state-federal vocational rehabilitation agencies now proffer the most comprehensive services in the United States. Medical rehabilitation has grown from its early concern with orthopedics and tuberculosis to every type of physical and mental disability. New professions have evolved—peripetologists, speech and hearing therapists, rehabilitation counselors. Depth has been added to those dealing with the blind, deaf and mentally retarded. Extensive pre- and post-employment training programs have been developed. The research literature has become so extensive that we need new computer techniques to keep current.

At this stage in the growth process, it is well to take a look at the present state of our knowledge. This volume represents an effort to show the variety of disabilities with which rehabilitation deals and the various facets of the process—physical, mental, social, vocational and economic. It deals primarily with physical disabilities for the sake of simplicity, leaving to others the area of mental disabilities.

It is hoped that the complexity of the rehabilitation process will come through clearly in this volume. That handicapped individuals do become restored to constructive community living is a tribute to the dedication of the professional and associated personnel who daily deal with these problems. But it is more a tribute to the courage and capability of the disabled themselves that they take their rightful place in society.

James F. Garrett
Edna S. Levine

CONTENTS

THE REHABILITATION SCENE

WILLIAM GELLMAN

FUNDAMENTALS OF REHABILITATION

THE HEALING AND HELPING DISCIPLINES are interwoven with our cultural history as man's responses to the continuing problems of disability and incapacity. The healing or therapeutic disciplines focus on the prevention, cure, or reduction of disability. The helping or restorative disciplines re-establish capacities which enable disabled persons to resume life's activities. Rehabilitation, primarily a helping discipline, is concerned with restoring disabled man to a productive role as doer and worker.

The concept of rehabilitation as the restoration of function appears in the early traditions of Western man. One could even interpret the story of the Garden of Eden as a metaphorical picture of rehabilitation. Adam, in a sense disabled by eating of the fruit of the tree of knowledge, is forced from the Garden of Eden. He is rehabilitated through the technique of work therapy and trained initially as a tiller of the soil. With time, Adam matures vocationally and becomes an agriculturist. When the story closes, he is engaged in farming, a socially desirable occupation with high prestige.

The tale of Adam, as retold here, outlines a typical rehabilitation sequence which is the model of rehabilitation used in this chapter. The occurrence of a disability results in a handicapping condition which limits ability to function. After vocational evaluation, treatment is initiated which facilitates vocational development. The treatment program

WILLIAM GELLMAN, PH.D., is Executive Director of the Jewish Vocational Service, Chicago, Illinois.

enables the rehabilitant to assume a productive role and to participate more fully in the life of the community. Work is both a means and an end in the process of rehabilitation.

This chapter follows the preceding sequence in discussing rehabilitation as a system of service to disabled persons. Section one describes the rehabilitation world, its background and current concepts. The second section discusses rehabilitation and its relation to other broad service systems. The third describes the rehabilitation process in terms of methodology, rationale, and theory, with emphasis on vocational evaluation. Finally, the fourth section discusses current issues in rehabilitation practice.

THE REHABILITATION WORLD

SCOPE OF DISABILITY

The disabled constitute a significant proportion of the population of the United States. Although there are various estimates of the extent of disability, the precise dimensions of the problem are unknown. In 1969 the National Health Survey reported that 53 million persons were injured in 1967 and estimated an average of about 26 disability days for each occurrence of an illness, impairment, or injury. Senator Dole estimated that some 42 million persons are handicapped in some way, although all of them may not have disabling conditions which restrict activities. The National Center for Health Statistics reported that in 1967 about 22 million persons, or about one out of every ten civilians living outside of institutions, had some activity limitation, and that close to 9 per cent of this group were restricted in their major activity (working, keeping house, school or preschool activities). The National Center estimated that 5 of the 18 million disabled adults between the ages of eighteen and sixty-four could benefit from vocational rehabilitation.

The incidence of disability is increasing because medical, biological, and technological advances are lengthening the life span. The change in life expectancy from 63 years in 1943 to 70.3 years in 1968 has increased the number of persons in our society prone to illness or injury. The National Health Education Committee estimates that improved medical knowledge saved eight million lives between 1944 and 1967 and that of the seven and a half million still alive, about 63 per cent are not working (National Health Education Committee, 1971). The latter are the actual or potential clientele of rehabilitation.

It should be noted that not all disabilities are handicapping. If the diminution in physical, mental, or emotional capacities resulting from disability is minor or temporary, the individual can resume his major activities. He is not handicapped. If the process of disablement is prolonged or if the disability is severe, the resulting impairment may handicap the person and force him to discontinue functioning in important life areas.

The processes of self-depreciation and social disparagement convert the disabled person into a handicapped person who suffers from a social disadvantage which makes achievement difficult. The person with a physical disability may see himself as unable to work and therefore as a worthless, useless human being. He may perceive himself as different or stigmatized. He may be barred from work or from normal social interaction by his own lowered self-esteem resulting from negative attitudes toward him. Changes in appearance, mannerisms, behavior, or performance may lead others to regard him as atypical or deviant.

The restrictions imposed by such handicaps diminish the person's capacity for effective performance in major cultural roles and make attainment of socially approved goals difficult. Whereas disability may be viewed as intraorganismic, handicap is considered a byproduct of society's biases toward the disabled.

The distinction between disability and handicap delineates two aspects of rehabilitation which reflect its role as a healing and a helping discipline: (1) enablement or the elimination or reduction of disabling conditions which cause handicap; and (2) potentiation or the shaping of abilities necessary for adequate role performance in important social realms in spite of handicap.

HISTORICAL BACKGROUND

The cultural web of institutions, customs, and interpersonal relations which routinize social living includes roles for the disabled and nondisabled and expectations about behavior appropriate to those roles. Cues learned in childhood serve as guides for distinguishing various types of handicapped persons and for developing socially accepted patterns of behavior toward them.

Different cultures foster different attitudes toward disabled persons, and vary as to the precision with which disabilities are defined. For example, Eskimos perceive a limited number of disabilities whereas we perceive many. Their language includes a few general terms for the handicapped while we use many differentiating terms, such as epileptic, orthopedically handicapped, cerebral palsied, mental retardate, emotionally disturbed, and more. In the same way, Eskimos have numerous names for different types of snow, while we have only one. India has always accepted the physically handicapped. France gave the blind a place of privilege during the late Middle Ages. The Eskimos left older persons to die. The ancient Greeks disposed of crippled children.

The development and use of rehabilitation is conditioned by cultural predispositions such as these. Jaques (1960) points out that "circumstances surrounding the onset of disability appear to be of importance in terms of social reaction and treatment." If disability is viewed as a natural event or as "the just retribution of the omnipotent God" (St. Augustine), the approach is fatalistic and nature is permitted to take its course with a minimum of medical care. However, if man is viewed as exercising power over nature and if the human being has value, then the healing and the rehabilitative arts are brought into play.

In the United States the approach to handicapped persons incorporates a wide variety of historical attitudes, among them the Greek belief that the physically impaired were inferior, and the preprophetic Hebraic idea that the sick were being punished by God; the early Christian belief that ministering to the handicapped leads to the acquisition of moral virtue; the Calvinistic assumption that the absence of material success resulting from handicap or disability is visible evidence of lack of grace; the Darwinian theory of the survival of the fittest; and the pre-World War I faith in the progress of mankind through science and technology.

This mixture of attitudes resulted in a marked ambivalence toward disability during the period spanning the close of the nineteenth century and the beginnings of the twentieth. The residue of social Darwinism led to the depreciation of the handicapped and the assumption that an obvious disability is a bar to productive living. On the other hand, the belief in technical progress strengthened humanitarian impulses to aid the poor and the sick. Individual philanthropy created voluntary social welfare agencies to help persons in need.

At approximately the same time, interest in rehabilitation was generated by a series of advances in medical care and treatment which increased survival possibilities for the ill and stimulated the development of physical restoration. In 1899 the Cleveland Rehabilitation Center established the first formal rehabilitation program using physical restoration to continue the gains made through medical care. The early rehabilitation programs were medically oriented and rehabilitation was defined "as the use of all those medical measures which expedite recovery" (Kessler, 1950).

The shift from a wholly medical approach occurred a few years later with the incorporation of the work goal in rehabilitation. In 1907 Pastur initiated this modern concept of rehabilitation by establishing a school in Belgium for the vocational training of people who were too disabled to be admitted to existing apprenticeships (Soden, 1949). The rehabilitation goal was thus extended to include improvement of individual earning capacity. The western European countries which adopted this approach to improving opportunities for the handicapped spoke of it as "re-education," the development of abilities and skills.

In 1918 the United States government initiated a national vocational rehabilitation program for disabled World War I veterans. The program emphasized the purchase of prosthetic appliances, training, and assistance for veterans seeking employment. Although the rehabilitation goal was a job for the disabled veteran, the Veterans Administration (VA) program still stressed the physical rather than the psychological aspects of disability. The major rehabilitation technique was physical restoration. The success of the initial program for veterans resulted in Congressional passage of an act in 1920 to develop vocational rehabilitation services for disabled civilians.

The World War II program for veterans was more comprehensive than its predecessor and reached a larger proportion of veterans. It marked a historical milestone for rehabilitation. As summarized by Oberman (1967),

In ten years of operation, ending in December 1953, over 600,000 World War II veterans were placed in rehabilitation training. Near 8,000,000 had entered other forms of training under P.L. 346. By 1947 a staff of over 28,000, including specialists in counseling, training, contract negotiations, and placement had been recruited and trained. Thousands of schools and training establishments had been evaluated and had entered into contracts with the Veterans' Administration to train veterans.

This strengthening of the vocational components of the Veterans Administration program opened new vistas for rehabilitation. The concepts of disability, physical impairment, and handicap were differentiated. The treatment of handicaps now involved a psychosocial approach which included contacts with the community. Education and rehabilitation counseling became important tools, with counseling using a one-to-one interpersonal relationship between the rehabilitator and the rehabilitant as a psychological tool to effect change. The goal of job placement took into account the veteran's choice of an occupation and provided for modifying the choice to meet changes in veterans' or the nation's socioeconomic condition.

The emphasis on vocational rehabilitation, with job placement as a major goal, extended the scope and broadened the concept of rehabilitation. For example, Kessler (1950) defined rehabilitation as "the restoration of the handicapped to the fullest physical, mental, social, vocational and economic usefulness of which he is capable." Rusk (1958) saw rehabilitation as "the third phase of medical care which takes the patient from the bed to the job." Soden (1949) echoed a similar theme when he stated that rehabilitation was more accurately rendered by the word reablement, primarily signifying "restoration."

The passage of the Vocational Rehabilitation Act Amendments of 1954 further reshaped the rehabilitation field. The Act, based upon the World War II experience of the Veterans Administration, strengthened the financial structure and the administration of the rehabilitation program for disabled "civilians." It encouraged the extension of rehabilitation facilities and workshops and authorized the financing of research and demonstration projects to provide new methods for improving the quality of rehabilitation service. The Act also provided for training programs to increase the number of professionally qualified rehabilitators, and permitted nonprofit voluntary organizations to participate directly in the nationwide public vocational rehabilitation program for civilians.

The 1954 amendments opened vocational rehabilitation to inputs from the helping professions and the behavioral sciences by way of the research-demonstration route and partnership with social and vocational agencies in the community. The concept of disability was broadened to include the idea that the effects of disability are persisting and long lasting, that disability is a process rather than a one-time event. Greater attention was paid to the vocational handicap resulting from disablement. Resources were extended to include the use of rehabilitation workshops for evaluating and modifying vocational behavior. The goal was expanded to include the concept of vocational adjustment as well as job placement.

Between 1954 and 1972, the civilian rehabilitation program continued to expand along the lines drawn by the Vocational Rehabilitation Act Amendments of 1954. The most striking alteration was in the changing composition of the population being served. The initial target population had been the physically disabled. It was now expanded to include the entire spectrum of persons separated from the work culture, whether for physical or psychosocial reasons.

The new rehabilitation population was defined as the vocationally disadvantaged, persons needing help to cope with the problems of assuming or resuming a productive work role (Gellman, 1966). The population thus came to include the dependent (persons with mental or emotional disabilities), the deviate (ex drug addicts, parolees, youthful offenders), the socially and economically disadvantaged (recipients of public assistance and residents of inner city or model city areas, including migrants from rural areas), and the disemployed (persons completely separated from the labor market as the result of prejudice, age, or lack of skill).

CURRENT TRENDS

The trend at present is to view the rehabilitation process as a form of social technology for facilitating change in a rehabilitant's vocational development and to serve as monitor. The shift in emphasis is from rehabilitation as a helping art, with the resultant connotations of therapy, to rehabilitation as an applied science which functions as a "change-agent" for vocational adjustment. This new viewpoint implies goal orientation, flexibility in the use of techniques, adaptability to the rehabilitant's needs, a multidisciplinary approach, and the ability to use community resources to deal with vocational as well as nonvocational problems.

Concurrent with the reshaping of the dynamic structure of the reha-

bilitation process in accord with the change-agent concept is the extension of the process in time and in space. Vocational development is
viewed as continuing through the rehabilitant's life span. With the acceptance of the possibilities of change occurring after the close of the
intra-agency rehabilitation process, service to the rehabilitant is being
extended beyond the placement period. Wright (1971) suggests that rehabilitants be placed in an "inactive" status after the period of initial
orientation on the job, and be maintained in that status until there is a
satisfactory vocational adjustment.

A similar process of extension is taking place in the growing use of a
variety of settings in nontraditional locations. The traditional model of
rehabilitation is office-centered, with a unidimensional decision-making
perspective. The newer approach is multidimensional, involving observational and experiential techniques in all types of nonagency settings.
Sociopsychological and sociocultural aspects are being incorporated into
rehabilitation through using community settings and by intervening in
familial, social, and work situations in which rehabilitants are involved.

The growing significance of the sociocultural approach to rehabilitation is leading to increasing emphasis upon environmental conditions.
Such factors as family, peers, social groups, co-workers, and subcultural
values are seen as shaping the rehabilitant's perception of himself and
of the forces influencing his life. Increasingly the combination of inner
and outer frames of reference leads to the inclusion in the rehabilitation
process of all the communities in a rehabilitant's life space. The rehabilitator sees the rehabilitant not only as an actual or potential member
of a work culture but also as a participant in other societal groups.

This sociocultural orientation brings in the wider community as a rehabilitation adjunct, with significant groups and individuals in the rehabilitant's life space as rehabilitation aids who can further the rehabilitant's progress. The rehabilitator now reaches into the community to
find disabled persons who should be rehabilitants, and rehabilitated individuals who have difficulties in adjusting vocationally. Implicit in this
approach is the occupational lattice concept, in which each position
held by a rehabilitant is considered temporary until he either reaches a
satisfactory level of vocational adjustment or is moved to another position which he is better capable of filling.

Paralleling the emphasis upon the social environment is the current tendency to de-emphasize psychotherapeutic counseling as a rehabilitation technique and to emphasize the use of rehabilitation workshops for evaluative and adjustive purposes. Methodologically, the workshop uses work as a situational tool to assess and modify working behavior and attitudes, and the psychosocial aspects of the work environment as a controlled stimulus setting in which to influence a client's work adjustment. The work done in such workshops is real work for which the rehabilitants are paid. Work activities are graded in terms of difficulty and success level, type of task, type of supervision, work pressure, work abilities, and monetary rewards. The psychosocial work environment in such settings is varied in terms of intensity and extent of client stimulation, anticipated success level, type of work role, participation in work group, and conformance demands. Technically, workshop rehabilitation services are interwoven with individual and group counseling, including on-the-job assistance, placement, and supportive programs.

The trends moving the rehabilitation process away from the counseling paradigm are modifying the gestalt of rehabilitation roles. Rehabilitation, the rehabilitator, and the rehabilitant are changing in response to emerging trends in rehabilitation and the socioeconomic scene. The mainspring for role modification is the concept of the rehabilitator as a dynamic of change (Chapple, 1970). The rehabilitator is viewed as a catalytic change manager who assumes the responsibility for bringing about change in the rehabilitant and directing change toward the rehabilitation goal.

The rehabilitant, on the other hand, is perceived as a participant-consumer. As a participant, he is included in the process of establishing his rehabilitation goal and of choosing the techniques to be used in his rehabilitation program. As a consumer, he evaluates the services received, the results obtained, and his satisfaction with the program. This transformation of the rehabilitant role is modifying the concept of the rehabilitant's family. They are now seen as intimately involved members of the rehabilitation team who can serve as rehabilitation aids by extending the process into the home.

This interrelated series of rehabilitation role-changes appears to be moving toward a picture of the rehabilitation process as modeled on the Italian commedia dell'arte of the Renaissance, which was unwritten and improvised (Burckhardt, 1958). Such plays used stock characters derived from widely known tales and a few stock situations. Although there is a plot, the players improvise as they go along and may even alter the original. While the plot lines and characters impose certain constraints upon the performers, each version of the play differs in the lines spoken and the situations chosen. The play reflects the individuality of the players and of their perceptions of the drama.

To continue the analogy, the rehabilitator is an actor-manager, a participant-observer in the rehabilitation play. As an actor, he interacts with the rehabilitant and with the other members of the cast in the rehabilitant's life space. As a manager, he guides the interaction toward the desired denouement—rehabilitation.

The rehabilitant plays the part of the lead actor who exercises a dominant influence in molding the play and in shaping the plot toward the denouement. As the protagonist, he enacts the epilogue, which critiques the drama and forecasts the future of the characters. The evolving set of roles for rehabilitation's dramatis personnae are rehabilitation as a change-agent, the rehabilitator as a change-manager, and the rehabilitant as a self-changer.

Three social welfare program-tendencies—active intervention, participatory democracy, and consumerism—are fostering this new concept of the rehabilitation process as a drama in which the dramatis personnae of rehabilitation—the agency, the rehabilitator, and the rehabilitant —are engaged together in acting as well as in writing the script.

REHABILITATION TERMS AND CONCEPTS

The rapid development of rehabilitation has brought new terms and fresh concepts into prominence and has changed the meaning of terms transplanted from other disciplines. The meaning of these terms is fixed in part by the rehabilitation context in which they are used. The more important ones are summarized here.

Rehabilitation. Current concepts of rehabilitation view the rehabilitation population as made up of persons who are emotionally, mentally, physically, or socially disabled, and who are limited in their capacity to function in some way because of the disability. Definitions differ, however, with respect to their conception of the rehabilitation problem and the rehabilitation goal.

Braceland's (1961) definition of rehabilitation takes an all-inclusive view of problems and goals. He states that "a handicapped individual has a right to be helped and to be restored, not only to as much usefulness and dignity as possible but that he also should be aided in reaching his own highest potential." For Braceland, all types of handicaps which restrict functional capacity are the concern of the rehabilitation field. However, his notion of potentiality suggests an ideal goal which is unreachable in practice, the emphasis being on the process of goal-seeking rather than on the endpoint.

Kandel's (1964) and Oberman's (1965) approach to the rehabilitation problem is similar to Braceland's in accepting all types of handicaps. However, their viewpoints differ from Braceland's in that they would restrict the goal to the ability to function in a limited number of social settings. Thus, Kandel defines rehabilitation as "that form of therapy which is primarily concerned with assisting the patient to achieve an optimal social role (in the family, on the job, in the community generally) within his capacity and potentialities." Kandel's use of the role concept adds an observable dimension to the goal.

Oberman defines rehabilitation as "that activity that is required to assist an individual to move from a status of inadequacy to a status of adequacy," and he pictures the rehabilitant's "life space" as a quadrilateral with the four sides being medical, psychological, social, and vocational. He also provides a basis for specifying and measuring the goal.

The present author defines rehabilitation as the process of improving inadequate role behavior in work settings. His definition limits the rehabilitation problem to vocational handicaps and the rehabilitation goal to vocational achievement. The problem is inadequate role performance in the vocational area. The goal is adequate functioning in work situations, with "adequate" being a cultural norm. The major objectives are vocational competence and economic self-sufficiency. The term "rehabilitant" includes all types of disabled or disadvantaged persons who exhibit a vocational handicap. The primacy of the vocational area in this definition implies that a vocational problem is a necessary element for the rehabilitation process, and that the effectiveness of the process is determined by evaluating vocational performance. The definition recognizes that the vocational sector touches other life areas and that services in these other areas are frequently needed for the rehabilitant to improve his work ability. Vocational rehabilitation is in this concept the basic model for rehabilitation practice, with the term "model" being used in Kuhn's (1970) sense as a paradigm that provides "model problems and solutions to a community of practitioners." Further, the results of the Wood County Project (Wright, Reagles, and Thomas, 1971) indicate the applicability of the vocational approach to the rehabilitation field. The Wood County Project report states that "the vocational rehabilitation process has been successful over the past fifty years in the United States in helping the medically disabled to alleviate their handicaps to employment and can also help culturally disadvantaged persons to realize their best vocational and personal potential" and is "ideally suited to help them change their dependent social and financial status to one of independence."

Rehabilitant. A vocationally disadvantaged individual receiving service from a rehabilitation agency in order to improve his performance in remunerative or nonremunerative work. The vocationally disadvantaged are persons who are handicapped because of an emotional, mental, physical, or social disability and who need help to cope with the problems of assuming or resuming a work role.

Rehabilitation Agency. A facility which provides or secures services for rehabilitating vocationally disadvantaged persons. The services include coordination and counseling and one or more of the following: evaluation, work adjustment, physical or occupational therapy, the fitting and use of prostheses, and job placement. Rehabilitation agencies comprise publicly supported state agencies, voluntary local agencies and units in hospitals, the Veterans Administration, insurance companies, workshops, rehabilitation centers, and speech and hearing clinics.

Rehabilitation Center. An agency which may be independent or part of a hospital which provides an integrated program of medical, psychological, social, and vocational services for rehabilitative purposes. The approach is multidisciplinary, rehabilitant-centered, and comprehensive.

Rehabilitator. A person with professional training in rehabilitation who is employed by a rehabilitation agency to provide services to rehabilitants.

Situational Technique. The use of a natural or lifelike situation to observe, assess, or modify the behavior of a rehabilitant introduced into the situation. The rehabilitator may allow the flow of events to proceed naturally or intervene to introduce problems or contrived events. The situational analysis studies people, places, and things affecting the rehabilitant's behavior in the situation.

Vocational. Characteristic of or related to the work subculture. Vocation refers to the work or productive role characterizing an individual at a given period of time.

Vocational Adjustment. The compatability of the work personality to the range of available work roles in the work subculture. Job adjustment, the more specific term, is defined as on-the-job work behavior and is measured by the relationship between the work personality and the work roles characterizing a specific position.

Vocational Development. A series of changes beginning in early childhood and occurring throughout life which result in the formation and modification of the semiautonomous work personality and the attributes and competencies necessary for functioning appropriately in a work or productive role.

Work. Goal-directed activity directed toward socioeconomic ends. In an industrial culture, most persons are paid for working and are related occupationally to the provision of goods or service through employment or self-employment. Unpaid, volunteer activity is deemed productive work if the individual (worker) and society consider it socially useful.

Work Personality. An integrated, semiautonomous part of the total personality which functions as a constellation of work behavior, attitudes, and values manifested in typical work or achievement-demanding situations. It is defined operationally as the set of behavior patterns exhibited in a work situation or the manner in which an individual enacts a work role.

Work Role. A comprehensive pattern of behavior and attitudes which is socially identified as an entity in a work situation and which is connected with an occupation, job, or task. The individual who is working is expected to play the appropriate role for his type of work, whether it be that of housekeeper, caretaker, volunteer, or civic-minded citizen. The work role requires the ability to work, the ability to secure work, and the ability to adapt to work. The productive role, a broader term, includes unpaid activities.

Workshop. A place of work operated by a rehabilitation agency to provide gainful employment for vocationally disadvantaged persons. Workshops are either (1) rehabilitative (using a controlled work environment and the work experience to facilitate the rehabilitant's progress to a productive vocational status) or (2) sheltered (furnishing vocationally disadvantaged persons who cannot compete in the labor market with paid work which they can do and which will maintain their capacity to work).

Work Subculture. The complex of manners, behavior, attitudes, values, and settings comprising the socioeconomic sphere. The work subculture is characterized by goal-directed, achievement-oriented value systems and activities. Work behavior results from a dynamic interaction between the work personality as manifested in a work role and the work subculture expressed through the work environment. The work subculture includes all types of productive activities, whether in the labor market or in other types of work settings.

Work Therapy. Treatment using work experience to change the work personality, so that the rehabilitant can function appropriately in a normal work situation. Work therapy presupposes the ability to control the work environment and to modify the behavior of coworkers and supervisors in accordance with the needs of the rehabilitant.

The preceding terms may be categorized with respect to the rehabilitation process as

1) *Characters:* rehabilitant, rehabilitator;
2) *Settings:* rehabilitation agency, rehabilitation center, workshop;
3) *Processes:* vocational adjustment, vocational development;
4) *Variables:* work role, work personality, work subcultures;
5) *Methods:* situational technique, work therapy;
6) *Descriptive:* vocational, work.

THE REHABILITATION SYSTEM
IN THE UNITED STATES

As previously noted, the rehabilitation system in the United States is based on a goal which is vocational in the broadest sense: to assist a rehabilitant to perform adequately in a productive role. This major objective involves developing the desire and capacity to function productively in either competitive employment or nonprofit work which contributes to the welfare of the community. Intermediate steps toward this end are self-care, increased work competence (the ability to function and adapt in a work setting), improved placeability (the ability to secure employment), and enhanced adjustability (the capacity for continued adaptation to a work environment). If the rehabilitant cannot bridge the gap to competitive employment, the rehabilitation goal becomes placement in a nonprofit work system or in productive work in the home.

The potential rehabilitant population served by the system includes disabled persons of any age who are vocationally disadvantaged or who will be vocationally disadvantaged because of physical, educational, psychological, social, or cultural handicaps. The primary settings in which such persons are served include rehabilitation centers, workshops, and agencies. Persons involved include the rehabilitant's family and any other groups with whom the rehabilitant interacts in vocational and social settings or spheres.

Structurally, the service system is a network of rehabilitation agencies (public and voluntary, national and local) and major service systems (health, welfare, manpower, and education) which relate to rehabilitation through a reciprocal referral process in the provision or use of service. The nodal points are the nationwide public and private systems, such as the Federal-State civilian vocational program, and such voluntary agencies as the National Easter Seal Society for Crippled Children and Adults. The Federal-State program influences the operating policies and programs of rehabilitation agencies at the local level through state vocational rehabilitation agencies in the fifty states, the Commonwealth of Puerto Rico, and the District of Columbia.

Federal and state funds are dispersed through the state rehabilitation agencies, which provide direct services for clients and purchase or procure from other public or private agencies such services as are not provided by the state agency. The typical state agency assesses applicant eligibility, accepts clients for rehabilitation services, evaluates rehabilitants for rehabilitation potential (with the aid of medical or rehabilitation facilities and workshops), provides counseling, training, or further education, and job placement either directly or indirectly. State agencies refer rehabilitants to and purchase services from medical institutions and physicians, vocational counseling agencies, rehabilitation centers, workshops, and educational facilities. The costs are met by the federal and state governments.

The private or voluntary portion of the rehabilitation system consists of vocational rehabilitation and guidance agencies, rehabilitation centers, and workshops, hospitals, and clinics. The medical agencies offer a diversified array of services ranging from specialized medical care to occupational training. The rehabilitation centers provide physical medicine and rehabilitation services integrating the medical, psychological, social, and vocational spheres. The workshops, of which there are more than two thousand in operation, use work activity as a methodology to provide vocational evaluation, work adjustment, and sheltered employment services. More than 400 speech and hearing clinics make up another large group providing rehabilitation service.

The rehabilitation service system interacts with other major systems, such as medicine and psychotherapy, welfare, education, and manpower, and it refers rehabilitants to the other healing or helping systems as well as receives referrals from them. In many instances the provision of services is multidisciplinary, involving a number of service systems and a team approach. The team may include those in any or all of the disciplines cooperating in the rehabilitation process, such as physicians, physical therapists, occupational therapists, social workers, rehabilitation counselors, speech and hearing therapists, psychologists, job placement specialists, vocational counselors, special educators, and vocational educators.

The axes of the rehabilitation system are: active case-finding; a coordinated multidisciplinary goal-oriented approach; the use of experiential methodologies; and follow-through to ensure optimal vocational adjustment. Active case-finding involves seeking potentially eligible recipients who may not know of rehabilitation services or who may not be in a position to come to an office. Such activity assumes that these services must be sold to potential rehabilitants as well as to the ultimate consumer—society. Rehabilitation services reach into the communities of the physically disabled, whether in institutions, clinics, or neighborhoods, to provide services when disablement or disadvantagement is apparent. The initial contact with the rehabilitant is designed to involve him as an active participant in the rehabilitation process.

Since rehabilitation services center on improving the rehabilitant and his social or work situation, the rehabilitator is called upon to play four major roles: psychological counselor; administrator; team leader; and coordinator of services. The proportion of time and effort devoted to each varies with program, agencies, and the needs of the rehabilitant. Gordon (1965) believes that the role of team leader of the professionals and paraprofessionals involved in the picture will prove to be most significant, and that the rehabilitator will be perceived as a person who "heads a team, trains people for the team, and supervises the activities of team members."

THE REHABILITATION PROCESS

The rehabilitation process includes the four following phases: initiating the process; vocational evaluation; treatment; adjustment to the community.

INITIATING THE PROCESS

Psychologically, the rehabilitation process becomes possible with the acceptance of loss, a process analyzed by Wright (1960) as the recognition that the effect of the impairment is limiting rather than total and that values are based upon abilities rather than disabilities. Acceptance also implies recognition by the physically disabled person that he is handicapped and will need assistance to reach his goals. The transition from the role of a patient to the role of a rehabilitant occurs when rehabilitation is accepted as a means for overcoming barriers to achievement. The stability of the role shift from patient to rehabilitant depends upon the rehabilitant's ego strength, the attitude of family members toward his rehabilitation, and the degree to which the rehabilitation programs meet his specific needs and generate satisfaction.

The rehabilitation process is initiated formally when the prospective rehabilitant comes into contact with the rehabilitation system. This, as Kandel (1964) states "can begin at any point and can be carried out concomitantly with other treatment modalities. It is not merely a post-hospital or post-treatment program. Rehabilitation can proceed in outpatient and inpatient settings, in day hospitals, or as part of the follow-up services for patients leaving hospitals." Ideally, however, the rehabilitation process should start as soon as possible after the onset of disablement. The earlier it begins, the greater the possibility of limiting psychic institutionalization and irreversible developmental changes.

During the intake period a number of processes take place simultaneously. The rehabilitator and the rehabilitant assess each other. The initial interaction is based on the facades presented by the rehabilitation agency, the rehabilitator, and the rehabilitant. Roles are reciprocally defined. The disabled person assumes the role of a participant in rehabilitation. The rehabilitator in turn chooses a role which enables the rehabilitant to proceed toward his rehabilitation goal. The rehabilitant learns what he is expected to do and what the agency can do and the rehabilitator learns what he can expect from the rehabilitant.

Exploration is the key to the initial phase of rehabilitation. A fluid situation and the maintenance of options is desirable. The rehabilitant clarifies his expectations for the future as the rehabilitator indicates possibilities for change without minimizing realistic barriers. The rehabilitator points out various pathways to goals and the steps to be taken, and begins the process of evaluation with a discussion of needed services and history-taking which focuses on continuing trends in the individual's work life. It can be assumed that without external intervention these trends would continue and shape the future work life. The rehabilitant examines the ramifications of the suggested rehabilitation possibilities and the constraints which the rehabilitant role imposes.

The intake process terminates with the fixing of roles between the rehabilitator and the rehabilitant. These roles, which may be explicit or implicit, provide the ground rules for this person's rehabilitation process. It is likely that the more clearly the two parties understand the roles the better the rehabilitation prognosis.

VOCATIONAL EVALUATION

The purpose of vocational evaluation is to develop a treatment plan that will forecast and pattern a client's future work behavior, with the initial objective directed to a formulation of predictions concerning the rehabilitant's future vocational behavior in various types of work situations. The predictions or hypotheses are stated as equations in the if-so-then form, detailing relevant personal, interpersonal, and situational conditions governing work behavior in work settings. These hypotheses constitute a preliminary map of the rehabilitant's realistic vocational possibilities.

The formulation of a vocational treatment plan is based upon (1) an estimate of the impact of the loss or injury resulting in the rehabilitant's need for rehabilitation, (2) knowledge of the individual's work personality, (3) consideration of the developmental possibilities of the work personality, (4) an appraisal of the rehabilitant's training capacity, and (5) a determination of the anticipated work-life pattern of the rehabilitant, that is, the level and type of work he will undertake. The specification of potential work settings requires knowledge of the work worlds and involves categorization on two levels: first, the type of work—industrial, office, service, agricultural, or manual labor—and the levels of participation, and second, the nature of the work—orientation toward people, data, or things (concrete, material objects).

The rehabilitant's work pattern is analyzed with an external and internal frame of reference. The external frame of reference presents the work behavior from the observer's point of view and provides a bench mark for forecasting the rehabilitant's work role performance. The internal frame uses the rehabilitant's perspective to analyze the factors which serve as compass points for his behavior in a work setting.

Vocational evaluation centers its analysis on the work personality, which is defined operationally as the rehabilitant's behavior patterns relevant to typical working conditions. The work personality operates at a number of levels. At the manifest level, it is observable as the behavior exhibited in a work setting and how it adapts to the demands of the work role. The facets of the work personality form a patterned gestalt so that change in any one aspect results in changes throughout the whole.

Vocational evaluation also examines the interaction of familial, social, and communal factors with the work personality since there is a reciprocal relationship between work and other significant life areas. Stresses of sufficient magnitude in the familial and social areas affect work personality and behavior. Problems in the work setting affect behavior in other social areas.

As to the techniques of vocational evaluation, they serve as means to various ends, the ends being to forecast a rehabilitant's behavior during treatment and his work behavior in the occupational world. There are no absolutes in the selection of assessment techniques. They vary with each rehabilitant. The choice of a technique depends upon the problems posed, the nature of the rehabilitant's work personality, the type of work situation the rehabilitant will encounter in the competitive labor market, available training resources, the possible treatment program, and the type of information required for assessment purposes. If sufficient knowledge is lacking, observational and preliminary assessments are used to formulate questions for a more detailed second-stage evaluation.

Evaluative techniques are classified as follows in terms of the appraisal objective:

1) *Determining work behavior and functioning capacities.* The techniques usually employed are observation of work behavior or work samples.

2) *Estimating learning capacity in a work situation.* Analyses of work history, tests, and situational techniques are used for this purpose. The situational techniques place the rehabilitant in a simulated or actual work situation in which he is confronted with work problems that require modification of work behavior or the work environment. The problems deal with impersonal and personal aspects in the work environment.

3) *Estimating the rehabilitant's capacity for acquiring work competencies or skills.* The most commonly used methods are tests, work samples, and work observation.

4) *Analyzing psychosocial factors influencing work behavior.* A variety of approaches may be used, including interviewing, review of the rehabilitant's work and social history, tests, and situational techniques.

The quality of service provided depends largely upon the accuracy of vocational evaluation because the treatment plan for the rehabilitant is based on inferences derived from vocational evaluation. Therefore, a discriminate and understanding use of vocational evaluation is a prerequisite to an effective rehabilitation program.

The following are suggested as guides to the use of vocational evaluation in the rehabilitation process:

1) Vocational evaluation is future oriented to enable the assessor to forecast the rehabilitant's vocational development and behavior. Evalua-

tions are stated as propositions of the if-then character which specify the sociocultural context for work behavior.

2) Effective vocational evaluation focuses on developing a treatment plan which is specific for the rehabilitant. The plan is defined by the objectives arrived at by the rehabilitator and by the rehabilitant's work personality and goals.

3) Vocational evaluation is a two-phase process. The initial exploratory phase leads to the preliminary formulation of questions necessary for the development of a treatment plan. The second or assessment phase provides the data necessary to answer the question raised in the first stage and to develop a treatment plan.

4) Vocational evaluation assumes that rehabilitants change during and after the active rehabilitation treatment phase, including the period of adjustment to work. Vocational evaluation is coextensive with the total rehabilitation process, beginning with intake and continuing until the rehabilitant reaches his realistic level of vocational adjustment.

5) Vocational evaluation is multidisciplinary, bringing into play the professions and personnel required to secure the data necessary for the vocational understanding of a particular rehabilitant. Psychologists, workshop specialists, social workers, physicians, the rehabilitant himself or members of his family or work groups—all may be brought into the process. It requires a thorough knowledge of the resources available to the rehabilitant in therapeutic, educational, and manpower systems.

TREATMENT

Treatment begins with direct services, support, and environmental manipulation, all of which are intended to achieve adequate rehabilitant performance in an appropriate work role. Service in turn is based on a vocational treatment plan developed during the evaluation phase. While the plan is individualized for each rehabilitant, there are certain common objectives: (1) to maximize the psychosocial factors that strengthen the work personality; (2) to increase the capacity to learn in a work situation; (3) to develop an acceptable work personality; (4) to prepare the rehabilitant for the type of work situation in which he will function; and (5) to stabilize or improve the rehabilitant's capacity to cope in other life sectors.

Treatment takes place on three levels: the individual, the family, and the community.

The Individual. This first treatment level includes the following important processes: counseling, preparing the individual to function in a productive role, social learning following Bandura's (1962) model, and client involvement as an active participant in the rehabilitation process.

1) Counseling is psychological in nature focusing on the problems hampering rehabilitation (Jaques, 1970). Samler (1966) believes that the general task of counseling is to help people prepare themselves for and function productively in work, and that in addition to the one-to-one relationship counseling can include a group approach. He suggests that counseling should be extended to embrace a wider range of activities, such as experiential, situational work techniques directed toward limited and specific goals. Observable behavior is his criterion for evaluating the outcomes of counseling.

2) Work activity is a primary tool for work adjustment as well as for vocational evaluation. Work therapy (or industrial therapy) is the use of work activity in a rehabilitation workshop or other work settings as a situational technique for evaluative, adjustive, and therapeutic purposes (Gellman, 1970, 1972). Black (1970) uses the term "in a generic sense to include all those rehabilitation and resocialization programs . . . (which) are utilized, mostly in a simulation of a true work situation." Work therapy involves productive work tailored to meet the rehabilitation needs of clients and which incorporates culturally approved values in a context that provides vocational goals acceptable to rehabilitants.

Methodologically, the workshop is used as a situational tool in work activity. The workshop permits simulation of a variety of work settings and working conditions. Its essence is the programmed modifiability of personal and impersonal aspects of the work environment. As previously mentioned, such factors as work pressure, the type of work, nature of coworker relationships, type of supervision, extent of client stimulation, anticipated success level, work pressure, participation in work groups, and conformance demands can be individualized and varied for each rehabilitant.

Work activity is real to the rehabilitant in terms of pay, hours, supervision, and quality control. Within the shop, foremen who are rehabilitators use rehabilitants as assistants. Among the problems which the client faces are increasing production, decreasing errors, assuming responsibility, maintaining quality standards, meeting quota demands, and dealing with supervisory pressures.

3) Situational techniques of three types are used for the workshop: the work sample; observation and manipulation of work behavior; and structured work problems such as are currently under development at the Chicago Jewish Vocational Service (Gellman, 1972). Structured work problems are a graded series of problem-centered work activities for groups of rehabilitants which permit the emergence of latent abilities and of reactions to work pressures, goals, and interpersonal relations. Each work problem involves interlocking work roles which require the rehabilitant to deal with the typical stresses of a work group.

Workshop situational techniques may focus upon work activity or upon problem-solving tasks similar to those used by the Office of Strategic Services during World War II (Fiske, 1954). The objectives of work therapy are similar in both instances—to determine the effects of variations in working conditions and the work environment upon the work personality and work adjustment and the factors which stimulate or inhibit vocational development.

4) Vocational adjustment levels vary inversely with the degree of divergence between work-sector requirements and the rehabilitant's handicapping restrictions. Where the divergence is great, the resolution of the rehabilitant's vocational problems requires a compromise between the satisfactions sought by the rehabilitant in productive activity and those afforded by vocational reality. The workshop enables the rehabilitator to determine the degree of vocational adjustment possible for a rehabilitant at different levels of the vocational adjustment triad—work demands, handicapping restrictions, and work satisfactions. Interwoven in the fabric of work adjustment programs are literacy training, education, and skill training. Achievements in training and remedial education are related to work competence by changing the rehabilitant's work tasks so that he can use his increased abilities to better his work performance. Workshop services are interspersed with individual and group counseling, including on-the-job assistance, placement, and supportive programs. Performance and situational tests supplement work therapy. Further, the workshop emphasizes the development of social skills and the ability to move freely in the community and operate effectively at work.

Projects involving the use of such community resources as trade schools, recreational facilities, and employment agencies are incorporated into the work adjustment program. Role playing is used as a preliminary step for such functions as job applications, dealing with on-the-job problems, securing psychological and medical services, and establishing appropriate behavior patterns in other social situations.

5) Rehabilitant participation is a necessary component in rehabilitation services on the individual level. The rehabilitant functions as a team member in all areas involving his present or future status and in the decision as to the success or failure of his rehabilitation program. In addition to taking part in establishing his rehabilitation goals, the rehabilitant should be given a realistic choice among alternative programs, and an opportunity to evaluate the rehabilitation program with the rehabilitator. He should be encouraged in self-evaluation and in assessment of his progress. The program needs to be flexible to permit reshaping those aspects which are unacceptable to the rehabilitant. If there is an option as to when a program can be taken, the rehabilitant should be permitted to decide on the time.

Family Service. This second level of service focuses on the individual in his family role. The rehabilitator visits the home to bring the family into the rehabilitation program and to obtain the flavor of the home and family constellation. The work of Spiegel (1959) and Levine (1965) illustrates the value of using home interviews to develop among family members supportive behavior which can help maintain the client in the rehabilitant role and prepare him for a work role. Family therapy helps to establish attitudes, values, and behavior patterns in the family constellation which further the rehabilitation process. Training family members to assist the rehabilitant to attain specific goals adds another dimension to service by extending the treatment program spatially and temporally.

Community Services. The third service level is concerned with smoothing the rehabilitant's entry or re-entry into the community and with facilitating his performance and adaptation in community roles. To ease the transition from the sheltering agency to the general community, rehabilitators are making greater use of small groups of rehabilitants who face similar problems. The group may be organized in the community or in a rehabilitation facility and later move into the community.

Fairweather (1964), in discussing the use of a group to ease movement out of the institution, points to the importance of establishing a context for change in the individual by creating a "total situation which requires similar behaviors and perceptions both within and without the agency work setting or institution . . . The reference will become the group to which the individual belongs and in which he has a well-defined and established role." During the first stage of transition, members of a self-help group may live together in halfway houses or use other types of congregate living arrangements. If the group does not live together, members may simply meet periodically to focus on the specific kinds of difficulties facing them. The functions of the group are mutual help and support in the handling of problems which create difficulties during initial orientation to the community.

ADJUSTMENT TO THE COMMUNITY

The next phase of the rehabilitation process centers upon the rehabilitant's actual adjustment in the community—his ability to function adequately in his vocational, social, and familial roles. Community adjustment services are ecologically oriented. A map of the rehabilitant's life space provides information about the type of individuals with whom he interacts, the role models available to him, and other environmental factors in the community which serve as paths or barriers to his goal. The community approach emphasizes the rehabilitant's frame of reference, perceiving the community as the rehabilitant does. The rehabilitant's perceptions of social situations in the community are related to his work behavior. In this service phase, the rehabilitator helps the rehabilitant learn how to cope with real life problems in an actual community setting and joins with key members of the family, social, and work groups to lower or eliminate barriers to adequate role performance.

If negative attitudes on the part of family members, friends, or workmates interpose blocks to adequate role performance, the rehabilitator intervenes to create conditions which make adjustment possible. The rehabilitator provides direct help to the rehabilitant in the form of counseling, psychotherapy, or the use of experiential, as contrasted with verbal, techniques to modify the rehabilitant's behavior. If the rehabilitant's problems reflect devaluating familial or social attitudes toward the disabled, service on a one-to-one basis may be insufficient. In such instances it may be necessary to attempt to change the attitudes of family members and leaders of social or work groups.

The problem of group attitudes based upon prejudice toward the disabled is one which must be dealt with on a large scale. The biases exhibited by employers, personnel men, and supervisors toward the physically handicapped is a major stumbling block in securing work for rehabilitants. A variety of job-placement techniques can be used to decrease discriminatory attitudes toward the disabled. These may be classified as follows: (1) changing public beliefs through a public relations program; (2) changing the public behavior of employer groups by citing employers who employ the handicapped or by having very capable disabled persons demonstrate their ability to do tasks deemed beyond the capacity of the handicapped; (3) convincing a potential employer to hire the handicapped for on-the-job training programs, which would give the employer an opportunity to see how the rehabilitant works out without making a permanent commitment, or by providing on-the-job coaching and other forms of assistance during the rehabilitant's orientation period; (4) helping the employer who might be unwilling to hire a disabled person because of fear he would be psychologically unable to release an unsuitable disabled person by having the rehabilitator agree to inform the rehabilitant that he is being fired; and (5) educating a specific employer by dealing with associations to which he belongs. For example, if a rehabilitant who can meet job requirements is refused a position in a retail store because of bias, the rehabilitator could shift his efforts to the retail trade association. He could ask officials of the retail association to convene a meeting on hiring the handicapped, or an association committee could be asked to issue a statement on hiring the handicapped and prepare a draft on model hiring policies for its members.

If the rehabilitant seeks competitive employment, he must be prepared for job interviews and be prepared through role playing and situational techniques to cope with prejudice. The process of job seeking involves active efforts by the rehabilitator-rehabilitant dyad to find a suitable position. A job is sought in which the rehabilitant would be productive and in which he would be accepted by the employer and work group. An analysis of the work environment may be necessary to determine if the personal and impersonal job factors will enable the rehabilitant to function and to derive satisfaction from work. Selective placement techniques are used which match the job to characteristics of the rehabilitant.

Rehabilitants who possess work competence but are unplaceable, that is, who are able to work but are unacceptable in competitive employment, may be placed permanently in a workshop which provides noncompetitive employment. The number of sheltered workshops offering work programs for the physically disabled is extremely limited in the United States. In contrast, Europeans provide more extensive programs for the employment of persons who lack the capacity to function at a level which permits employment in industry. For example, Remploy, Inc. in Great Britain operates a number of factories which employ handicapped persons whose work capacity is insufficient for competitive employment (Black, 1970). Work settings such as Remploy which produce goods for the market on a large scale appear to be better adapted for partially productive individuals than are sheltered workshops in the United States. The factory atmosphere and the more structured work orientation provide a greater sense of reality and a feeling of participation in the labor market.

The follow-up phase, which concerns work adjustment, continues after placement, whether the rehabilitant is involved in remunerative or nonremunerative work. The rehabilitator aids the rehabilitant by furnishing job coaching and counseling and assistance for problems in the family and social sectors. Placement is treated as one step in a continuing process of vocational development which may involve the rehabilitant in a number of job replacements and occupational changes. The agency may make services available to the rehabilitant for a stipulated period after placement, usually one year. Thereafter, service may still be provided if the rehabilitant experiences major vocational problems because of altered socioeconomic conditions or significant modifications in the work personality.

ISSUES IN REHABILITATION

The questions which a science seeks to answer are primary determinants of its theory and methodology. The problems for which a helping profession seeks the answers play a similar role in shaping its goals and techniques. Thus, rehabilitation objectives and methods are a function of the formulation of the problems the profession seeks to resolve. Objectives and methods change with problem-reformulation.

THE OBJECTIVES REFORMULATED

When rehabilitation began as a helping discipline, the emphasis was on medical problems. With the realization that physical restoration was insufficient to enable the severely disabled to cope with the demands of daily living, preparation for day-to-day activities became part of the rehabilitation problem. As the disabled learned to function in the home and to move about in the community, the difficulties of finding employment became more apparent. Job placement became a primary task for rehabilitation. With increasing knowledge of the psychological and sociocultural bases of work, rehabilitation reformulated its core problem as enabling the rehabilitant to function adequately in a productive role either in industry or the home. This reformulation strengthens rehabilitation's emphasis upon the social problems faced by the rehabilitant as a member of society. Focusing the problem on role performance adds a specific criterion for evaluating the effectiveness of rehabilitation services.

Associated with this reformulation is the growing use of vocational rather than medical or psychological classifications for rehabilitation clientele, together with the use of such concepts as vocational development, work personality, and work role. The concepts are interrelated. Vocational development creates a work personality which, if adequate, enables the individual to enact a culturally approved work role. An adequate work personality provides the building blocks used to construct the work role and includes (1) work competence, or the ability to function in a productive setting; (2) placeability, or the ability to secure work; and (3) adjustability, or the capacity for continued adaptation to a work environment. Turner's (1968) definition furnishes the parameters of the work role: "it provides a comprehensive pattern for behavior and attitudes; it constitutes a strategy for coping with a recurrent type of situation; it is socially identified, more or less clearly, as an entity; it is subject to being played recognizably by different individuals; and it supplies a major basis for identifying and placing persons in society."

Reformulating the problem both socially and vocationally has broadened the base of rehabilitation to include the socially disadvantaged as well as the physically disabled. Frequently, the disadvantaged also face situations of social dislocation and deprivation which modify normal vocational development and result in atypical performance of work roles. In terms of rehabilitation, the disabled and disadvantaged may both be viewed as members of demarcated subcultures which exert pressure upon their members to engage in conduct judged nonconformist by society's standards (Merton, 1968). Merton further believes that the significant determinants of conformance or nonconformance are the compatability of subcultural goals and pathways to their counterparts in the majority culture. The rehabilitant will conform vocationally if his goals are compatible with culturally defined goals, and if his work-role enactment is consonant with socially accepted modes of reaching vocational goals. The preceding analysis leads to the classification of the vocationally disadvantaged as shown on page 32. A vocational classification system based upon empirical variables which relate evaluation data to treatment methods and outcomes provides a mechanism for evaluating the effectiveness of treatment techniques. The classification serves also as a framework for modifying work behavior which is deemed inappropriate and for matching characteristics of work situations with a rehabilitant's anticipated work-role performance (selective job placement).

With the broadened scope of rehabilitation in our industrial society, the subculture has now become the operational realm of vocational rehabilitation. The use of the word subculture in understanding the problems of the individual as well as the possibilities open to him resembles Quine's (1961) emphasis upon the growing significance of the context-of-occurrence in making variables in the physical sciences more meaningful. Thus, the work sector context, including rehabilitation workshops, is differentiated from such other specialized social contexts as home, school, or recreation. The context is operationally characterized by goal-directed, achievement-oriented, productive behavior which is based upon culturally acquired patterns and skills. Within this demarcated subcultural context, the vocational development process shapes and fashions work personalities in consonance with the demands of the various work roles. In turn, the work personalities shape the work roles which define the particular job. Thus, each work setting is characterized by a pattern of work roles which limits the kinds of work personalities that can function effectively in that particular context.

CLASSIFICATION OF THE VOCATIONALLY DISADVANTAGED

	Vocational Development	Orientation of Goals and Work Personality	Enactment of Work Role
Vocationally Arrested	Limited but able to progress	Subculture and dominant work culture	Unable to function on a protracted basis due to inner goal conflict
Vocationally Maladjusted	Complete	Subculture	Unable to function due to goal conflict with work culture
Vocationally Displaced	Complete	Dominant work culture	Unable to function due to loss of occupational skill
Vocationally Nonadjusted	Limited but unable to progress	Goals of dominant work culture. Work personality partially formed, from dominant work culture	Unable to function due to lack of vocational development

Changes in the formulation of rehabilitation objectives also involve a change in rehabilitation theory and methodology, since practice and theory are joined into a unifying process by systematic correlations (Northrop, 1966). The movement from descriptive variables to empirical constructs provides a framework for converting rehabilitation service experiences into treatment theory. The more important constructs are vocational development, the work personality, vocational adjustment, and the work sector or subculture. These have been previously considered. They constitute a foundation for restructuring practice methodology and for redefining the rehabilitation service process in terms of: (1) demonstration of the applicability of the methodology of vocational rehabilitation to the range of rehabilitation clientele and problems; (2) the formulation and specification of empirical constructs related to the work sector; and (3) the evaluation of a treatment methodology.

THE EXPANDED SCOPE OF REHABILITATION

The rehabilitation process is becoming more comprehensive. Involved in both theorymaking and practice is the recognition that vocational adjustment occurs in a social medium. The rehabilitator does not deal with isolated vocational problems. He helps people handicapped by interactional problems which reflect discrepancies between the demands of the occupational world and the limitations imposed by disability. Mayo (1945) regards adherence to group standards of behavior as an important element in survival on the job. Menninger (1955) believes that more jobs are lost because of personal or social difficulties than because of lack of job skills or of inability to meet job specifications. These beliefs are reflected in the increasing use of situational techniques in diagnosis and treatment.

This growing awareness of the significance of the psychosocial approach in the rehabilitation process is strengthening the emphasis on environmental conditions. Factors such as family, peers, social groups, coworkers, and subcultural values are seen as shaping the rehabilitant's perception of himself and of the forces influencing his life. Increasingly, the rehabilitator sees the rehabilitant as an actual or potential member of a work culture as well as of other groups in society.

The scope of rehabilitation depends on the degree of specificity of the problem of concern and on the attainability of the goal. If the problem and goal are vocationally oriented, rehabilitation deals with vocationally disadvantaged individuals who are helped to achieve adequate performance in productive roles. But if the rehabilitation goal is improvement in other types of roles as well, then the function of rehabilitation is to foster potentiation of all persons who are functioning at less than maximum effectiveness. Such broadening of problem and goal has the effect of immeasurably increasing the scope of rehabilitation. Careful decisions must be made in order to understand and control future expansion and development.

REHABILITANT CONSUMERISM

The transformation of the rehabilitant from a passive consumer of services to a participant consumer poses a core issue for rehabilitation. Can the field provide effective service to clients who exercise autonomy during the rehabilitation process?

In practice, accentuation of rehabilitant self-direction produces role conflict in the rehabilitant and the rehabilitator. As the rehabilitant proceeds, he discovers that the rehabilitation process is fluid and unstructured. He becomes aware that he is unacquainted with all the roles of the game and can learn only a few. As he makes decisions about the type, timing, and sequence of services, he discovers that his control over the process is illusory and that the alternatives are limited. The information presented to the rehabilitant tends to determine his choice. As he experiences success in his rehabilitation, he finds that he is being molded by the rehabilitation system into a client dependent upon the system (Scott, 1969).

The rehabilitant's role of participant-consumer generates severe stresses for the rehabilitator and the rehabilitation agency. The new rehabilitant role implies a reciprocal role of advocate-facilitator for the rehabilitator. Jaques (1970) believes that it is difficult to play an advocacy role under present conditions. She feels that "the counselor particularly will need the help and support of his professional colleagues when the role of advocate 'goes against the grain' of society." It is equally difficult for the rehabilitator to function as a facilitator for more than a limited number of clients. A myriad of duties and the demands of other rehabilitants prevent the rehabilitator from paying full attention to the needs of any single client. The rehabilitator's role as a professional may be threatened or negated by rehabilitant decisions. If techniques of behavioral control such as operant conditioning are deemed necessary, is the rehabilitator placed in the position of the philosophers in Plato's ideal Republic? What are the implications for rehabilitation if the rehabilitator eschews controls?

Jaques' discussion points up the conflict between the totality of client needs and the limitations of agency structure and function. She believes that the traditional agency authority structure prevents rehabilitators from meeting client needs. The issues posed when the rehabilitant assumes a participant-consumer role affect all aspects of rehabilitation. Full acceptance of this role may involve extensive and radical changes in the rehabilitation system by giving the rehabilitant the ultimate power to determine and evaluate his rehabilitation program. Is the field ready and able to undertake a thoroughgoing reformulation and reorganization of roles, methodologies, competencies, and agencies?

If the agency takes up the challenge of advocacy, of playing an active role in trying to meet the needs of the client, it moves into realms of social action which may run counter to the attitudes of the wider community. Concepts which may encounter resistance include the belief that the amount of service should be dependent upon the individual's needs rather than on his chances of securing employment; the belief that every handicapped person who cannot enter the competitive labor market should be provided noncompetitive employment; the belief that the rehabilitant should be free to make decisions which may lead to problems with influential figures in his family or work lives.

REHABILITATION AND THE COMMUNITY

The treatment of the rehabilitant as a person-environment configuration follows Lewin's dictum that behavior is a function of the person and the environment (1966). The rehabilitation goal of adequate role performance in the productive sector of life poses the issue of rehabilitation's relationship to the community in terms of intervention and prevention.

The employment field is an example of an area in which active intervention by the rehabilitator is necessary if the rehabilitant is to secure an opportunity to enact a significant role. Many personnel men and businessmen misunderstand and fear disability in themselves and in others. Uncertainty, fear, and prejudice create unwillingness to hire a disabled person. The decision not to employ may reflect an unwitting bias rather than an analysis of the rehabilitant's capabilities. Similar barriers and hurdles exist for the disabled and disadvantaged in familial, social, or communal life sectors. The family may not be able to accept the rehabilitant as a nondisabled person. Public gatherings may not provide for inclusion of handicapped persons in wheelchairs. Schools are often unwilling to provide services to older, handicapped youths or accept severely disabled children.

The existence of such impediments to the rehabilitant's effective role performance necessitates intervention by the rehabilitator in social and community situations to change the attitudes and behavior of significant individuals in the rehabilitant's life space. Such actions may be helpful to the individual rehabilitant, but seldom deal with the roots of general problems. It is necessary to go beyond ameliorative measures and on to community action for the elimination of handicapping conditions. Through community action, Kandel (1960) believes that "rehabilitation may also be viewed as tertiary prevention . . . reduction in the prevalence of disabilities resulting from disease."

Society exhibits a great deal of prejudice toward the disabled, the dependent, and the deviant. Many individuals are handicapped only because society's attitudes turn the biases of the nondisabled into handicaps for the disabled. However, social action to eliminate or reduce prejudice will lead to friction with those segments of society which are threatened by change. The question is whether rehabilitation is a healing discipline in the preventive sense as well as a helping one. Is rehabilitation a compound of professional competence plus community action? The pressing issue for rehabilitation to resolve is whether taking action to eradicate social conditions that create disablement and disadvantagement is appropriate to its goals and functions.

SUMMARY

This chapter has presented an overview of the rehabilitation field and discussed rehabilitation practice, trends, and issues. The theme is the evolution of rehabilitation from a helping art to an applied discipline. The focal point is the change toward a sociopsychologic approach. After two decades of growth and expansion of techniques, rehabilitation is entering a new stage which combines the development of treatment theory with advocacy, and which unites service to the individual with the creation of an open community in which the disabled and disadvantaged can use their abilities proudly and productively.

REFERENCES

Bandura, Albert. 1962. Social learning through imitation, in Marshall R. Jones, ed., Nebraska Symposium on Motivation. Lincoln, University of Nebraska Press, pp. 211–69.

Black, Bertram. 1970. Principles of industrial therapy for the mentally ill. New York, Grune and Stratton.

Braceland, Francis. 1961. The restoration of man. Acta Psychiatric Scandinavica 141:378–86.

Burckhardt, Jacob. 1958. The civilization of the Renaissance in Italy. New York, Harper & Row.

Chapple, Elliot. 1970. Rehabilitation, dynamic of change: an anthropological view. Ithaca, Cornell University Center for Research in Education.

Fairweather, George. 1967. Methods for experimental social innovation. New York, Wiley.

Fiske, Donald. 1954. Why do we use Situational Performance Tests? Personnel Psychology 7:464–69.

Gellman, William. 1970. Adapting the rehabilitation workshop to the needs of the disadvantaged, in William N. Button (ed.) Rehabilitation, sheltered workshops, and the disadvantaged: an exploration in manpower policy. Ithaca, Cornell University Press, pp. 199–210.

———— 1966. New perspectives in vocational rehabilitation. Bulletin, Division 22, Psychological aspects of disability, American Psychological Association, 13:3.

———— 1972 Vocational rehabilitation trends and issues (in press).

Gordon, Jesse. 1965. Project Cause, the Federal Anti-Poverty Program and some implications of subprofessional training. American Psychologist 20:334–43.

Jaques, Marceline. 1970. Rehabilitation counseling, scope and service. Boston, Houghton Mifflin.

———— 1960. Treatment of the disabled in primitive cultures, in C. H. Patterson, ed., Readings in rehabilitation counseling. Champaign, Ill., Stipes, pp. 8–14.

Kandel, Denise and Richard Williams. 1964. Psychiatric rehabilitation: some problems in research. New York, Atherton Press.

Kessler, Henry. 1950. Principles and practice of rehabilitation. Philadelphia, Lea and Febiger.

Kuhn, Thomas. 1970. The structure of scientific revolution. Chicago, University of Chicago Press.

Levine, Louis. 1965. Implications of the Anti-Poverty Program for education and employment. Vocational Guidance Quarterly 14:8–15.

Lewin, Kurt. 1966. Principles of topological psychology. New York, McGraw-Hill.

Mayo, Elton, 1945. The social problems of an industrial civilization. Cambridge, Harvard University Press.

McGowan, John, ed. 1960. An introduction to the vocational rehabilitation process. Washington, D.C., U.S. Government Printing Office.

Menninger, William. Spring, 1955. The psychological key to success. Menninger Quarterly.

Merton, Robert. 1968. Social theory and social structure. New York, Free Press.

National Center for Health Statistics, U. S. Department of Health, Education and Welfare, 1969. Current Estimates for Health Interview Survey, U. S. 1967. Washington, D.C., U. S. Department of Health, Education and Welfare.

National Health Education Committee. 1971. Facts on the major killing and crippling diseases in the U.S. New York, National Health Education Committee.

Neff, Walter. 1968. Work and human behavior. New York, Atherton Press.

Northrop, F. S. C. 1966. The logic of the sciences and the humanities. Cleveland, World.

Oberman, C. Esco. 1965. A history of vocational rehabilitation in America. Minneapolis, Denison.

Query, Richard. 1968. Towards a definition of work. Personnel and Guidance Journal 47:3, 223–27.

Quine, Willard Von Orman. 1964. From a logical point of view. Cambridge, Harvard University Press.

Rusk, Howard. 1958. Rehabilitation medicine. St. Louis, Mosby.

Samler, Joseph. 1966. The counselor in our time. Madison Lecture on Vocational Rehabilitation. Madison, University of Wisconsin Press.

Scott, Robert. 1969. The making of blind men. New York, Russell Sage Foundation.

Soden, William. 1949. Rehabilitation of the handicapped: a survey of means and method. New York, Ronald Press.

Spiegel, John. 1959. Some cultural aspects of transference and countertransference, in J. E. Masserman, ed., Individual and family dynamics. New York, Grune and Stratton.

Turner, Ralph. 1968. ROLE: Sociological aspects, in David L. Sills, ed., International Encyclopedia of the Social Sciences 13:552–57. New York, Macmillan and Free Press.

U.S. Rehabilitation Service Administration. 1972. Information Memorandum IM-72-49, 1972. Washington, D.C., Rehabilitation Service Administration.

——. 1972. Vocational Rehabilitation Agency Fact Sheet Booklet—Fiscal Year 1971. Washington, D.C., U. S. Department of Health, Education and Welfare.

Wright, Beatrice. 1960. Physical disability: a psychological approach. New York, Harper & Row.

Wright, G. N., I. W. Reagles, and K. T. Thomas. 1971. The Wood County project: an expanded rehabilitation program for the vocationally handicapped. International Labor Review 104:1–2.

EDITH F. LYNTON

THE PHYSICALLY HANDICAPPED CITIZEN: A HUMAN RIGHTS ISSUE

IN DECEMBER 1968 the New York City Human Rights Law * was amended to include discrimination against the physically handicapped in housing, public accommodations, and employment under the jurisdiction of the City Commission on Human Rights. This was a signal event, an explicit recognition of the difficulties faced by the thousands of physically handicapped New Yorkers in leading fulfilling, self-sufficient lives. Because of prejudice, ignorance, or arbitrary policies that permeate the fabric of our society, thousands, perhaps as many as 12 per cent, of the city's residents who are handicapped are intentionally or unwittingly either excluded or have only limited access to essential services and activities.

The Commission is fully aware, and its experience with other minority groups has proven, that legal guarantees of rights are not automatically translated into effective protection simply by the passage of an amendment to a statute. Ingrained attitudes and policies are neither dispelled nor reformed swiftly or easily. Furthermore, it is unrealistic to place total reliance on the assertion of newly guaranteed rights by

EDITH F. LYNTON is a member of the staff of the Hearings and Research Division of the New York City Commission on Human Rights. This essay is from the first part of her Report of a Conference Sponsored by the Commission, June 10, 1971.
    * Administrative code of the City of New York, Section B1-1.0-Ba-12.0

those long inured to their very denial. For a host of reasons, lack of knowledge of the law, timidity, fear of confronting authority figures, individual claims of discrimination on the part of members of a group that formerly has been unable to protest, or who may have come to accept less than equitable treatment—all of these come only tentatively and hesitantly at first. The physically handicapped are no exception. Indeed, the nature of their handicaps may intensify the diffidence and unassertiveness characteristic of others who have been accorded minority treatment in the past. The individual claims made represent only a tiny fraction of the inequities the law intends to correct, voiced by the most vocal among the group. Predictably, the claims made under this most recent amendment of the Human Rights Law have been few.

The Commission is not content to limit its activity to protecting the few who have sufficient political awareness and perseverance to file and follow through the prosecution of a claim of discrimination. To do so, in the case of the handicapped, would be a dilution, if not a perversion, of the intent of the Law and the Commission's mandate. Reliance on the time-honored concept that it behooves citizens to know their legal rights would render this important amendment relatively meaningless. In time, handicapped people, it is hoped, will know their rights and how to assert them, and the public will become aware of its responsibilities. But that time has not yet arrived.

To fulfill its mandate to assure equal treatment of the handicapped, the Commission believed it necessary to take steps to heighten public awareness of this expansion of the Law and to develop a fuller understanding of the nature of discrimination than was disclosed by a limited number of individual claims. The Commission must know what policies or processes are exclusionary or restrictive, and how and by whom they are made. And it must also understand what gives rise to these policies or procedures, whether personal prejudice, institutional structures, or social, economic, or political postures. Such an understanding is essential for the fullest application and maximum utilization of the law and the Commission's powers within that law. And in the Commission's view it is impossible to obtain sufficient understanding without open and full communication with the members of the very group the Commission is intended to serve. A Human Rights Law mandate, broadly construed, makes it incumbent upon the Commission to not only process the claims brought to its attention but also to call attention to the problems beyond the scope of its particular and limited jurisdiction, so that all other city agencies and state and federal bodies will be sensitized to the needs of the handicapped.

As a first step, the Commission determined to hold a conference to give the handicapped themselves, as well as organizations that represent or work with them, the opportunity to discuss the whole range of issues involved in enabling them to become full participants in New York City life. Accordingly, a day-long conference on "Governmental Approaches to Discrimination Against the Handicapped" sponsored by the New York City Commission on Human Rights was held on June 10, 1971, with the cooperation of the Mayor's Advisory Committee on the Handicapped. More than 300 people attended, the majority of them handicapped. Also included were members of a wide range of related service organizations, government agencies that determine policies for essential services, both in general and in direct relation to those with physical handicaps, and individuals with special knowledge and expertise.

THE CONFERENCE FORMAT

The conference was designed as a working session, divided into day-long workshops focused on a particular life function. Topics for individual workshops were housing, public accommodations, transportation, employment, education, health, and social welfare. The design itself represents a departure from traditional conference plans that generally group participants by type of handicap. Workshops cut across disability lines; and although individual preferences were solicited, each workshop was constructed so as to include a cross-section of the various handicaps represented together with representatives of the range of agencies, both voluntary and governmental, in attendance. Each workshop operated under the guidance of a moderator and consultants, among whom were officers of such groups as the Eastern Paralyzed Veterans Association, the State Division of Employment, the AFL-CIO, United Cerebral Palsy of New York, Disabled in Action, the Public Service Council, and the Office of Public Housing. Staff members of the Commission participated in each group. In addition, a special panel moderated by Councilman Mario Merola, co-sponsor of the 1968 amendment that added the handicapped to the City Human Rights Law's protection, focused on the provisions of the law itself.

THE OBJECTIVES

Chairman Eleanor Holmes Norton, in her opening remarks, set forth the Commission's perspectives and objectives for the conference as follows: *

In 1969 an historic and unprecedented bill sponsored by Councilman Mario Merola forbidding discrimination against the physically handicapped was passed by the City Council. The New York City Commission on Human Rights was given the power and the duty to construe provisions banning discrimination in employment and in the sale or rental of housing and commercial space to cover the physically handicapped, where consistent with the nature and extent of the handicap. This city thus took an historic step in extending the tradition of New York pluralism to recognize and give official status to this important group of our citizens.

Only a few months after my appointment to the Commission, I became intrigued with the possibilities the law afforded the commission to affect the lives of the physically handicapped in an important and exciting way. For this statute departs from the law's tradition of segregating out the physically handicapped as abnormal people. Instead it places the handicapped alongside blacks, Puerto Ricans, Jews, Italians, and every other ethnic group in the city, as well as women and older workers. It is hard to overestimate the potential effect of this governmental recognition that a physical handicap is often of no greater relevance than skin color, sex, or age.

Considering that estimates of the physically handicapped in our city run as high as 12 per cent, it should not surprise anyone if the handicapped emerge as the largest new minority group in the city. Still, indications are that the handicapped have yet to come to full consciousness of their legal and actual status as a discriminated-against group.

Indeed, I first decided upon this conference after learning of the small number of complaints that had been filed by handicapped complainants since the law was passed. I was particularly concerned that without more complaints the Commission would not be able to build up the expertise that can only come from investigating and adjudicating actual complaints. This

* *Remarks of Eleanor Holmes Norton, Chairman of the City Commission on Human Rights, delivered at the conference on "Governmental Approaches to Discrimination Against the Handicapped" at the Jewish Guild for the Blind, 15 West 65th Street, New York City, on Thursday, June 10, 1971.*

in turn would affect the vitality of the new law and ultimately the handicapped themselves.

Still, the small number of complaints filed thus far is consistent with the way every new group to be covered by the antidiscrimination law has reacted to that coverage initially. Despite group pressure to be included under such protection, individuals in the group traditionally come forward only slowly to claim the available protection. For it takes a bold set of mind to become a combatant in a law suit, whether you are a handicapped person, a black person, or an older worker.

Nothing illustrates how typical is the reluctance of the handicapped than the close similarity between their initial reaction to inclusion in the Human Rights Law and the initial reaction of women. Although women have been included under our law since 1965, there were only one or two complaints a month when I first came to the Commission, and this in the face of the most widespread, overt, and intentional discrimination against the largest group in the city. There, as here, the Commission decided to summon the target group to a public hearing which would educate them and the public to the problems faced and which would incorporate their active participation. If the significant, stepped-up flow of complaints that followed our women's hearings is any indication, we will be hearing much more from the handicapped following this conference.

This word must get to the handicapped if this law is to reach its obvious potential: A free, committed, and sympathetic attorney expert in the Human Rights Law is available to every complainant who comes to the Commission. And there are no court costs or other expenses. A phone call may save a trip to the Commission since free advice concerning discrimination can be provided by phone. There is the right to file a complaint, to full consideration of the grievance, to conciliation if discrimination is present, and to a full hearing if conciliation fails. This entirely free mechanism to correct discrimination could change the lives of handicapped New Yorkers every bit as much as it has changed things for black people in this city.

The fact is that this country has always had blacks of many colors. For skin color is not the only symbol that has been irrationally used to treat people unfairly. Nor has race been the only condition to be misunderstood by the public.

Handicapped people pursuing their right to live as ordinary free citizens are in the great civil rights tradition of blacks and other minority groups. They are only the latest group of deprived Americans to step forward to claim their due. They provide us with yet another test of our willingness to accommodate to the diversity we proclaim so proudly. Even though other groups are welcomed into society's mainstream, if we draw the line at the handicapped, we give the lie to our principles of full equality and justice. But we do not have ten or twenty years to begin to see significant change for the handicapped. We have set ourselves the goal of one year in which to see substantial changes under way. If we at the Commission and the Mayor's Advisory Committee have our way, if the handicapped and those who serve them have their way, if the best in the city's tradition is given its way, we shall surely meet that goal.

CONFERENCE ISSUES

For the rest of the day the conference participants were free to explore the issues related to their workshop topic as extensively or intensively as they wished. Moderators were provided only with a few general questions to serve as a suggested framework for group discussion. They were:

1) What are the specific problems faced by persons with various physical handicaps in the area your workshop is discussing?

2) In the areas covered by the Human Rights Law (employment, housing, and public accommodations) what guidelines should the Commission promulgate to implement the law? (E.g., can a restaurant refuse service to a person in a wheelchair or an individual with a guide dog, claiming lack of space or sanitary reasons?)

3) How should the current narrow definition of "physically handicapped" in the Human Rights Law be realistically expanded?

4) Aside from the Human Rights Law, what other laws affecting the handicapped—federal, state, or city—should be modified or introduced? How can this be accomplished?

5) What rules, regulations, and procedures should other governmental agencies adopt to aid the handicapped? (E.g., how should the Civil Service Commission change its requirements and procedures for physical examinations to accommodate the handicapped?)

6) How can the Commission on Human Rights (as well as other governmental agencies) and organizations working with the handicapped help each other in preventing discrimination against the handicapped? (E.g., can organizations screen and refer discrimination cases to the Commission?)

The plan, designed to impose only that degree of structure that would stimulate and focus discussion rather than formulate a precise agenda, was adopted because the Commission believes that the handicapped themselves have had insufficient opportunity for across-the-board discussion. And their opportunity to transcend the boundaries of particular handicaps and focus instead on the common problems that affect all those with some form of physical limitation has been especially limited. The usual pattern of organizing groups around a particular physical disability has resulted in very little knowledge among the handicapped themselves of the problems they share with others who have different disabilities. This is perhaps in part the reason why the general public is largely unaware of what constitute barriers for handicapped persons, except in relation to individuals or relatively small groups. The Commission believes that not only are there many common denominators, but also that only a broader basis for approaching these problems is likely to yield workable solutions.

GENERAL TENOR OF THE WORKSHOPS

The assumptions underlying the basic conference plan apparently were justified, for discussion in each workshop was lively, spirited, and participated in by virtually every member of each group. For many of the handicapped present, it was clearly the first, or one of only a few opportunities, they had had to express opinions, protest against felt inequities, or recommend changes in public and private sector policies. Indeed, many told the Commission staff that the conference represented a new experience for them. As one participant put it, "We blind are accustomed to talking only with others who are blind and it becomes a general commiseration session. We never get away from the individual sad stories."

The value of this opportunity to discuss common problems that occur in essential life functions was apparent not only in the responsiveness of the groups, but also in the evident development of their ability to deal with the topics assigned. For despite the fact that the workshops operated very differently—some were entirely free-flowing interchanges, some were partially structured by moderators, and one followed a carefully preplanned format—it is possible to trace a pattern of progression in each. Although the pace was different, the directions were remarkably similar. They moved from statements of problems, that upon closer examination proved to be only symptoms of larger problems, to formulating solutions for the major issues. Perhaps the most significant development was the progression from the individual case history approach, through the discussion of the needs of a particular type of disability (the blind, the deaf, or the orthopedically handicapped) to identifying the common or generic issues and broader-based strategies for remediation.

All of the workshops found it somewhat difficult to handle their assigned topics as a discrete entity. Admittedly, the topics were thoroughly interdependent. It is difficult to decide whether housing is a more basic need than transportation, or whether employment opportunity depends more on access to education, to transportation, or to rehabilitation services, than on the number and quality of job openings. Thus, in each workshop there were areas of overlap. But in the main they held well to the focus assigned them. Differences in the degree to which they were able to formulate problems and devise solutions are attributable largely to differences in the complexity of the topics. For example, it is easier to recommend innovative forms of transportation or other essentially practical services than it is to formulate a whole city-wide educational policy. And one can more readily suggest immediate remedies for what were identified as inequitable provisions in health insurance or in public assistance regulations than for the desperate shortage of appropriate housing.

Reviews of each workshop are indicative of the areas of agreement and disagreement and furnish the principal recommendations made that relate directly to the topic assigned. The problems identified run a wide gamut, ranging from specific examples of physical or regulatory impediments to broad philosophical or theoretical policy questions. The recommendations made include suggestions for legislative action, for further research and investigation, and for the development of effective political constituencies.

AN OVERVIEW OF WORKSHOP DISCUSSIONS

Notwithstanding the broad scope of the conference, an overview of the discussions is not only possible but also extremely useful because of the similarities in major concerns. Underlying the specific barriers to full participation in each area are numerous common, fundamental issues. Indeed, the parallel lines of discussion and the consistency in the types of action recommended can be taken to indicate that in each workshop the essential and most important elements to be dealt with to improve the position of the handicapped were identified.

Developing a plan for reorganizing basic societal arrangements to better serve any group requires first a careful analysis of problems in order to separate symptoms from causes, and myths from realities. It requires selecting the direction of change likely to provide solutions, and choosing tactics and strategies for action likely to provide movement toward the goals. Furthermore, it is necessary to identify the individuals, groups, or coalitions of groups that can best serve as agents of implementation.

At the conference, all four aspects of social problemsolving were approached, separately in each workshop, and jointly in the concluding session. One day is obviously insufficient to formulate a total package in detail, but considerable strides were made, especially in the primary areas of identifying what constitutes basic problems and in reaching agreements on the key elements.

PRINCIPAL AREAS OF AGREEMENT

Not all issues raised could be resolved. Among the recurrent themes in all workshops, some were clarified by discussion and can be considered consensus views. Others remained unresolved, but emerged as important areas for further study and consultation.

The areas of basic agreement, broadly stated and in somewhat simplified terms, are nevertheless important as the foundation for the principal recommendations. They are:

1) The current New York City Human Rights law is limited in immediate effect because it is either unknown to or misunderstood by both the handicapped themselves and by those who control the designated areas of protection. The law is limited in potential impact by its ambiguous language and by its restricted definition of what constitutes a handicap. Nonetheless, the concept of legal intervention in relation to discrimination against the handicapped, new to jurisprudence, is symptomatic of an emerging view that the handicapped can and should be part of the functioning society. Therefore, this law must be utilized to its maximum.

2) Restricted access to and participation in all aspects of major life

functions requires a careful reexamination of institutional structures, both physical and organizational. Many of the problems lie outside the scope of the Human Rights Law and demand other forms of action.

3) Discrimination against the handicapped is largely attitudinal. It is less a problem of overt and intentional exclusion or specific physical or organizational barriers, and more a reflection of apathy to and ignorance of the needs and capacities of the handicapped on the part of the total society.

4) Despite the proliferation of agencies that serve the handicapped, there is little adequate data upon which to base sophisticated planning. What is needed is an accurate estimate of the numbers of physically handicapped, basic demographic characteristics, socioeconomic status, physical and intellectual capacity.

5) Essential services for the handicapped are fragmented and disorganized, and channels of information and referral are unclear. Both the ability to reach the handicapped and the impact on those reached is diminished by the unavailability of comprehensive knowledge of what exists, and by the methods of service distribution and delivery.

6) The handicapped themselves must come out of hiding and become a visible, articulate, and organized group, capable of effectively presenting their needs and asserting their rights. They must move from concern with individual problems to the larger issues common to the greater number. Those attending the conference are but a fragment of the total handicapped population, the small number who have been able to overcome the timidity and immobility characteristic of the majority. The larger numbers that are now unseen and unheard must be reached.

UNRESOLVED ISSUES

Underlying the basic areas of agreement and complicating the search for remedies are two fundamental issues, both unresolved in the course of discussion—one concerning the problem of defining and delimiting the handicapped constituency and the other the question of that constituency's underlying objectives.

Defining an effective constituency presents the choice of either opting for size to gain political impact by merging around the broadest conception of common interests with other groups such as the mentally handicapped, the poor, and the aged, or limiting the constituency to the physically handicapped in order to avoid diluting or subordinating their concerns.

The problem of objectives is how to integrate the handicapped within the total fabric of society, allowing them maximum participation in all activities, and yet provide for them the special accommodations, treatment, and intervention they need for self-sufficient and productive lives.

Both issues are critical and complex, and to date neither has been resolved satisfactorily by any minority group. In essence they are the crux of the problem for minorities—how to achieve a balance between integration and self-identity.

The principal recommendations flow directly from the six areas of agreement, and take into account, as well, the two major unresolved issues. The recommendations of individual workshops reflect the details of these general considerations: the actions and policies required to combat discrimination, reorganization of service delivery systems, development of adequate knowledge, and mobilization of effective organizational capacity.

THREE LAYERS OF DISCRIMINATION

The first three of the areas of agreement can be conceptualized as three layers of discrimination against the handicapped. The first layer is the overt denial to individuals of jobs, apartments, or access to public accommodations—a denial attributable directly to their being handicapped. It is to this layer that the Human Rights Law is primarily addressed. The second layer consists of the barriers that result from architectural design or formulation of regulations or policies in a host of public and private institutions or activities that are not intended to be discriminatory, but in effect are. Some may be construed to be within the jurisdiction of the Commission, others may fall beyond its scope, and still others may not be susceptible to solution by legal remedies. The third layer, the general indifference to and the misconceptions about the handicapped that prevail, is the most difficult to counter. Because these attitudes give rise to a sense of alienation among those who are in some way disabled, they tend to be self-perpetuating by isolating the handicapped and rendering them silent and almost invisible. Public disinterest thus continues undisturbed, and the policies this disinterest engenders remain unchallenged. The conference, itself, was an initial attack on this fundamental layer.

The three layers of discrimination are interrelated, and in essence form an indivisible whole. But separation permits a more detailed analysis of their component parts and a sharper assessment of potential solutions. Such separation makes it clear that no single approach will suffice.

THE FIRST LAYER

The most immediate concern, and indeed, the primary focus for discussion by the workshops, was the current Human Rights Law. Each workshop was directed to give particular attention to the problems of applying the Law. Interest in the current Law, predictably, was more intense in workshops assigned to areas now covered by that Law. But other workshops also assessed the Law and considered ways to make it more effective. Workshop discussions, together with the findings of a special panel designated to coordinate and synthesize the various workshop views, fall into two parts: first, how the Law in its current form can be utilized to its maximum, and second, how the Law should be amended, expanded, and its enforcement provisions strengthened. This two-part approach reflects Chairman Norton's statement to the special panel on the Law:

The New York City Law is unprecedented in the country, and, therefore, there is little prior experience on which to rely. The specificity of the problems delineated by the conference is helpful to the Commission. Some problems may require additional statutory amendment, but many, perhaps, can be handled through regulations the Commission can issue pursuant to the law, as enacted. Therefore, let me ask you to consider your recommendations for change in two categories, first, the specific problems that come under the Law and that require promulgation of regulations, clarifications, or special attention, and second, problems that relate to areas not now covered by the Law but that should be covered, and therefore require realistic expansion of the Law or careful study to determine how best these areas can be encompassed.

The principal barrier to the full use of potential guaranties under the Law was believed to be the lack of awareness of the existence of the Law on the part of the general public and those primarily affected—

landlords, employers, government officials, and especially the handicapped themselves. One answer was felt to be an intensive publicity campaign to alert all citizens to the Law's provisions, focusing in particular on those groups most directly involved. Many suggestions were offered, including the preparation of literature to be disseminated, and posting the Law in all places of work, residence, and in all public facilities. Use of the mass media and the development of a series of conferences or special symposia for employers, landlords, and other affected groups were discussed. Who should sponsor and develop this publicity, admittedly a sizeable task, was difficult to determine. The problem of disseminating information is magnified when so many of the handicapped are conceded to be virtual shut-ins, isolated from contact with other handicapped persons and unrepresented by the range of special service agencies. Many saw dissemination as the Commission's responsibility but, mindful that current budgets scarcely allow for massive and continuing public education programs on the part of the Commission, suggested that this now should be the responsibility of the voluntary agencies serving the handicapped.

Some of the participants thought that the type of publicity likely to have the greatest impact would be exposure of the Law in relation to violation and enforcement. They wanted all complaints publicized, irrespective of outcome; and some even urged publicizing complaints before they were processed and investigated. But, in discussion, it was conceded that neither would be consistent with sound public policy. Some suggested that vigorous enforcement would be equal to or perhaps more effective than generalized publicity. But, one participant commented that publicizing the Law without amplifying its capability of enforcement might result "in the Commission losing its credibility for doing service to the handicapped."

The difficulties with enforcement were identified as twofold: first, the problems inherent in relying on individual complaints from those unaccustomed to asserting their rights, and who, because of physical immobility or financial insecurity, "find it difficult to initiate, let alone endure the complex procedures"; and, second, the difficulties of determining what constitutes discrimination against the handicapped in the absence of well-defined guidelines understood by both handicapped people and by those on whom they depend. To help individuals assert claims, several recommended that complaint forms be distributed to all agencies serving the handicapped, and that personnel in agencies be designated and trained to encourage and assist with filing complaints. Agencies should develop handicapped members to serve as ombudsmen to help clients identify and process claims.

The second problem, that of guidelines for landlords, employers, and managers of public facilities, is obviously an area for continuous and long-term study. A specific proposal for immediate action, enthusiastically endorsed by the entire group, was that the Commission request funding to employ handicapped persons to work with the problem. If the Commission were able to employ handicapped persons as key personnel in the provision of service to the city's handicapped population, some of the principal recommendations made at the conference would be fulfilled. First, it was unanimously agreed that it is important for a public agency to set an example, to both the public and private sector, in the employment of handicapped people in appropriate and responsible roles. Second, the Commission's capacity to formulate guidelines would be facilitated and strengthened by inclusion on its staff of those likely to be most sensitive to the ways in which discrimination against the handicapped manifests itself.

However, the group was aware of certain realities, namely, that the Commission's budget and staff would need to be increased to permit intensive publicity and investigation and to engage in outreach activities. Indeed, it would require additional funds to establish a special department assigned to work with the handicapped. The group further recognized that it behooves handicapped citizens to press for adequate budget allocations to the Commission commensurate with the demands of expanded jurisdiction. As one participant said, "It's up to us to see that the Commission has the clout to do a job for us." Augmenting the Commission's capacity is necessary not only to enforce the Law as it now stands but, even more, to broaden the Law's coverage.

The conference participants were keenly interested in expanding the Law. Although they recognized, as Councilman Merola stated, that limitations in the Law are the result of compromises made to assuage opponents and assure its passage, the majority believed that these limitations should not be allowed to continue for long. They were aware that the watering down that takes place as a temporary expedient too often becomes a permanent fixture, continuing long after anyone remembers why the compromises were adopted.

Among the problems to be dealt with in amendments by the Council is the obvious ambiguity of the language of the Law. The Law states that the handicapped are those "who may depend" on a device or appliance. The word "may" is itself unclear. Does it mean "may" in a sense of possibility under certain circumstances or at certain times, or does it mean only those who do in fact depend on devices or appliances? The devices enumerated are "brace, crutch, cane, seeing-eye dog, hand-controlled car, or such other device or appliance." What are "such other devices"? Can they be construed to include an ordinary car, considered by many to be virtually a prosthetic device for those unable to manage public transportation? What about those with visual, hearing, or orthopedic limitations who do not use any mechanical aid, as for example the legally blind who can manage without a seeing-eye dog or a cane? It was the consensus that definitions based on reliance on devices inevitably would be ambiguous and limited, given the rate of progress in rehabilitative techniques.

In addition to ambiguities of language in the Law, also left unclear is the extent to which landlords, employers, or others can be required to alter structures to meet the needs of handicapped persons. At present there are no court decisions that are strictly relevant to this question, and it remains an area for serious study and future testing in the courts.

The major defect detected in the Law, however, is not its ambiguity but the narrow and arbitrary definition of what constitutes a handicap. That definition, it is generally agreed, excludes large categories of neurological, cardiac, pulmonary, and other physical disorders capable of control by medication, therapy, or by compensation through rehabilitation. It also excludes those who differ physically from the norm, such as people of abnormally small stature. And it makes no mention at all of mental handicaps.

It was unanimously agreed that the definition of what constitutes a handicap needs rethinking. A new definition should clearly encompass all types and degrees of physical disability. Whether to include the mentally handicapped was a topic of discussion. Many believed that the mentally retarded should be included, and perhaps also those with specific mental illnesses controlled by therapy. But the issue was beclouded by the difficulty of defining mental or emotional problems with precision. Uncertainty about whether or not to include intellectual and psychological limitations is probably attributable to the fact that conference participation was limited in the main to the physically handicapped. Participants were not only unable to specify other handicaps but were also concerned that combining both physical and mental handicaps in one legal provision might prove to be a disservice to either or both groups, with their so completely dissimilar problems.

Conference opinion on the definition was perhaps best expressed by one participant who stated that, "Legal protection should be expanded to the maximum feasible in terms of current ability to specify the nature of a disability or its susceptibility to compensatory treatment and control."

An underlying concern voiced by many was whether the Human Rights Law guaranty could move away from dependence on individual assertions of damaging discrimination to issues of broader group concern—issues not so likely to be called into question by individual claims.

Regarding the first layer, it was recommended that: (1) The Human Rights Law, in its application to physically handicapped persons, must be vigorously enforced; and (2) that steps must be taken to rectify the deficiencies in the Law's provisions, both in its language and its coverage.

The conference was a first step toward the accomplishment of both objectives. Token enforcement and "gerrymandered" coverage tend to breed cynicism concerning the efficacy of the legal process.

It is gratifying that several complaints were filed with Commission staff investigators during the day of the conference; and since the conference, new claims have been filed at an increasing rate, claims that evidence a greater range of issues. Through the heightened awareness of those who participated, and particularly the many who are members or staff of public and voluntary agencies, information will spread.

The Commission also has been active in examining how to improve the existing statute. In consultation with groups of physically handicapped persons and with the Mayor's Advisory Committee, Commission staff has been working on drafting a new definition of handicap. All existing definitions used by public agencies and in other statutes

have been gathered and studied. The intent is to formulate a new definition that will be sufficiently precise and yet inclusive. A new definition,
when ready, will be proposed to the City Council, and will require
broad-based support.

In addition, the Commission is seeking funding for the establishment
of a special division, within its organization, to deal with the problems
of the handicapped. The aim is not only to process complaints, but also
to study the complex problems involved in formulating guidelines and
issuing regulations to clarify what constitutes discriminatory practice
and what accommodation can realistically be required. It would be the
Commission's goal to include in this division personnel who are themselves physically handicapped.

Of considerable value will be the findings of a census of all handicapped city personnel, initiated by the Commission on October 15,
1971, and soon to be completed. The data compiled, covering the job
titles and salary levels of physically handicapped employed by type of
handicap, should serve as a basis for understanding their current status
in city agencies.

THE SECOND LAYER

The second layer is a network of stumbling blocks, both literally and
figuratively. Major components are physical obstructions: doorways too
narrow for access by wheelchairs; inadequate or poorly located wash-
rooms, parking space, or dining facilities; spikes in supermarket exits
designed to prevent the removal of shopping carts; educational and
recreational buildings served only by stairways; narrow aisles in
shops and theaters, and many more. Some constitute barriers in and of
themselves. Others become the justification for policies of exclusion
when the proprietor or manager of a shop or restaurant prefers to avoid
patrons in wheelchairs.

But stumbling blocks in the form of regulations or policies governing
various institutional arrangements, not necessarily directed at the handicapped but which nonetheless inhibit their access, pose problems that
may be even more critical and more pervasive in effect. Among these
are insurance policy provisions that attach high-risk costs to participation by handicapped persons, health insurance coverage tied to institutional care at the expense of outpatient or home service, school policies

that place children in unnecessarily specialized settings, welfare provisions and income eligibility standards for public housing determined without reference to the financial needs and higher living costs of handicapped people, fire laws that prohibit wheelchairs in theater aisles, and restricted parking facilities.

The problems within this layer are manifold. It is difficult to determine realistically how seemingly simple physical obstacles can be removed. Some, for example, the supermarket spikes, probably could be replaced by another method of handling the stores' problems. Situations of this type might be resolved in negotiation. Widening doorways and installing ramps or elevators, however, might necessitate alterations too costly to, in all reasonable expectation, be made voluntarily. Inducements in the form of subsidies or tax relief suggest themselves, and also intensify the need to restudy building codes and to press for wider application, once enacted. The fundamental defect in most legislative remedies with respect to physical structures is that they deal only prospectively, applying only to those structures built after adoption of new codes. But another defect is the tendency to exempt large segments of construction, especially the private sector, and to govern only partially the facilities housing public agencies. Pessimism over the ability to provide immediate solutions has diminished effective support for legislative remedies. As a result, new building codes are often watered down in the legislature in the face of objections voice by vested interests in the construction industry. The housing workshop, in particular, deemed it important for handicapped citizens to mobilize support for new legislation, even if its impact would not be immediate.

The presence of physical impediments is symptomatic of insufficient concern for disabled people. But the use of such impediments as the basis for excluding or segregating people with handicaps by individual managers and proprietors of buildings, airline personnel, or even school principals who wish to avoid "problem" enrollments, often in a totally idiosyncratic manner, suggests some underlying prejudices. The same can be said of the issue of insurance costs. Some participants claimed that the insurance problem, as used by landlords and employers in turning down the handicapped, is essentially a "straw man." Clarification of the impact of insurance probably would help to eliminate this barrier, if indeed it is genuinely the product of misunderstanding.

Health insurance, welfare regulations, and school policies are in different ways issues to be settled in the political arena, and appear likely to yield only to the application of pressure at appropriate and sensitive points. But their effect needs documentation in precise measures of the waste incurred by hospitalizing those who could be cared for less intensively, of the counterproductivity of welfare rules that discourage rather than offer incentives for employment, and of school costs of conducting specialized programs for those who could be better served in the regular classroom. All of the existing standards need to be scrutinized to assess the impact on the handicapped population, for most were designed without regard to the needs of the handicapped.

It was recommended that a series of working task forces should be organized, to (1) review all existing and proposed building codes to ascertain their effect on handicapped persons; (2) review regulations promulgated by all public agencies including the social services administration, federal, state, and local health agencies, especially those governing medical insurance and school systems; and (3) study the questions of insurance costs and comparative building costs, as well as the cost of modifications to all existing structures, both residential and public.

In essence, all of these problems devolve upon the political process. Indications are that handicapped persons are becoming increasingly politicized, and are gaining spokesmen. It is noteworthy, for example, that Councilman Merola has introduced legislation before the City Council to expand parking privileges for the handicapped by mandating privileges to all who need them for any reason, personal, social, or recreational, on the basis of a physician's certificate. Currently, parking permits are extended at the discretion of the Traffic Commissioner to those who need cars for work or school. Success in enacting this legislation, in the face of questioning on the part of traffic authorities, will be one index of the ability of the handicapped to organize effectively. For parking was an issue of considerable concern in workshop and other group discussion concerning the transportation needs of the handicapped.

Effective political action will depend on the ability to specify needs and document their significance, especially through sophisticated cost-benefit analysis, and to muster sufficient support for action. And because many regulations and policies that ignore or injure handicapped citizens emanate from state or federal authorities, it would appear desirable to seek statutory protection, similar to the City Human Rights Law coverage, in both higher jurisdictions.

THE THIRD LAYER

The ultimate complication is that many of the elements found in the second layer are intertwined with a general indifference to the needs of handicapped people. This constitutes the third layer. This layer, however, is manifest not only in limitations on the use of facilities and services that do exist, but also, and perhaps even more injuriously, in the nonexistence of much that is essential. It is exemplified by doctors who do not make home visits or who are unwilling or unable to treat the handicapped, by architects who design buildings in complete innocence of their impact on the handicapped, by school policies that make little attempt to look beyond a handicap to the individual learning capacity of the child, by transportation systems that are either totally unusable or prohibitive in cost for daily living, and by the fact that the police are often unaware of handicapped citizens' special protective needs, even of the existence of the Human Rights Law itself.

Those attending the conference recognized that their preoccupation with the first two layers of discrimination was essentially unrepresentative of the problems that the majority of handicapped persons face. However, the very fact of their attendance at the conference indicates considerable progress on the part of numbers of handicapped individuals in surmounting obstacles. Unlike many of their counterparts among the city's handicapped residents, those in attendance are alive to the issues and able to participate in programs. Their participation represents an adjustment to the world of work and a degree of personal commitment. For the handicapped person who is homebound, isolated, and financially and physically dependent, the problems of explicit denial of an apartment or job are irrelevant, and the difficulties in entering a theater or parking a car remote and rather esoteric concerns. As one participant stated,

We at the conference are hearing only the feelings, concepts, and philosophies of the more vocal of the disabled. There are countless thousands out there who could not be here today because they did not know about the conference, or because they didn't have the twenty-five or fifty dollars to get here with specialized transportation. I think it is imperative that, in addition to asserting the needs of the vocal disabled, we try to reach those in the woodwork.

Public prejudice—for indeed there is prejudice even if it is not characterized by hostility to handicapped people, but rather by what one participant called a "cosmetic problem"—exists because few able-bodied have any direct contact or involvement with disabled persons. They are separated from each other in school at the outset, and the separation continues as handicapped people become increasingly unable to participate in social and vocational activities. And the isolation compounds itself. The handicapped are doubly disabled in their attempts to move out into the mainstream. They are handicapped first by physical difference, and second by their self-perception and the way they are perceived by others. The "they don't apply" rationale is perhaps even more accurate for the physically handicapped than it has been for all other minorities. How to break this self-perpetuating cycle is a major problem, for society at large is unlikely to respond unless the handicapped make their needs felt. And unless handicapped people are better able to negotiate the system they will continue to be ineffectual in voicing their needs. Major commitments of public and private resources will be required to build more than the pitifully few apartments now available to handicapped people. Appropriate and reasonably priced systems of transportation must be developed, and education refocused so as to integrate handicapped children into the school system. Comprehensive social and health services with sufficient reach must be supplied, and handicapped people trained for responsible job opportunities. Unless these primary objectives are attained, the likelihood is that the majority of the handicapped will continue to be neglected.

What the conference participants would like to see is a massive educational program directed not only toward those who are the providers of basic human services, but also toward the handicapped themselves to assist them to develop as a political constituency. Each workshop concluded that key personnel—doctors, teachers, architects, and other professionals—should, as an integral part of their vocational preparation, be exposed to the handicapped and given at least a basic understanding of how professional attitudes condition or even control the lives of those who are in any way physically limited. An important adjunct is that the handicapped themselves be actively recruited to be developed as professionals in basic service fields.

Mindful that it is a cliché that conferences recommend more conferences, the participants nevertheless considered this conference a ground-breaking experience, and one that should be followed with a series of planned consultations. Future conferences may need to be decentralized, with smaller groups meeting in many neighborhoods to permit involvement of a broader representation. Additional major citywide conferences could provide time for analysis and consultation with larger numbers of employers, landlords, and public agency officials to formulate policies for affirmative action in specific areas.

Therefore, the conference recommended that:

1) Public education programs should be developed to reach the public at large, and especially those segments whose policies have particular impact on the life-style of physically handicapped people—owners and managers of housing and public facilities, employers and personnel directors, legislators and public officials.

2) A basic understanding of the problems and potential of physically handicapped persons should be included as an integral component of the educational preparation for all relevant professions—architecture, medicine, social work, teaching.

3) Physically handicapped personnel should be actively recruited and developed for managerial and policymaking roles in public and voluntary agencies serving the disabled population.

4) Outreach techniques should be utilized to contact the many handicapped people generally unreached.

Public education is a popular panacea for all social problems. Indeed, it would be unthinkable to oppose any activity that increases public consciousness of conditions that demand attention. The question is, what constitutes effective public education? Skepticism concerning the value of an educational approach to solving social problems was expressed in many of the workshops. In the employment workshop, for example, some participants had little patience with "educating employers," believing that this has been a traditionally ineffectual tactic. But the past failure appears to be attributable to a "good works" approach, experience proving that promoting altruism generally results in token or peripheral reactions. Economic inducements or legal sanctions tend to have a speedier and more pervasive impact.

What the workshops agreed on, and what experience in civil rights, anti-poverty, and other social movements substantiates, is that little meaningful learning occurs in the abstract. Public ability to understand the capabilities and aspirations of handicapped people will best develop through direct contact in specific situations. This underlines the importance of developing handicapped personnel to higher levels of responsibility in organizations that have important relations with social and economic policies in the city. Assuredly, it is the responsibility of those agencies now serving the handicapped, and who therefore should know their capability, to rethink their hiring and promotional procedures so that more handicapped individuals operate in key roles.

The same is true with respect to professional preparation. While teaching architects, doctors, and others about the handicapped is certainly to be endorsed, still better would be the inclusion of more persons with physical handicaps within the ranks of the professions. All of the foregoing calls for redesign of job specifications, personnel practices, training and educational techniques, and entry criteria. And if this process is not to result in an intensive "creaming" of a select few, outreach activities will be needed to broaden the base of participation in all institutions and urban affairs on the part of handicapped people. Too many are now isolated and out of contact. Better use should be made of media, of group work, of neighborhood and local activities, and of home visiting techniques.

INFORMATION, RESEARCH, AND
REORGANIZING SERVICE PROVISIONS

The conference identified two principal gaps in current knowledge that inhibit the devising of ways to overcome major problems facing handicapped people. One is the lack of any comprehensive information about the nature of services now available. The second is the absence of basic data descriptive of the city's handicapped citizens. From conference discussions, it was evident that even those intimately involved seldom have accurate, current information as to the nature of all existing services, their location, or for whom they are designed. At the conference, participants frequently exchanged information unknown to each other before the face-to-face meeting. A first step is the development of a clearing house of information for use by individuals and agencies. This is a role now partially fulfilled by the Mayor's Advisory Committee on the Handicapped, but the job requires substantial increases in budget and staff.

The fragmentation of service in both public and voluntary settings into small specialized units devoted to a single handicap, or a single type of service, results, it is believed, in wasteful duplication and significant gaps in what is offered. Thousands are not served at all. Many individuals are clients of several agencies, and some services are underutilized because of poor communication or ineffective outreach techniques. In addition, attitudes on the part of potential clients must be understood. For example, in the health workshop it was noted that much of the city's rehabilitation service is located in municipal hospitals to which free transportation is available. But because municipal facilities suffer from a negative image, they are utilized most often only by the very poor or the elderly. Underutilization, however, is probably less of a problem than inadequate amount of service or inappropriate mode of delivery. A critical element for a target population whose mobility is impaired is the location of facilities, the ease of transportation, and the availability of outpatient or service in the home.

Obviously a clearing house is only a beginning, but it is an important step. The conference members were certain that availability of information would provide an overview that could lead to better planning, paving the way also for more cooperation and collaboration among public and voluntary agencies. According to some, a kind of factionalism now exists, intensified as agencies compete for private and public financial support. Impartial evaluation of the outcome of differential types of service or alternate uses of available funding is unlikely in the absence of interagency cooperation. Information-gathering might reveal, for example, that, as alleged by some participants, a major share of current vocational services focus on those considered most employable, or conversely, that medical rehabilitation concentrates on the most "interesting" medical problems. If these allegations are correct, they imply a selectivity based on professional judgments and interests that merit more objective appraisal. In a different direction, comparative studies might accelerate the move from a case-work approach to group work or community organization, a trend apparent throughout social service practice. But that is warranted only if research evidence indicates that individual remediation has only limited outcomes. Perhaps it is unrealistic to expect this much research and planning to flow inevitably from the establishment of a clearing house. But any step that stimulates communication between the multiplicity of agencies is to be endorsed.

Planning in any sophisticated sense, it was agreed, is unlikely to develop in the absence of good and reliable data about the handicapped. Census figures are rudimentary and agency records fragmentary. Neither, for example, offers sufficient information for the development of a useful transportation system. The Mayor's Committee, in the absence of funds for a complete demographic study, is gathering data from a 5 per cent sample of the 1970 census. It is also submitting proposals to the Department of Health, Education and Welfare and to the Department of Transportation for feasibility studies of local livery services. Basic data are to be gathered by distributing questionnaires to voluntary and public agencies. But these calculations obviously omit the homebound or those not known to agencies. Comprehensive data is not only vital to planning of specific programs, but essential also to document the magnitude of the need for the whole range of services and facilities for the handicapped. Reliable data can be a powerful tool in the development of political influence, for few legislators currently know the size of the potential constituency among handicapped citizens.

It is recommended that:

1) research capacity be developed to compile statistical data on the numbers of handicapped citizens and their basic characteristics;

2) current facilities for centralized service information be improved; and

3) a series of pilot programs be established to test the relative merits of different patterns of service delivery.

The three recommendations constitute the essential minimum of activity demanded. Without better information and some basic research and evaluation, it is difficult to consider with any degree of precision how to restructure service delivery systems.

The experience of the conference strongly indicates the value of meetings that cross disciplinary lines, and especially those that bring together individuals and agencies that represent different types of handicaps. Moreover, the various voluntary and public agencies with similar functions should meet to coordinate their approaches to program development. Nowhere is this need more apparent than in housing, where city, state, and federal agencies operate with overlapping jurisdiction and sometimes conflicting policies.

As in many other fields, medical knowledge—the ability to mitigate the effects of physical handicaps, control progressive disorders, and provide mechanical or chemotherapeutic compensation for disabilities—has far outstripped the social arrangements for the satisfactory delivery of medical service itself, and for permitting those benefited by this service to function to the full extent of their increased capacity. Moreover, scientific and technical progress inevitably increases specialization, and with increasing specialization there is a need for concerted, conscious planning to avoid splintering of services. The current development of multiservice centers and comprehensive service approaches is especially needed in the field.

There is a question that needs exploring as to whether to concentrate all service to the handicapped within special units or to structure service functionally. For example, is job development for physically handicapped persons likely to be best handled by a center catering to all the needs of the handicapped, or by a center that acts as job developers for all people who seek employment? The former way would most likely have greater familiarity with transportation and other practical problems and the latter probably would offer wider coverage of the job market. Such questions are likely to be answered reliably only through practical experience. The number of similar problems to be tested by demonstrations is large. Many are specified in the individual workshop summaries. Ultimately the choice of patterns involves not only testing for measurable effects, but also depends on the ideological considerations discussed below.

DEVELOPING A POLITICAL
CONSTITUENCY

Chairman Eleanor Holmes Norton, addressing the plenary session at the conclusion of the day's discussion, stated that "Government reacts to a constituency that is broadly organized. There is an acknowledged need for concerted and systematic pressure, and monitoring of all agencies on behalf of all of the handicapped citizens of this city."

The need for an effective political force, and the belief that the handicapped themselves must take the initiative to develop organizational capacity, was perhaps the single most important conclusion reached in each workshop. Indeed, the plenary session focused almost exclusively on this issue. The role for handicapped citizens is a dual one, involving both individual initiative and group participation. These are manifest in the statements of two participants; one who said, "We must come out and be seen, use the facilities, demand to be served, and apply for the jobs we know we can do"; and the other, "We must learn to see beyond personal problems, but find the largest common denominator."

In all likelihood, the ability of individuals to overcome their unassertiveness will best develop through group action directed toward common problems, for most of the problems discussed emanate from societal structures and policies, rather than from individual action. Individual behavior reflects public attitudes. In any event, inclusion under the guarantees of the Human Rights Law affords recourse against discriminatory action by specific individuals. The larger aspects of social change may require legislation at every jurisdictional level as well as restructuring of major public and private sector policies.

Therefore, the issue is how to develop an effective constituency, not only in size, but also in skill and commitment. Not all those who participated in the conference were able to think beyond the confines of a specific handicap, although many broadened their perception of problems in the day's exchange of ideas. Building a cohesive force that encompasses all physical handicaps will demand continued activity. But an even more difficult issue raised by several participants is whether or not the physically handicapped should seek to strengthen their position through alliances with other groups. Only the transportation workshop was ready to join forces with another group—the aged—and this is attributable to the need for federal appropriations for new transportation systems. In addition to the reluctance to join forces with the mentally handicapped, as already discussed, there was a recurrent opposition to linking with the culturally handicapped, or with the poor. The resistance to municipal hospital services and to the specially constructed apartments in low-income housing projects are symptomatic of this attitude. In a few instances this resistance was made explicit as a problem of status, for some stated that physical problems do not carry with them any stigma of personal failure, while poverty apparently does.

The majority recognized, however, that many of the handicapped are disadvantaged in other ways. Many are also poor, undereducated, black, members of other minority ethnic groups, aged, or mentally handicapped as well. In addition, many specific needs are common to other groups. But the question is whether the political influence required to achieve the goals of the physically handicapped would be aided through a coalition with other disadvantaged groups, or whether in such combination the needs of the physically disabled would be subordinated and minimized.

In all probability there is a need for both forms of organization, for special groups to represent the physically handicapped in particular, and for coalitions with other groups to strive for common needs. The education workshop evidenced concern with the development of community control and its application to the physically handicapped, indicating a potential third level of organization, the neighborhood.

For the present, the challenge of building a cohesive force of physically handicapped citizens alone appears to be a demanding one. And the majority opinion was that handicapped individuals must fulfill the leadership roles. Nevertheless, it was acknowledged that this organization must also include outside experts, especially those professionals who deal in rehabilitative and social services. Expert participation is needed to deal with the many practical and technical problems encountered. Professional involvement, it was believed, would engender a commitment to the broader social goals of handicapped people, enlarging the professional viewpoint beyond the strict confines of a particular discipline. As one participant stated, "What good is it if doctors are able to perform medical miracles but their patients are still unable to move out of the hospital into the world."

A major problem for a newly formed organization is the problem, as yet unresolved, of how to integrate those with physical handicaps into society without denying them special accommodations, treatment, financial assistance, or any other service they need. Most workshops vociferously opposed any form of separatism. Separate housing units, specialized education, or work settings ran counter to the basic goals. Yet, it was recognized that specific forms of intervention might be required and that their absence might be even more discriminatory in the long run. The issue is dramatized, for example, in considering how best to educate deaf children, when regular classrooms depend almost entirely on oral instruction and discussion.

Within a general framework that has as its guiding principle the minimization of physical differences, a host of specific conceptual and practical problems remain. The first is to identify those aspects of separatism that are purely arbitrary, as, for example, school assignments contingent on physical attributes of school buildings rather than on the learning needs of the child. The second is to assess the individual and the social consequences of separation versus integration. For it may better serve some handicapped individuals to omit certain aspects of curriculum, live in less than perfectly adapted apartments, or work in offices not optimally arranged, than to be isolated from others in ideal physical surroundings. Educators, manpower specialists, social workers, and other professionals have relatively little knowledge of what arrangements would maximize satisfactions for handicapped people. Obviously, the precise arrangements must be flexible if they are to adapt to different types and degrees of handicap as well as to individual aptitudes and interests. But merging whatever special intervention is required within the total societal fabric relates more to a commitment to objectives than to technique.

Shifting objectives from the creation of protected settings for those who are disabled to the facilitation of their movement into the society at large would cause major changes in the design of sheltered workshops or special educational programs. And it would be the most powerful stimulus for building interdisciplinary approaches and for transforming the social service focus from one of assisting individuals to adjust to prevailing conditions toward mobilizing action directed at social change.

It must be recognized, however, that not all who participated accepted as a basic principle the need to do away, to the extent possible, with all manifestations of special treatment. Many will continue to require or prefer particularized treatment or settings. Indeed, some aspects of "separatism" may be essential for some, at least for the present. The debate in the education workshop over the relative merits of the regular classroom and special classes or home instruction, moreover, indicates the need for systematic research on this fundamental issue.

Ultimately, the effective constituency for action in the political arena will depend on whether the majority wish to press for special tax features, welfare provisions, health insurance, training facilities, and the like, for the physically handicapped alone, or whether they will opt instead to consider all basic policy questions in the light of their effect on all who are disabled by any handicap, physical, mental, cultural, or economic. These are, of course, the extremes, and many midpoints do exist from which it is possible to operate both as a separate entity and in combination with other groups. Increasing political sophistication on the part of the physically handicapped will probably suggest how best to combine their special needs with the larger social good. Joint efforts with other groups, such as those concerned with the development of transportation systems to serve the aged, will aid in reconciling some apparent conflicts in interest.

Finally, it was recommended that an effective organization be developed and funded for organizing physically handicapped people, developing leaders, recruiting and educating memberships, and for basic research to clarify objectives and determine specific goals within the broader objectives.

A likely pivotal force in New York City can be found in the already established Mayor's Advisory Committee on the Handicapped. But to have political impact, the organization must be relatively independent. And it will need a secure financial basis in order to engage in ongoing organizational development activities and to promote, channel, and monitor the research that it determines necessary to clarify and achieve its goals. Whatever form is initially adopted should be designed to allow considerable latitude for flexibility. Given the state of knowledge and the lack of organizational experience on the part of the majority of those with some physical disability, it would be a disservice to freeze a new structure into a predetermined form.

THE DISABILITIES

THE HOMEBOUND

ELIZABETH BARRETT BROWNING personified the Victorian image of the homebound person—tragic, appealing, and thoroughly romantic. Despite epochal social changes in the ensuing years, this percept of homeboundness continued to dominate the Western world, and to some extent, still does. As nostalgic old-timers will remember, the golden years of radio during the 1930s were marked by "shut-in" programs. Under the aegis of chatty and infinitely sympathetic smooth-talking men and women, homebound persons became a prime target population of daytime shows that oozed with sentimentality. As one listened to these programs one could readily envision the shut-in audience as consisting of little old ladies who lived from one spring to the next so that they could observe the nesting behavior of their "feathered friends."

Although Americans are generally more knowledgeable today, many still cherish the "shut-in" stereotype. Lack of close and continuing contact with homebound persons leaves unchallenged such misconceptions as: the homebound are essentially helpless; their central need is for friendly visitors; they lead rather wistful, bittersweet lives that are somehow tinged with a romantic quality.

Those who work with the homebound know homeboundness in different terms. They see homebound persons as an isolated and disadvantaged minority, among whose members are some of America's most poverty-stricken citizens. They see the homebound as one of the most

HERBERT RUSALEM, ED.D., is Professor of Education, Teachers College, Columbia University, New York City.

underdeveloped manpower sectors in the nation, a resource that lies continually idle and fallow. In the hard world of reality there is little that is romantic about the empty and unproductive lives led by most of America's homebound citizens (Federation of the Handicapped, 1968, 1969, 1970, 1971).

Perhaps the most cogent factor in the current situation is that most homebound persons are invisible. Confined to their residences, institutions, and neighborhoods, they rarely venture into the domain of the opinionmakers of the community and, thus, generate little anxiety and concern for their condition. The enveloping apathy that surrounds most homebound persons is confirmed by the fact that few rehabilitation agencies, public or voluntary, provide services for them. Indeed, most agencies function as though the homebound didn't exist. So well concealed is this client population, that no one really knows their incidence in the American population and no one has proposed a commonly accepted definition for their condition that would facilitate enumeration (Rusalem, 1967).

From a rehabilitation viewpoint the tragic dilemma of the homebound is the fact that there is ample evidence at hand that almost all of them who are vocationally motivated can benefit from rehabilitation service to the point of becoming at least partially self-sustaining. Yet, such evidence has not been assimilated by the large majority of rehabilitation administrators and practitioners. As a consequence, little organized programming exists for the homebound. Yet, when Public Law 565 was passed in 1954, Congress was astute enough to create a commission under the terms of the Act to study the problems of homebound people in America (U. S. Congress, 1954). The reports of the public hearings conducted by this commission express much well-meaning concern but contain few facts, bearing testimony to the limited information about the homebound that was then available. Most of the remarks made at that time by distinguished rehabilitation leaders reflected the widespread belief that the homebound constitute a neglected segment of the disabled population and merit stepped-up services. However, even the most knowledgeable witnesses were able to offer few concrete suggestions about how better service delivery systems for this group could be organized. But, this was no more than should have been expected, because very few agencies in the United States in the mid-1950s could speak from direct experience in providing day-to-day rehabilitation services to homebound persons. Consequently, in its recommendations the commission confined itself to a series of general proposals that provided little impetus to rehabilitation programming for the homebound (U. S. Office of Vocational Rehabilitation, 1955). In fact, more than ten years passed before the next major step was taken to bring homebound clients into the rehabilitation mainstream.

Then, in 1967, moved by a perceptive recognition of the service gaps that existed in rehabilitation service to homebound persons, the Social and Rehabilitation Service of the United States Department of Health, Education and Welfare awarded a Programmatic Research Project Grant to the Federation of the Handicapped, a comprehensive rehabilitation facility in New York City. This facility had pioneered in the early 1950s in industrial homework programming for the homebound in cooperation with the New York State Office of Vocational Rehabilitation (Cohen, 1956; Cohen, 1956a; Katz, 1961).

Unlike previous more limited research and demonstration projects in the area of homebound rehabilitation, which had focused narrowly upon local problems, this Project undertook the mission of encouraging communities, states, and regions to expand their programs for the homebound through such means as special community organization interventions, administrative and staff training, grant incentives, the personal impact of project personnel upon individuals and groups in the community, and demonstration services. As will be noted in detail later in this chapter, the impact upon services in this field of the Programmatic Research Project on the Rehabilitation of Homebound Persons has been considerable.

Perhaps the nature of this impact is best encapsulated in the remarks made by Edward Newman, Commissioner of the United States Rehabilitation Services Administration, in striking the keynote for the First National Conference on the Rehabilitation of the Homebound. "I suggest here that it is time for the homebound to receive higher priority. I see in the rehabilitation movement the capacity to accept this long-neglected responsibility, and I see in the sheltered workshop the natural focus of such programs . . . I am confident that together we can devise workable solutions to the problems of serving the homebound disabled." (Rusalem, 1971).

This hopeful statement would have been difficult, if not impossible, to make in 1967 when the Programmatic Research Project was first launched. At that time, the first outcome of the Project, a state-of-the-art paper (Rusalem 1967), summarized current rehabilitation opportunities for the homebound as follows: "From the point of view of the homebound client in most states and communities in this country, the available services are less than satisfactory. . . . Although estimates vary, the number of homebound persons in the United States probably exceeds one million. A large majority of these people have not received adequate rehabilitation service."

Stripped of all ancillary details—the attitudinal components, the apathy of many communities, the lethargy of many members of the rehabilitation establishment, the misconceptions about the cost and effort required to rehabilitate homebound persons, and the paucity of good experimental evidence concerning this group—the central issue for rehabilitation workers today is that feasible rehabilitation techniques for the homebound have been demonstrated for more than twenty years by such agencies as the New York State Office of Vocational Rehabilitation, the Federation of the Handicapped, the Wisconsin Division of Vocational Rehabilitation, and a number of other state and local agencies. Despite consistently favorable results, the experience of these agencies has not yet been translated into nationwide programming.

In response to this deplorable situation, the Programmatic Research Project not only generated relevant research findings but as quickly as possible also converted these findings into viable rehabilitation programs. For example, as part of this demonstration effort the Federation of the Handicapped initiated its Higher Horizons for the Homebound Program, which, after undergoing careful evaluation in a "spin-off" demonstration, now operates as an innovative free-standing ongoing service conducted by the Federation in cooperation with the New York State Office of Vocational Rehabilitation.

The width and the depth of the chasm between what is known about the rehabilitation of the homebound and everyday clinical practice is extraordinarily large. Thus, although the homebound are qualified both legally and by reason of existing research and experiential findings to participate in rehabilitation activities, for the most part they are excluded from such services by man-made barriers. It is neither simple nor inexpensive to serve homebound persons. On the contrary, the process is usually long, difficult, and complex. It is nevertheless wholly possible in most cases. The barriers that exist do not reside exclusively in the extreme limitations imposed upon homebound persons by their obvious disabilities. Rather, the really impenetrable barriers for this group are those that exist in the minds of the men and women who have been charged by our society with the task of delivering rehabilitation services to disabled citizens. Notwithstanding the continued frustration that such barriers create, the outlook is brightening.

In concluding an updated version of the previously cited state-of-the-art paper on the homebound, Rusalem (1971) observed:

A ferment seems to be developing in the rehabilitation of the homebound . . . [which] is expected to result increasingly in real accomplishments in providing comprehensive rehabilitation services to homebound persons. Important evidence of this can be noted in the number of agencies serving the homebound, the growing body of research, the strong interest in the field expressed by the Social and Rehabilitation Service, the Rehabilitation Service Administration and state and voluntary rehabilitation agencies, and the innovative approaches to the life problems of homebound persons now being tested. A firm foundation for future development in this field was laid during the period 1960–1970. The decade of the 70s should prove to be the turning point in the rehabilitation of homebound persons. Perhaps, by 1980, the homebound will have achieved rehabilitation parity with other disability groups in the United States.

DEFINITION, INCIDENCE, CLASSIFICATION

One of the evidences of neglect in homebound rehabilitation is the absence of a commonly accepted definition of this client group. As an operational foundation for subsequent material in this chapter, the definition formulated by the Programmatic Research Project has been adopted. Within this definition a homebound person is one whose physical, intellectual, emotional, and/or social disabilities are so limiting that he cannot regularly leave his place of residence with the use of available transportation to participate in community-educational, rehabilitation, social, or employment activities.

Although this definition, like others, is not fully acceptable to everyone, it does focus upon the critical environmental variable. This distinguishing characteristic is that, in most cases, rehabilitation services have to be brought *to* the homebound individual where he lives in contradistinction to more conventional rehabilitation service delivery patterns in which the individual is required to reach out to some central source of assistance to obtain the benefits of rehabilitation.

During the 1950s authorities tended to favor the statistic of 1,000,000 persons as a reasonable estimate of the homebound population (U. S. Office of Vocational Rehabilitation, 1955). But, then, as now, wide variations in the definition of homeboundedness and the inaccessibility of homebound persons for ready enumeration made this claim rather tenuous. Even today, no one is quite certain about the size of the group and one estimate is about as inaccurate as the next. For its part, the Programmatic Research Project on the Rehabilitation of Homebound Persons, basing its estimates on sample surveys of urban neighborhoods, "guesses" that about two-million Americans fall under the umbrella of its definition of homeboundedness. However, the more intensively one engages in community organization activities in this field, the more one is persuaded that even this estimate constitutes an understatement of the size of the group.

Among other enumeration problems is the fact that the homebound are difficult to count because they are such a heterogeneous group. One general classification of the various homebound subpopulations is as follows:

1) Long-Term Community-Based Homebound Adults. The long-term community-based homebound adult is a member of the traditional shut-in group. These are the severely limited persons, ages twenty-one years and over, who live in the community but who cannot regularly leave their homes with available resources to participate in community activities. At one extreme are those who are bedbound and who rarely leave the room in which their beds are located. At the other extreme are those who can leave their homes but who do so infrequently or to a limited degree. Between these extremes are those who can move about their residences to some extent but who only occasionally leave their homes.

2) Long-Term Community-Based Homebound Children. These individuals under the age of twenty-one are restricted by reason of their physical, emotional, intellectual, or social conditions to the extent that, if they receive educational services at all, such services are delivered to them at home. Rehabilitation workers are most concerned with the teen-age segment of this population since, like others in their age group, they are at a crucial stage of social and vocational development which may well determine the shape of their adult lives. Although many of these children receive educational and vocational services in their homes, others do not.

3) *Short-Term Community-Based Homebound Persons*. The members of this group have physical or emotional conditions which render them homebound only for a period of some six months or less. Examples include students who are recovering from skiing accidents, persons who are recent dischargees from medical and psychiatric institutions, those who are in the process of having architectural barriers removed from their homes and schools, and individuals who are responding to rehabilitation treatment so favorably that early transition to fuller community participation seems likely. Experience indicates that some of the members of this group do, in time, become long-term homebound persons if they fail to respond to treatment procedures or if their homeboundedness becomes reinforced by prolonged isolation and experience deprivation. An important subsample of this category consists of individuals who are under the care of outpatient clinics and visiting public health nurses. Suitable outreach rehabilitation programs reaching these clients in the early stages of illness can effectively prevent or shorten the homebound condition for many members of this group.

4) *Institutionalized Homebound Persons*. The largest subgroup of homebound persons consists of individuals who are residents of institutions for the mentally retarded, the emotionally disturbed, the aged, the chronically ill, the sensorily impaired, and the socially limited (such as narcotics addicts and alcoholics). Limited to their residences as much as the members of the community-based group, institutionalized homebound persons generally have greater access to the services they need from the institution itself but, concurrently, suffer from those deprivations that institutional life commonly imposes, including loss of privacy, lack of nuclear family relationships, bureaucratically determined living conditions, monotony of stimuli, and lack of opportunities to develop and maintain a sense of personal worth and integrity.

5) *Sheltered Living Homebound Persons*. Still small in numbers but

growing in significance are those homebound persons who cannot remain in ordinary community residences but are not in institutions. They live in "halfway houses," hostels, or other types of special residences which combine some of the elements of both community and institutional life. Persons in this group usually retain a greater measure of self-direction than those in institutions but the degree of shelter and control that they receive exceeds that normally found in unsheltered community living. Although they are partially segregated, their segregation is not as all-encompassing as in most institutions and is tempered by more frequent contacts with the community.

6) *Therapeutically-Oriented Homebound Persons.* Members of this group are rendered homebound, temporarily at least, by having been isolated from the rest of the community for therapeutic purposes. Examples include residents of narcotics treatment centers, inpatient rehabilitation centers, residential schools for the blind and the deaf, convalescent centers, residence facilities attached to outpatient rehabilitation agencies, and transitional residences for those who are in the process of being evaluated for either community-based or institutional programs. By definition, the duration of therapeutically-oriented homeboundedness is short-term and, it is hoped, results in successful treatment that frees the individual from his homebound status. However, this does not always occur, and some individuals in this group move from this category into long-term homeboundedness.

7) *Neighborhood-Bound "Homebound" Persons.* Many of the members of this group, consisting mainly of aged persons, are marginally homebound, if at all, but are included because they constitute a high-risk segment of the population who could, without proper rehabilitation service, become homebound in time. Generally, they are individuals who are not strictly confined to their homes as much as to their immediate localities. Either public transportation does not exist or cannot be used as a practical means of gaining regular access to community-wide facilities. Restricted as they are to what is available in their neighborhoods, they usually receive very little rehabilitation service. However, unless prompt and effective service is forthcoming, many of them enter a retrogressive process through which increasing isolation occurs, resulting, in some cases, in long-term homeboundedness.

The above classification system fails to reflect the true diversity of homebound persons. Indeed, the homebound group crosses all customary age, disability, social, and psychological groupings. Although intellectual factors are rarely considered of major importance in the homebound condition, mental retardation accounts for much more homeboundedness than is generally supposed, much of it concealed by family shame and community indifference. The intellectual component enters the picture in still another way. Some homebound persons who are clearly not mentally retarded to begin with may subsequently test in the mentally retarded range in conjunction with having spent extended periods of time in home or institutional isolation. Longitudinal studies conducted by the Programmatic Research Project on the Rehabilitation of the Homebound suggest that there is probably a linear relationship between the duration of homeboundedness and the degree to which intelligence test scores become depressed, an effect especially apparent in the institutionalized group.

In another dimension, it should be recognized that the physical and mental conditions accompanying advancing age precipitate a high incidence of homeboundedness. Regardless of whether this homeboundedness is induced primarily by social or physical factors, disengagement from the environment does occur with some frequency among aged persons as they advance in years. In many instances, this process culminates in institutionalization or homeboundedness, either of which can be prevented or remediated in many instances through early rehabilitation intervention. Avoidant attitudes toward older persons and a single-minded emphasis upon a youth culture seem to foster unnecessary decline and homeboundedness among older persons. This decline is only partially due to physiological causes. Thus, studies conducted at the Federation Employment and Guidance Service confirmed the fact that involvement in a vocational rehabilitation experience and subsequent remunerative employment retard deterioration among vocationally-motivated older disabled persons and reverse retrogressive processes leading to neighborhood- and homeboundedness (Rusalem, Baxt, and Barshop, 1967).

THE HOMEBOUND ENVIRONMENT

The inclusive group of homebound can be regarded as the universe of disabled persons in microcosm. No one is exempt from being homebound by reason of age or disability and no one can escape it by reason of social class, type of community, occupation, or social affiliation. It is a condition that is described most accurately not by the limitations endured by the individual but by his relationship to the environment in which he is required to function. This constricting environment has for the homebound person, regardless of his other relationships, the following characteristics:

1) It restricts the individual from enjoying the range of experiences that he might be expected to have otherwise.

2) It renders him more dependent upon others than would normally be the case.

3) It deprives him of experiences that are generally considered in our society to be growth-inducing and stimulating.

4) It separates him from essential services that are designed to help disabled people who are not homebound to realize their potential.

5) It *progressively* limits the individual, extending the effects of the disability cumulatively far beyond the original precipitating loss. Rusalem (1967) has described this phenomenon as a narrowing circle.

6) It endows the individual with lower social status and deprives him of opportunities to exercise essential human rights enjoyed by other citizens in our society, such as formation of groups for mutual social action, access to appropriate employment, and even such political rights as participation in community movements.

COMMON CHARACTERISTICS

The diversity of the group and its lack of visibility and mobility have made the benefits of group identification impossible to achieve. Indeed, the homebound experience imposes such a degree of isolation upon homebound persons that they cannot physically interact with each other and are thus rendered powerless to form pressure groups through which they could negotiate with cultural institutions and instrumentalities. Group membership is made all the more difficult because individual differences abound in all the personal dimensions by which homebound people are measured. This raises difficulties for practitioners and researchers in making valid generalizations about the group. Yet, despite their endless variations, members of the homebound group do have the following characteristics in common (Federation of the Handicapped, 1968, 1969, 1970, 1971).

Economic Deprivation. A substantial proportion of homebound persons are on welfare and/or are recipients of social security disability benefits. Many have been impoverished by the back-breaking costs of diagnosing and treating their illnesses. Most are unemployed and, thus, have no current earnings. And, almost all cope with one or more additional expenses of living, such as transportation, special equipment, telephone costs, and the inability to shop economically. Therefore, their current incomes are almost uniformly low, and they also have fewer options in using whatever income they have to purchase goods and services on the most economical terms.

Social Isolation. As the duration of chronic illness and disability lengthens, old prehomebound social relationships tend to wither away and new ones become increasingly difficult to form. In contrast to the changing world outside, the world of the homebound person remains monotonously the same. In time, he becomes disengaged from the social environment, unable to keep pace with emerging trends. He finds it more difficult to sustain his own interests and the interest of others in him. Almost inevitably, loneliness and segregation from others replace previous interpersonal involvements and, although he may hunger initially for more contacts with others, recreational studies (Federation of the Handicapped, 1968–1971) indicate that, in time, even this hunger becomes suppressed and the homebound person becomes progressively more withdrawn and depressed. Although the rate with which this occurs varies from person to person, apathy and hopelessness usually dominate the homebound person's outlook, until in time he appears to the casual observer remarkably unmotivated to participate in social as well as in rehabilitation activities.

Family Tension. The central support which enables long-term homebound individuals to stay in the community despite serious limitations and multiple adjustment problems is a supportive, interested, and competent family. So long as strong family ties can be maintained, the prognosis for continued residence in the community continues to be favorable. However, even under the best of conditions, a high emotional price is usually exacted from both the family and the homebound person as the cost of sustaining the individual in the community rises. The special care, expenses, and companionship required to succor the homebound family member almost always affect the degree of self-fulfillment that his nondisabled relatives are able to achieve. However dedicated relatives may be, resentment and hostility can be aroused when family members find their own freedom restricted by responsibility for the homebound person.

In exploring such relationships, the Programmatic Research Project discovered that serious family disruption was present in more than two-thirds of the homebound people in its longitudinal sample. Stress appears even in family groups which, prior to the occurrence of homeboundedness in one of its members, had been characterized by unity and happiness. Rare, in fact, was the family that was so durable that it could withstand the unrelenting pressure of having a homebound relative in its midst. Almost all of the community-based homebound persons studied in the Project were sensitive to the delicate balance that existed in their family relationships and were conscious of the ever-present risk that any significant shift in this balance could well lead to their being moved out of the home into some type of congregate living arrangement. As a consequence, few felt entirely secure and stable vis-à-vis their families.

Loss of Competence. As the months spent as a homebound person lengthen into years, and as the quantity and variety of stimulus input decline, existing social and vocational skills begin to deteriorate. Evidence of such declines in competence begin to appear not only in the interpersonal and vocational areas, but also in general coping and adjustive behaviors. Personality brittleness and emotional fragility increase, and the capacity for enduring change and displacement lessens. In the intellectual area, intelligence test scores show a decline over time.

In the course of the Programmatic Research Project's psychological studies, a linear relationship was found between duration of homeboundedness and degree of depression in performance on measures of intellectual ability. When the duration of homeboundedness extends beyond a few years, there is a mounting danger that negative changes in functioning level may become largely irreversible. In that event, the individual's promise for rehabilitation is correspondingly reduced and, in cases of very prolonged deprivation, the individual may become so socially disengaged that he cannot participate in the rehabilitation process at all. Fortunately, this extreme reaction is rare. In confirmation of the fundamental durability and toughness of the human personality, the Programmatic Research Project found that all but a few of its community-based homebound participants achieved at least partial reversibility of their homeboundedness-induced losses when they became engaged in rehabilitation service.

Emotional Status. Programmatic Research Project findings indicate that more than 60 per cent of the homebound sample studied had mental health problems so severe that early therapeutic intervention was recommended. Another 25 per cent had emotional problems which, while not as critical, were expected to become exacerbated if prompt treatment were not provided. Apparently, the stresses of living as a homebound person, the absence of adequate environmental supports, the ever-present foreboding that the family or institutional staff might abandon one at any time, the lack of suitable channels for the expression of anger and disappointment, and the expressed or implicit blame borne by the homebound person for depriving the family of important satisfactions—all combine to raise the anxiety level. Outlets for relieving tension, such as physical activities, involvement in new social relationships and experiences, changing one's residence, taking on a new job, travel, or escaping physically from troublesome interpersonal relationships are all less feasible for homebound persons than for others. As a consequence, from a mental health viewpoint the homebound should be considered a high-risk group. Many of them are in a precarious position, with the emotional demands of living often exceeding the adjustive capacity of the individual and the readiness of the environment to support him.

Lack of Vocational Direction. Homebound persons who retain a desire to participate in vocational activities are usually perplexed about the means of achieving vocational objectives. With a history of out-of-home employment activities behind them, confinement to the home seems incongruent with the world of work. Quite often, they cannot conceive of any vocational activities whatsoever in their field of interest which can be practiced within the four walls that surround them. It is almost as though their previous contacts with work are now simply too irrelevant to be of any value to them. Beyond stating a general interest in work, they typically are unable to specify personal and vocational objectives and plans. To a degree, vocational paralysis is reality-based, since job opportunities for the homebound are few in number and since even those that do exist are probably outside the experience of most lay persons. In actuality, the vocationally-motivated homebound person doesn't know where to turn. If left to his own devices in the vocational area, he is likely to be frustrated and blocked at every turn in seeking some form of suitable remunerative work that he can perform at home. After a while, he abandons whatever vocational aspirations he may have had and accepts his inactivity as inevitable.

Neglect of Health Care. The Programmatic Research Project found that a proportion of homebound persons does not have regular access to needed health care. As a matter of fact, some members of the project sample had not seen a physician for years, even for decades. Frequently the precipitating condition which had caused homeboundedness had been reinforced by additional and, often, correctable secondary disabilities. In a few instances, the original illness had long since responded to treatment and was no longer the major factor in prolonging the homebound status. In these cases, other disabilities had become sustainers of homeboundedness. In a number of instances, even the "unaffected" aspects of the homebound persons's health had suffered as a result of his lengthening inactivity and, thus, personal health resources that once had been available to him were no longer as useful as they had been. In general, it may be expected that a large proportion of the homebound persons in any caseload will have serious problems in the dental, audiological, ophthalmic, systemic, and digestive health areas in addition to their major disabilities.

REACTIONS TO REHABILITATION INTERVENTION

Although the pattern of losses suffered by homebound clients in the economic, social, emotional, vocational, and health domains varies from one individual to the next, some losses in each of these areas invariably occur. In combination, these losses may seem, at first glance, to be so overpowering in their limiting effects upon the individual that his feasibility for rehabilitation seems doubtful. However, initial evaluations of homebound clients should be very tentative since, once the overlay of neglect and disuse is removed, rehabilitation-related strengths generally will become apparent in the personality structure. Thus, in an unselected sample of fifty-nine community-based homebound individuals it was possible for the Programmatic Research Project staff to devise rehabilitation interventions for fifty-six of them. Fifty-three (94.6 per cent) of these homebound persons, all of whom had previously been declared unfeasible for rehabilitation service, accepted these interventions.

Wherever possible, the rehabilitation potential of the homebound should be measured in terms of "hard" outcome data. Thirty-four out of fifty-three members of the Programmatic Research Project Homebound Intervention Sample entered Higher Horizons for the Homebound, a specialized rehabilitation program conducted by the Federation of the Handicapped in cooperation with the New York State Office of Vocational Rehabilitation. Another four achieved immediate entry into homebound employment. The other fifteen were given combinations of mental health, recreation, housing, welfare, and transportation services. At the time of the most recent project follow-up survey, some twelve to eighteen months subsequent to the initiation of the rehabilitation intervention, 60.8 per cent of these fifty-three homebound persons were in employment or were engaged in vocational rehabilitation processes designed to lead to employment. With the exception of four cases, all had benefited from rehabilitation to the extent that they had become more independent in their daily living tasks and more capable of meeting adult family responsibilities.

On the basis of these intervention data and concurrent supporting clinical evidence obtained from demonstrations and samples of blind, arthritic, and institutionalized homebound persons, the project staff arrived at the following generalizations in regard to rehabilitation intervention (Federation of the Handicapped, 1968, 1969, 1970, 1971):

1) Despite severe and multiple limitations, most homebound persons —even those who have failed previously to benefit from general rehabilitation programs—retain sufficient vocational and social potential to make constructive use of specialized rehabilitation programs established for the homebound.

2) When suitable rehabilitation services are offered to them, the large majority of homebound persons accept these services and make progress toward greater independence and self-support.

3) At least half and, under favorable environmental conditions and creative agency programming, perhaps as many as three-quarters of the homebound can be helped to enter some form of remunerative employment.

4) The rate of rehabilitation case closure achieved in this group is equivalent to the rate commonly found among the members of other groups of severely disabled persons.

5) Among those who cannot benefit substantially from vocational services, possibilities still exist for social and personal rehabilitation leading to greater autonomy and personal happiness. When appropriate rehabilitation services were delivered to the members of this subgroup, most of them emerged from rehabilitation as more effective and self-directing family and community members.

6) The positive findings reported by the Programmatic Research Project do not reflect the unique unreplicated experience of one agency. On the contrary, at the first National Conference on the Rehabilitation of the Homebound in 1971, a dozen different agencies located in different parts of the United States reported similar outcomes for specialized services that they had established for the homebound. Beyond confirming the Programmatic Research Project findings, these reports suggested that the parameters of rehabilitation potential of homebound clients is not a function of any single program, agency, or location, but of reasonable attempts to meet the needs of this population. The potential is there and is waiting only for suitable rehabilitation services to energize it (Gersten, 1968; McKenna et al., 1967. Thus, it may be said that potential homebound rehabilitants are all around us but professional

rehabilitation workers who are ready to help them are not; at least, not yet.

THE REHABILITATION PROCESS

INITIATING THE PROCESS

Case-Finding. Homebound clients are referred to rehabilitation by many sources. These include physicians, hospitals, clinics, visiting nurse services, friends, family members, welfare, housing, and health agencies, and other community organizations. However, the proportion referred is relatively small. Limited in their mobility, homebound persons obviously have fewer encounters with potential referral sources. Even when such encounters do occur, professional agency personnel generally consider the homebound as more or less "hopeless," and, in accordance with such perceptions, are disinclined to make rehabilitation referrals. Furthermore, homebound persons who have rehabilitation experiences often emerge from them frustrated and disappointed. Most of them report a history of ineffective service that did little but raise initial hopes that were rarely realized. In some instances, the pattern of defeat recurs a number of times, leaving the homebound individual cynical and embittered. Thus, at first contact, homebound persons tend to be understandably skeptical about and reluctant to engage in rehabilitation activities.

Almost everything about the homebound makes them a relatively inaccessible rehabilitation population. As may be expected, programs that wait for homebound clients to take the initiative in applying for service at a central agency office are likely to enroll few homebound clients. The limited number of such voluntary applications often leads to the ingenuous and erroneous generalization that few homebound persons reside in a particular catchment area or that those who do are really not interested in rehabilitation. Neither of these interpretations is accurate. The fact is that, like certain other special rehabilitation caseloads, the homebound are not in a position to apply for service at central facilities, and a differentiated case-finding procedure will have to be established if they are to become more fully involved in existing services.

The Programmatic Research Project conducted an innovative special-

ized demonstration of case-finding in the Greenwich Village-Chelsea
area of New York City. This investigation found more than 100 neglected but rehabilitatable homebound persons in a comparatively com-
pact neighborhood by using the following outreach techniques: (1) educating professional community workers to recognize and refer
homebound persons; (2) distributing to community residents handbills
about the case-finding project printed both in English and Spanish; (3)
asking local storekeepers to serve as points of initial contact with the
homebound; and (4) enlisting the aid of volunteer community action
groups to inform residents about the need to identify and refer homebound persons.

Although the specific case-finding techniques that should be used in
various geographical areas will vary in accordance with local conditions, it may be safely assumed that a commitment to rehabilitate homebound persons requires a special case-finding effort of some sort. Without it, large numbers of homebound persons inevitably will get "lost in
the cracks." (Federation of the Handicapped, 1968, 1969, 1970, 1971).

Initiating Interview. It is usually desirable to conduct the intake interview in the client's home even if transportation to the agency can be
arranged safely and economically. Such an interview communicates to
the rehabilitation worker more clearly than any office interview the
flavor of the home setting, the interpersonal relationships that prevail
there, the resources and problems of the family, and family attitudes toward the homebound person. Intake interviews conducted in the client's
home are like other interviews of their type in that an effort is made by
the worker to develop a working relationship with the homebound person and his family. The client and his relatives are given an orientation
to the rehabilitation program, opportunities are provided for them to
describe their problems and to express their feelings, and a foundation
is laid for subsequent case action. In reference to the homebound condition, however, the rehabilitation worker should attempt to determine the
psychosocial factors that are contributing to client isolation, the meaning
of homeboundedness (including its adjustive value) to the client, the
environmental conditions that seem to be reinforcing the individual's
helplessness, and the possible dynamics (such as illness, financial distress, or family disorganization) which are probably precipitating
apparent movement toward consideration of rehabilitation at this time.

Taking precedence in the interviewer's mind, however, is the possibility of reducing or eliminating the client's homeboundedness.

The rehabilitation worker who is untrained to work with homebound persons is likely to be unduly discouraged and, at times, dismayed by what he finds in the initial interviews. More likely than not, the homebound rehabilitation applicant appears to be beyond repair. Upon his original disability has been built a handicapping superstructure composed of apathy, deteriorated skills, self-doubts, social ineptness, and extreme dependence. Extended periods of stimulus deprivation invariably have left him with few obvious competencies. It is easy to understand why first impressions, focusing as they usually do upon the more superficial aspects of the personality and those superimposed by isolation experiences are not very hopeful. Unless the interviewer has the disposition and skill to penetrate these layers of debilitation, there is little likelihood that he will find the rehabilitation potential that lies underneath.

In this context, it may be noted that one of the most serious shortcomings of existing rehabilitation services for homebound persons is their tendency to provide for only casual observations of the homebound person, focusing narrowly upon the presenting individual. All too often, that is as far as the rehabilitation worker goes, and the rehabilitation process stops abruptly at that point. Having cursorily identified the client as a detached and, perhaps, poorly motivated individual, some counselors conclude that rehabilitation potential is exceedingly modest and that the effort required will be far greater than warranted by the expected rehabilitation outcome. In almost all cases, this is a serious miscalculation. Quiescent, almost dormant in most of these people, lying beneath the facade of withdrawal and debilitation, there usually is a person with far more rehabilitation potential than initial impressions would lead one to believe. The task of the rehabilitation worker, therefore, is to uncover and mobilize these strengths (Federation of the Handicapped, 1968, 1969, 1970, 1971).

Preliminary Planning. As a result of earlier service disappointments, the homebound client is likely to have ambivalent feelings about an offer of rehabilitation assistance. Unless the homebound condition and the consequent deprivation have been so prolonged that client movement toward independence is highly improbable, the homebound individual usually feels a desire to improve his generally bleak situation. Simultaneously, however, a fear of the unknown and apprehension that he may be exposed to still another failure generate feelings of avoidance. When such ambivalent feelings toward rehabilitation appear in the homebound person the rehabilitation worker must be extremely skillful in understanding them and in reinforcing client tendencies that are rehabilitation oriented. At this point, rehabilitation motivation can be exceedingly fragile and readily annihilated by insensitive or unsympathetic counselor behavior. Thus, it is imperative for the worker to be highly supportive, interested, concerned, and nonjudgmental in coping with these early ambivalent reactions. Unwarranted and precipitous case action before the client is ready for it can heighten his anxiety and cause him to retreat from rehabilitation. Those who work with the homebound should be prepared to move forward slowly with the client, and, if necessary, move back temporarily with his motivational ebb and flow until the client has developed confidence in his worker and in himself and has thereby acquired some stability in his feelings about his rehabilitation program.

Since rehabilitation for most homebound persons does not follow a straight line, counselor patience and understanding are required. The fact is that the homebound do not ordinarily produce quick rehabilitation case closures for an agency. On the contrary, greater counselor effort and longer periods of service time are the rule rather than the exception. Not infrequently, the family has feelings that are as ambivalent as the client's, if not more so, about his entry into rehabilitation. Families, too, can be maddeningly indecisive or apparently irrationally vacillating in relation to the rehabilitation service offered. In view of this possibility, counseling becomes as important a service for family members or institutional surrogates as for the homebound client himself.

With few exceptions, preliminary planning for the homebound person centers upon preparing him for admission to an appropriate evaluation process. The reasons for this are twofold: (1.) prolonged observations of the client in an action setting usually enable rehabilitation personnel to assess more accurately the person beneath the overlay of isolation and neglect; and (2.) participation in rehabilitation activities can be an essential service intervention in that it re-establishes reasonable expectations in the mind of the homebound person and enables him to test out emerging and almost forgotten aspects of himself under controlled and sheltered conditions that are engineered to promote feelings of self-worth. Even so short a time as a week spent in a rehabilitation evaluation process often results in surprising changes in the homebound individual. Participants in the Programmatic Research Project's experimental evaluation experience which was conducted in a rehabilitation facility to which they were transported daily underwent a dramatic alteration in outlook, goals, and plans. The effects were still apparent months and, in some cases, years after termination of the evaluation procedure.

Individuals who have been homebound for shorter periods of time, perhaps a year or less, may not require an evaluation that is as extensive and encompassing as that for the more deprived subgroup. In selected instances, the former may move from intake directly into restoration, training, or placement. However, because of the nature of homebound experience, such cases occur infrequently. Therefore, a rehabilitation program that purports to serve unselected homebound rehabilitation clients in a state or a community should make provision for a formal evaluation experience that includes conjunctive transportation and psychosocial, short-term residence services that support the evaluation process.

EVALUATION

Medical Factors. Persons who are physically or emotionally homebound often have a history of medical neglect. It is not uncommon for homebound individuals with severe physical limitations to have had their more recent health evaluation many years before the current agency contact. In such instances, consideration should be given to the possibility that recent advances in medicine that have not come to the attention of the homebound person and his family may be of substantial benefit if made part of comprehensive rehabilitation treatment. Beyond the major disability, additional health conditions acquired since the person became homebound may be equally important in defining and prolonging the homebound condition (Federation of the Handicapped, 1968, 1969, 1970, 1971).

These factors suggest the necessity of arranging for a thorough medical assessment of the homebound person as early as possible in the rehabilitation experience. Since the medical configurations in homebound clients are complex in their own right, and are made more so by contributing emotional and intellectual components, the medical evaluation should be conducted, whenever possible, in a well-equipped interdisciplinary facility at which the interrelationships among these conditions can be studied. When a client cannot possibly leave his home because of the severity of his medical or psychological limitations, such examinations must be conducted at his residence. As may be expected, home examinations are not only more difficult to arrange but also the results are less complete and less functional, even when an attempt is made to be as comprehensive as possible in the medical and psychosocial areas. In evaluating the results of medical assessments, priority should be given to the possibilities of restorative treatment which may render the client more self-sufficient and more socially and vocationally competent.

In addition to expecting the examining physician to provide the usual diagnostic, therapeutic, and prognostic information required for rehabilitation planning, the rehabilitation worker should seek information from him relating to such questions as: (1) Is the extent of homeboundedness found in this individual consistent with his medical condition? (2) Can medical intervention reduce the degree of homeboundedness? (3) Are out-of-home rehabilitation activities medically approved if proper transportation or living conditions can be arranged? (4) Can the physician suggest aids, appliance, treatments, medications, or other assists that may render the person more independent? In accordance with general rehabilitation policy, recommendations for physical or emotional restoration should take precedence over the delivery of other rehabilitation services. In view of the neglect suffered by homebound persons, many clients who enter the rehabilitation process bound to their homes emerge from it better equipped to enter community activities as a result of the restorative services received. Conversion of a homebound individual into a community participant constitutes superior rehabilitation, indeed.

Psychological Factors. The Programmatic Research Project staff found that mental health problems are among the most serious consequences of prolonged homeboundedness. When coupled with evidence of intellectual deficit, these findings indicate that psychological evaluations (coupled with psychiatric and social work assessments) have a key role in service to homebound rehabilitation clients. They are essential, for example, in evaluating intellectual ability. As in the case of other client groups, psychological evaluations of the homebound help to describe educational and vocational status and development, suggesting, in addition, the estimated degree to which stimulus deprivation has impaired cognitive functioning. Since reduced intellectual performance due to deprivation has been shown to be remediable to some extent, the psychological examiners' judgments about this variable can suggest the possible level of accomplishment homebound clients may reach when they are introduced to a stimulating rehabilitation environment designed to foster intellectual "recovery." Consequently, psychologists working with the homebound must be exceptionally sensitive to individual potential for growth as well as to current levels of functioning. For rehabilitation purposes, their emphasis should be upon underlying intellectual abilities rather than upon superficial evidences of current mechanisms for coping with tests. Intelligence test scores analyzed by the Programmatic Research Project indicate that most homebound persons test at or below the low-normal range, with the depression of test scores being especially marked in the institutionalized subgroup. Even though the project reports are hopeful in indicating that an exposure to a stimulus-rich environment promotes a degree of "recovery" in intelligence test performance, it should be remembered that some of the losses suffered during the homebound experience tend to persist, even after participation in a suitable rehabilitation program (Federation of the Handicapped, 1968, 1969, 1970, 1971).

Turning to *personality evaluation,* it was found that personality tests administered to the homebound reveal a high incidence of mental health difficulties. Evidences of constriction, a rich inner fantasy life, passive aggression, and a pervasive sense of helplessness are among the common symptoms found in this group. Interestingly enough, "emotional breakdown" was not common in the sample studied. Most of the symptomatology represented more or less successful attempts on the part of homebound persons to cope with exceedingly difficult personal and family situations. The projective measures used by the Project, including the Rorschach Ink Blot Technique and the Thematic Apperception Test, indicated that most of the mechanisms employed by these homebound individuals to deal with the multiple stresses of severe social limitation originally were relevant for the homebound condition, although not consistently gratifying. However, these apparently functional mechanisms soon became barriers for the homebound person who entered rehabilitation since they failed to provide as much autonomy and flexibility as rehabilitation required. Responses which had been appropriate for confinement in the home were grossly incongruent with the daily demands of treatment situations.

Evidences of personality problems in the homebound should be viewed with caution and restraint, since symptoms in this group are often situational responses to a way of life which denies the individual warm peer contacts and a sense of self-worth. The Programmatic Research Project studies revealed that homebound persons are not characterized by any distinctive adjustment pattern. They respond individually to their problems with varying degrees of effectiveness and adopt as wide a range of adjustive mechanisms as any other group. Their selective approaches to life problems seem more related to the pre-homebound personality than to the specifics of the homebound condition itself.

In the Project's family assessments it was found that family disruption is common in the lives of homebound persons. The time, cost, and effort of caring for a homebound person can become so burdensome for some relatives that they attempt to disengage themselves from their responsibilities by changing their residence, institutionalizing the homebound individual, or absenting themselves from home as often as they can. In other instances, family members, motivated by feelings of guilt that they cannot rationalize or otherwise control, devote almost their entire lives to the homebound person and become martyrs who sacrifice themselves for his welfare. In still other cases, the families of homebound persons become punitive and subject the homebound person to interpersonal stress, even to the point of precipitating recurring emotional crises. Although no single pattern of family response predominates, serious adjustment problems are commonplace when relatives are called upon to cope with the homebound condition for a protracted period of time.

In evaluating the family situation, the social worker or counselor should be aware of any family dynamics that sustain or intensify the dependence of the homebound individual. It is by now clear that rehabilitation services for this caseload are rarely effective without family involvement and support. The entry of a homebound person into a rehabilitation process sometimes upsets delicate interpersonal balances and exacerbates family problems. Unless such problems are dealt with promptly, client benefits from the service may be minimal. In focusing on the family, the rehabilitation worker must identify and buttress family strengths and, if possible, shore up family weaknesses. As in other types of casework, counseling with individual family members should be supplemented by group counseling with the family as a unit.

In *psychiatric assessments,* the mental health problems observed among members of the homebound group by the psychiatric staff of the Programmatic Research Project were generally considered to require either short-term treatment or environmental therapy. Institutionalization was virtually never needed by the subsample with serious emotional problems. On the contrary, institutionalization needs were aroused primarily by social, not psychiatric, conditions, and became a factor when essential family supports were withdrawn so markedly that requisite physical care could no longer be delivered to the homebound person.

In addition to making his customary diagnosis and prognosis, the examining psychiatrist working with the homebound should shed light on the emotional readiness of the client to withstand the demands of a rehabilitation experience, the extent to which the dependence life style has been incorporated into the personality or character structure, the secondary gains which have resulted from being homebound, and the estimated capacity of the individual to sustain the interpersonal relationships required in a rehabilitation experience. If immediate psychotherapeutic interventions are recommended, it follows that they should be provided prior to, or in conjunction with, other rehabilitation services.

Special multidisciplinary diagnostic procedures for the homebound should be conducted outside the home at sites where facilities and equipment are likely to be useful in arriving at a more accurate assessment of the individual. As may be expected, the home contains many pitfalls for the diagnostician. Family members may try to participate inappropriately; lighting, ventilation, and other physical features of the environment may not be fully satisfactory; the person's behavior may be different in the home than it would be in an external millieu; excessive staff time and energy may be spent in merely traveling to and from the client's residence; and some homebound persons may reside in neighbor-hoods hazardous to outsiders.

Experience in the Programmatic Research Project indicates that within a rehabilitation facility, test responses and interview behavior change as the homebound person progresses in his rehabilitation pro-gram. As a result, findings obtained shortly after intake may differ from those obtained after participation for a time in the rehabilitation milieu. The careful counselor will accept the data of examinations performed early in the process as tentative indicators of client competency and po-tential, to be confirmed by subsequent observations and re-examina-tions. Knowing that it is risky to exclude homebound persons from re-habilitation on the basis of initial psychological and mental health evaluations, the counselor will rarely make a case decision on the basis of first, or even second, impressions. As an example, apparent apathy toward remunerative work and reluctance to consider out-of-home ac-tivities are often replaced by unabashed enthusiasm for both. A hunger for the outside environment begins soon after a rehabilitation facility experience starts.

In some cases, the homebound person is almost literally "reborn" during rehabilitation. This rebirth requires those who serve the home-bound to take a developmental approach to their clients. Such an ap-proach necessitates a relatively long-term process with many guidance in-puts. Consequently, examiners and interviewers are urged to assess homebound clients in the context of an extended time dimension, a pro-cess that calls for the re-evaluation of the homebound individual at stip-ulated intervals and which uses the test and interview results gathered at any point as one in a series of steps leading toward an evolving diagnosis.

Although the customary short-term assessments in the psychological and vocational areas have some relevance for homebound clients, their value as conclusive screening devices for determining whether a home-bound person should be accepted or rejected for service is doubtful. Thus, rehabilitation workers are encouraged to exclude no homebound individ-ual from rehabilitation on the basis of initial test and interview findings. As the victims of long-term neglect and isolation, homebound clients re-quire an opportunity to emerge from their socially imposed cocoons and to test themselves in a rehabilitation experience which strips away layer after layer of home-induced defenses. No matter how skillful the examiner and how reliable the instruments and techniques used, generalizations about the homebound client should be reserved until most of the returns are in.

Sociocultural Factors. While homebound persons come from every stratum of society, most of those who enter rehabilitation are poverty-stricken persons with a middle-class outlook. Relatively few inner city or rural poor homebound persons enter rehabilitation because such persons tend to be ill-informed about rehabilitation. They generally have less access to all services, are not encouraged by others to seek assistance, and, as confirmed by the Programmatic Research Project, the homebound poor in the inner city more often enter institutions for long-term health care than their more affluent peers. This selective factor and its motivational corollaries endow homebound caseloads with attitudes that augur well for rehabilitation success. Having decided to undergo rehabilitation, homebound individuals tend to be guided by a middle-class value system that views the pursuit of vocational "success" in positive terms. Much less is known about the special problems of homebound clients residing in inner city areas. This suggests that research studies are needed to determine the incidence of homeboundedness in such areas, the unique problems that confront inner city homebound persons, and the services and procedures that hold the greatest promise for rehabilitating them.

Economic poverty is a fact of life for most homebound persons, regardless of their cultural heritage. More than 90 per cent of the Programmatic Research Project longitudinal study sample were on welfare or receiving social security disability benefits at the time of survey. Living at or below the poverty margin, these individuals not only lacked the wherewithal to pay for needed medical care, transportation, and appliances, but most also lacked the funds for such basic comforts as books and magazines, arts and crafts supplies, favorite foods, and telephone service. Along with all other arguments favoring homework programs for homebound persons who are vocationally motivated is the fact that even the most modest earnings make a vital difference to them. Such earnings give them access to funds which they can spend as they like. In most instances, this means obtaining those things that can make life a little more pleasurable.

Socially, homebound persons have virtually no status as a group. Separated from and unknown to each other, they find it impossible to organize themselves for social and political purposes. Their minority status is unique in that, as minority group members, they are unaware of each other. Consequently, they function as individuals rather than group members, drawing little strength or satisfaction from interaction with each other. Experiments now being conducted by the Programmatic Research Project are testing conference telephone hookups as a means of bringing homebound persons into each other's psychological fields for community action, adult education, socialization, mental health, and vocational preparation. Early pilot efforts in this regard have generated positive results.

The acute isolation suffered by most homebound persons indicates a need for social-cultural alternatives. As an example, consideration is being given to the provision of congregate but independent living quarters for some homebound persons in special apartment houses or hostels which contain facilities for social and vocational activities. Although entry into such facilities would require movement out of the family residence and the familiar neighborhood, it would constitute for some a major step toward achieving a more useful and independent life. Currently, American opinion generally does not favor segregated arrangements of this type except in extreme cases. Yet, observations of those who choose to enter such enriched environments confirm the supposition that it is possible in such residences for homebound people to lead a far richer life than they have known in the homebound experience, especially if the program is developed so as to maximize their personal autonomy and self-direction.

Vocational Factors. Homebound persons vary widely in their vocational interests, abilities, and aspirations. Beyond the fact that they tend to be more severely limited and to have more acute mobility problems than other clients, they require vocational evaluations that are comparable to those set up for rehabilitation clients in general. Such evaluations should be multifaceted in character, providing for interactions between the client and a variety of worksamples and remunerative work situations. When brought into an established vocational evaluation center, the homebound are able to follow the general evaluative schedule established for other clients when the following factors are given due consideration:

1) During the early stages of vocational evaluation, and sometimes

thereafter, homebound individuals are likely to have limited physical and emotional work tolerance. Thus, the evaluation program should be highly flexible, accommodating clients who have as little as one hour of initial work tolerance, including travel time.

2) Many homebound persons suffer from orthopedic and neurological conditions which place low ceilings upon their manual dexterity. Consequently, they tend to score low on such tests as the Purdue Pegboard and the Crawford Small Parts Dexterity Test. These low scores can be misleading since, when given opportunities to adapt to work challenges at their own pace, some homebound persons attain unexpected levels of productivity. The same might be said about work simulations. Initial observations of homebound persons performing such tasks may be discouraging. Yet, when helped to develop substitute means of coping with such tasks, some homebound individuals show remarkable gains in performance.

3) Homebound persons vary in their vocational interests. Some enter rehabilitation with a blue-collar orientation and readily accept repetitive manual work assignments. On the other hand, some homebound persons reject such activities, expressing a preference for white-collar work assignments or more highly skilled manual operations. When a homebound person elects to enter types of work that are not represented in agency evaluation, training, and employment programs, a challenge is presented to the vocational rehabilitation worker. Programmatic Research Project vocational data indicate that homebound individuals have for too long been restricted to arts and crafts and low-skill industrial homework. Other opportunities do exist, many just waiting to be developed for the homebound. Therefore, evaluation procedures, even those including a wide range of occupational activities, should be supplemented by custom-designed evaluative experiences keyed to the needs of an individual client, even if considerable time and effort is required to engineer such experiences.

4) An evaluation procedure for the homebound should take into account their need for a longer period of adaptation to a new vocational environment. Consequently, provision should be made for extended service so that the homebound person may be observed developmentally over a longer-than-usual period of time, giving his work-related competencies ample opportunity to change.

5) Homebound persons tend to have a multiplicity of problems in

such areas as housing, income, family adjustment, recreation, interpersonal relationships, and education—problems which influence vocational performance. Unless such problems are recognized and dealt with during evaluation, the ever-present risk of client discontinuance or failure will be increased. Consequently, evaluation programs set up for this group should include supportive services which aim at alleviating or eliminating possible interferences with vocational functioning. The vocational evaluation problem becomes even more complex for a homebound client when, for whatever reason, he cannot leave his home. In the past, rehabilitation workers were content to rely exclusively for data upon interviews with the client and his family and, to a certain extent, psychological tests. Although these evaluation approaches have their uses, they usually reveal the homebound person in only partialistic terms. As evaluative adjuncts, some state and local rehabilitation agencies have devised informal portable work samples that are brought into the client's home for evaluative purposes. Through observing the client performing these tasks, the counselor assesses potential that might not be revealed by tests and interviews. Unfortunately, these work samples lack standardization and norms and do not provide opportunities for the adaptation process to come into play. As a result, their value is still limited. There is a strong current need for carefully structured evaluation "kits" which can be used in the home and which, over a period of time, can differentiate areas of preference and competence.

VOCATIONAL TRAINING AND EMPLOYMENT

Because homebound persons have so few employment opportunities, the tendency has been to train them for types of work that normally are available in a particular geographical area. Thus, some communities train homebound persons exclusively for industrial homework, typing, or arts and crafts. Admittedly, any employment can be better than none. Yet, occupational stereotyping can have deleterious effects in terms of loss of client interest and the squandering of potential skills. But present realities dictate that rehabilitation workers will have to consider stereotyped occupational areas to some extent. This should not, however, preclude a continuing search for "unconventional" homework activities that are more congruent with individual client interests and capacities.

Nationally, this search has only begun. Experiments conducted by the Programmatic Research Project, Abilities, Incorporated, and George Washington University indicate that American technology and emerging industries offer promising leads for new occupations for the homebound. A number of these have been identified in such diverse areas as computer programming, the handling of insurance claims, checking corporation records, serving as a telephone "clerical pool" typist, functioning as a telephone communication center for schools, agencies, and other institutions, and operating a wide variety of electronic business machines.

If the client can be transported to a rehabilitation facility, prevocational and vocational training for the homebound will follow the usual instructional pattern, with the exception that homebound clients frequently need additional time, more personal and individualized instruction, special jigs and aids, closer supervision, and more supportive services. The training problem is most acute when the homebound client cannot leave his place of residence. Under such conditions, training must be brought to the client, a process that involves considerable staff time and effort and relatively high transportation costs. Since it is usually impractical to assign a full-time staff member to work with the client in his home for weeks at a time, the general practice in both prevocational and vocational training is for the staff to provide one-to-one initial instruction and to make periodic visits thereafter to monitor client progress and to provide additional instruction. Although there has been some movement toward the preparation of self-instructional materials for this purpose and the wider use of nonprofessional aides, these approaches are still in an early stage of development.

When clients are targeted for entry into home industry of some sort, skills training generally is related directly to the types of work to be performed at home. In these instances, training is interwoven with employment, since both are almost identical in content and conditions. Under these circumstances, remuneration is sometimes provided during training and, of course, is continued in home employment. Whether skills training occurs at a rehabilitation facility or in the client's home, the goal is early and reasonably stable employment. Unfortunately, available home employment opportunities for homebound persons are still too few in number and, in many cases, too simple and too repetitive to challenge many homebound individuals.

Arts and crafts have been a home industry mainstay for several generations. In some instances, the homebound person is required to sell his products locally, usually not a very satisfactory arrangement since his homebound status mitigates against reaching any sizable market. On the other hand, stronger arts and crafts employment programs distribute home-manufactured products through thrift shops, profit-making and non-profit marketing groups, mail order houses, displays at places where large groups of potential purchasers congregate, such as business meetings, conventions and the lobbies of office buildings, and Christmas and holiday sales.

Industrial homework usually comes in the form of raw materials to be assembled, packaged, or fabricated under the terms of contract between a private firm and a homebound person or a rehabilitation agency. In the latter case, the agency distributes the work to a roster of homebound clients and takes responsibility for establishing liaison with the employer. Parts are delivered to the homebound person's residence and stored there until he fabricates or assembles the product. After the client has performed the work task, a family member, a representative of the employer, or a staff member of the cooperating agency delivers the completed work to the employer who then places the product in the proper commercial distribution channels. Industrial homework plans of this type have been the vehicle through which some of the large home-employment programs, such as that sponsored by the Federation of the Handicapped, have operated for many years.

Beyond arts and crafts and industrial homework, relatively few jobs are currently available for the homebound. Of course, gifted professionally trained homebound persons, such as writers, researchers, and music teachers, can continue to function in their respective fields to a certain extent after they become homebound. But they are exceptional. Selected homebound white-collar workers in small numbers do engage in such occupations as monitoring television programs, telephone selling, performing follow-ups on delinquent accounts, or operating small mail order businesses. In view of the still limited occupational opportunities for the homebound, a large-scale investigation is needed to identify and develop broader and more varied jobs for the homebound. Perhaps, the whole field of homebound rehabilitation will not advance significantly until this is accomplished.

With the possible exception of the relatively small number of professional and technical jobs open to the homebound, homework usually generates modest earnings. Although theoretically mandated by federal and state wages and hours legislation to receive the same rate per piece or per task as other workers in industry doing the same work, the clients' severe disabilities, the unsatisfactory nature of the home as a place of employment, the clients' isolation from the stimulation of other workers and supervisors, the high costs of delivering the service, and the fact that homework often is the least remunerative work in the community—all these factors tend to keep homeworkers' earnings at a low level. Although some homebound persons do earn the minimum wage and more, many do not, an obvious source of dissatisfaction both for homebound clients and for those who rehabilitate them. As things stand now and until more satisfactory jobs can be developed for them, some homebound clients must either accept earnings that, in some cases, are as low as $5 to $10 a week or remain unemployed. Unfortunately, some homebound persons who could really benefit from a work experience understandably choose to remain unemployed, because the proposed remuneration is so low.

Agencies that sponsor homework programs have their problems too. Transporting raw materials to the homeworker and the finished goods to the employer is exceedingly costly, as are instruction of the client in his home, supervision of his work activities, and the provision of supportive services throughout the employment experience. The problem is made even more complex because such agencies undertake a long-range responsibility to the homebound client for which fees cannot be paid by state vocational rehabilitation agencies. As a consequence of this financial bind, many rehabilitation agencies are reluctant to undertake long-term employment programs for homebound clients.

As indicated earlier, rehabilitation agencies have acted as a temporary matchmaker for homebound clients and homework employers, helping to establish the relationship and them stepping out to allow the two to conduct their business independently. Although there are instances in which this has been successful, the frequency has been low. Many employers are unwilling to assume the day-to-day responsibility for transporting raw materials and finished goods to individual workers, are not equipped to engage in specific job training and supervision, and dislike having to cope with the provisions of state and local homework and wages and hours laws. By and large, an arts and crafts or an industrial homework program ordinarily depends upon the services of a mediating rehabilitation agency which assumes the major burden of coordinating all employment activities, as well as rehabilitating the client and sustaining him in the long-term work program. This task is so demanding that, up to the present, few rehabilitation agencies have seen fit to enter this service field. Yet, the fact that it can be done is evident. The Federation of the Handicapped and other agencies are demonstrating daily that homework programs can be administered successfully by imaginative and committed rehabilitation workers.

Despite their faults, industrial homework and arts and crafts employment programs for the homebound are needed in ever greater numbers. But, if they are to grow accordingly, special financial incentives to sponsoring groups will be required. Among these may be higher state rehabilitation agency fees for evaluating, training, and employing homebound persons, long-term subsidies for each homebound person employed in the program subsequent to rehabilitation, special research innovation and demonstration grants, and expanded local philanthropic support. With such aid, many more rehabilitation agencies will be better able to bear the costs of homebound rehabilitation programs, thus rendering them less resistant to initiating such services.

SPECIAL REHABILITATION GROUPS

Employment can have beneficial results for almost all homebound people. An income, little matter how modest, can take the edge off poverty, provide the client with the social status of a wage-earner, fill the time vacuum that creates unending boredom, and reinstate the homebound person as an equal member of the family and the community. Yet, for all this, remunerative work is not the answer for all homebound persons. Members of the subgroups listed below have vital nonvocational needs that should be the concern of rehabilitation workers.

The Homebound Homemaker. The homebound condition rarely contraindicates successful functioning as a homemaker, for both severely disabled men and women. Most vocational rehabilitation agencies consider homemaking preparation as a legitimate and desirable career alternative to remunerative employment, especially if the enhanced independence of the disabled homemaker frees another family member from home tasks so that he can enter employment. Homemaking training usually is accomplished in model apartments as well as in the home itself. In both instances, instruction should be provided by a team of occupational therapists, homemaking counselors, nutritionists, child care specialists, and nurses. Under favorable circumstances, homemaking can be a suitable occupation for selected homebound persons because it enables the client to structure his own environment, work at his own pace, operate within the home, use all the supports that are built into one's residence, and have access to needed assistance from family members and friends. Despite all these advantages, homemaking does have the drawback of generating no additional income.

The Homebound College Student. Access to a college education for the homebound is not as difficult as it once was. Indeed, many of the barriers that kept severely limited persons from obtaining preparation for professional careers have been swept away by college administrators and rehabilitation workers. Such institutions as Long Island University in New York, Southern Illinois University, the University of Missouri, the University of Illinois, and the University of Arizona have been conspicuously successful in removing campus architectural and attitudinal barriers and have set up special programs for severely handicapped students. By moving the homebound student from his community to a college residence, many institutions of higher education have neutralized students' mobility problems and, with the aid of special support services, have enabled students to obtain the benefits of college preparation. In this process, state and local rehabilitation agencies help handicapped students to obtain the environmental prostheses that they need for campus living, such as tape recorders, special typewriters, and battery-operated wheelchairs. Aided by such supports, many homebound students are able to function as well academically and socially as others enrolled in the same institution. With growing acceptance on the part of the colleges, students with limited self-care abilities, and even those who need such ongoing treatment services as physical therapy, are no longer automatically excluded from the campus. On the contrary, if the college knows that a rehabilitation agency is assuming responsibility for the student in a cooperative educational effort, such students may actually be warmly welcomed. At present, however, very few institutions are following the lead of Long Island University to offer college training to the homebound student through such media as recorded tapes, home-to-college telephone communication, and correspondence study. Thus, although institutions of higher education have become increasingly flexible in recent years, facilities for the student who is bound to his home are still rare. Since a college education and graduate study open numerous social and vocational doors for the homebound person, a high rehabilitation priority should be given to bringing a college education into the home of every qualified homebound student.

The Institutionalized Homebound Person. Most hospitals and homes for the chronically ill and disabled lack sufficient rehabilitation facilities to serve their residents adequately. If nothing else, such institutions should have the services that would make it possible for their residents to derive greater benefit and gratification from the institutional environment as it now is constituted. Beyond this, it should be recognized that most of the institutional environments in America constrict the human spirit and impoverish human potential and motivation. Insensitive to human needs for independence, self-direction, and self-fulfillment, all too many of these institutions demand rigid conformity, provide daily monotony, and offer devitalizing programs, all of which reduce the person to less than what he could be. In the current climate of social action, it is no longer adequate for rehabilitation workers to sadly shake their heads in despair over institutional conditions. Those who care about the homebound will work aggessively for change.

Some institutions have revitalized their programs so that many of their residents can have a more exciting and satisfying experience, but they are in the minority. An especially significant aspect of this movement has been the installation of sheltered workshops and on-site work stations which provide residents with an opportunity to assume a worker-patient role. Institutions that add vocational rehabilitation components to their existing programs experience dramatic changes both in the institution and its population. A new sense of movement and involvement seems to pervade the institution, with residents acquiring a new purpose for living and a more meaningful role in the life of the institutional community. As yet, relatively few institutions maintain vocational rehabilitation programs, but the number is growing. Homebound persons who enter the relatively few rehabilitation-oriented institutions are likely to escape the additional personal and social losses that have been associated traditionally with institutional life, and some may even return to their communities. This possibility is highlighted by the Programmatic Research Project finding that up to 25 per cent of the residents of the long-term institutions studied have the potential for leaving the institution if proper rehabilitation services and living arrangements are made available to them.

The Aged Homebound Person. Mounting physical and emotional problems combined with societal indifference contribute to progressive disengagement and ultimate homeboundedness among the aged. The physiological losses that the aged suffer are insufficient to account for this. Tens of thousands of older disabled persons become homebound each year because they do not receive suitable local rehabilitation services. A series of studies on the older disabled worker reported by Rusalem, Baxt, and Barshop (1967) and undertaken by the Federation Employment and Guidance Service (FEGS) demonstrated beyond question that participation by vocationally motivated older persons in a vocational rehabilitation program devised expressly for this group enables many of them to stave off homeboundedness, and, in a striking number of instances, to reverse the disengagement process. FEGS reported that numerous older disabled individuals who were on the brink of entering institutions or becoming either confined to their neighborhoods or homebound were able to continue functioning as useful and far more effective citizens after being helped to re-enter the world of work.

When an older person does become homebound or institutionalized, the current tendency is to "write him off" as unfeasible for rehabilitation. Yet, FEGS studies found that homebound older persons were able to make constructive use of rehabilitation services to the degree that they underwent a marked change in health, outlook, family status, and independence. These investigations suggest that, regardless of age, homebound persons can be rehabilitated into useful employment if service is delivered to them promptly so that they can re-enter employment as soon as possible after homeboundedness sets in.

SERVICE DELIVERY IN A REHABILITATION PROGRAM FOR THE HOMEBOUND

Much misunderstanding surrounds rehabilitation programming for the homebound. For example, many professional workers believe that rehabilitation services for the homebound differ substantially from those for other client groups. The fact is that, whether the client is home-bound or not, the same service components make up a rehabilitation program. In this frame of reference, the central problem for the home-bound client is not the precise services he is to receive, such as intake, evaluation, counseling, training, placement, and follow-up, but how those services are to be delivered to him. Since most rehabilitation agencies still function on a centralized basis and require clients to come to them on the agency's terms, they are ill-adapted to serve the home-bound. If proper programs for the homebound are to be developed, re-habilitation will have to devise more effective means of bridging the gap between homebound clients and the services they need.

In the past, when rehabilitation seemed less complex, some rehabili-tation equipment could be carried about in a counselor's pocket. In fact, during the 1930s and to some extent the 1940s, the counselor often constituted an itinerant rehabilitation facility. Lacking substantial re-course to established local rehabilitation centers, sheltered workshops, community rehabilitation agencies, and similar institutions, he brought with him into the client's home, whether the client was homebound or not, some of the tools that then were thought to be essential for rehabil-itation. His stock in trade occasionally included small worksample tasks, some paper and pencil tests, arts and crafts materials, and even homework items. In today's more frenetic and sophisticated rehabilita-tion world, there is a relative plethora of rehabilitation facilities con-taining elaborate evaluation and training systems, and counselors have fallen out of the habit of being self-contained rehabilitation facilities. As dependence upon rehabilitation centers and workshops grows, coun-selors seem to express less confidence in informal evaluation techniques. Thus, unless transportation can be arranged to such facilities, the home-bound client may be neglected. This is particularly so when there is a widespread reluctance to engage in rehabilitation planning with a client in the absence of a formal evaluation report.

In most homebound rehabilitation programs, the emphasis, wherever possible, is on bringing the homebound client to the facility. For example, the Iowa Easter Seal Society, in a pioneering demonstra-tion, found that it could transport many homebound clients to a summer campsite and use the consequent group experience to train homebound individuals to become skillful workers. On the other hand, the reverse procedure, that is, bringing the program to the homebound individual, has been found helpful in working with an institutionalized group. Thus, in Los Angeles, Industrial Services, Incorporated, a local sheltered workshop cooperating with the Programmatic Research Project, found that delivering services to a central location where homebound persons reside is a feasible design for reaching some severely limited clients.

Since many homebound persons reside in individual residences distributed randomly in urban, suburban, and rural communities, the institutional model described above is inapplicable except in special cases, regardless of the fiscal economies and social advantages it offers. One alternative to the continued isolation of homebound clients is to develop congregate rehabilitation living situations for those whose family and home environments are exceedingly unsuitable, a measure that is undesirable for those who prefer to remain with their families. Another alternative is to devise transportation systems which overcome the massive physical and cost barriers that currently characterize this field. At present few transportation systems meet the criteria of consistent comfort, dependable scheduling, and moderate cost. Consequently, the search for an innovative transportation network that will liberate homebound persons from geographical restraints goes on. Until it materializes, existing local service delivery systems of all kinds should be fully utilized and improved, insofar as possible. Inadequate as they may be, they constitute the only hope in some communities for the rehabilitation of homebound persons.

SPECIAL COUNSELING PROBLEMS AND TECHNIQUES

The disappointments that homebound people have had in the past and their current expectations of failure tend to generate conflicting feelings about entering the rehabilitation process. The resolution of such conflict often depends upon their developing a warm and trusting relationship with a rehabilitation counselor. Thus, as in all forms of rehabilitation service, the role of the counselor is crucial in shaping the homebound client's attitudes toward, and subsequent participation in, rehabilitation. Homeboundedness has, for many of them, become a shield and a haven. Abandonment of the homebound status involves an unusually high degree of risk which requires a sharing of the experience with a trusted counselor.

This profound need for a professional counseling relationship has built-in risks for the counselor, as well. Adoption of an initially highly protective and almost parental role in relation to a homebound client sometimes fills personal needs for the counselor, perhaps at a cost to the client. The client's need to be protected may coincide with the counselor's need to protect, enhancing the possibility that both may work together to perpetuate the client's dependence. When this occurs, rehabilitation into autonomous functioning may be slow in coming. Thus, unless the counselor who has such needs controls his relationship with the homebound client and uses that relationship therapeutically, not personally, he may substitute dependence upon him for other forms of dependence, increasing the risk of rehabilitation failure.

In other respects, counseling for the homebound parallels counseling for clients with other disabilities. However, there are certain special points of counseling emphasis that characterize working relationships with homebound clients. The following are particularly noteworthy:

1) Since the client's relatives play a key role in the rehabilitation of homebound persons, counselors serving the homebound should devote more than the usual amount of effort to family counseling.

2) In view of the finding that homeboundedness is to a large extent, a psychosocial condition, counselors should be prepared to make frequent referrals to mental health facilities in conjunction with the delivery of other rehabilitation services.

3) In some instances, homebound clients are required to endure continuing long-term confinement to the home and, possibly, ultimate institutionalization. In these instances, skillful counseling is often needed to help homebound clients and their families to accept realistic limits on their expectations and to prepare them for long-term sheltered living arrangements.

4) Many areas of client adjustment are usually involved in the rehabilitation of homebound clients. Consequently, the counselor usually finds himself coordinating an interdisciplinary team which draws upon the resources of a multiplicity of resources, including health, housing, welfare, rehabilitation, and recreation agencies.

5) Since home visits are time-consuming and, in some instances, troublesome, the counselor serving the homebound may have to find substitutes for multiple home contacts with clients. Among these substi-

tutes are, wherever possible, arranging transportation for clients to central rehabilitation facilities, conducting telephone interviews with them, and using volunteers or nonprofessional workers to make the necessary home calls as representatives of the rehabilitation agency.

6) After rehabilitation service in the conventional sense has been completed and a rehabilitation case closure has been effectuated, serious adjustment problems may continue for the homebound person, requiring recurrent, perhaps lifetime counseling. Since rehabilitation plans ordinarily have finite time limits and rehabilitation counselors generally provide service only during the "intensive" phase of rehabilitation, other provisions should be made for long-term counseling for rehabilitated homebound persons. Typically, this problem is handled by interesting other community agencies, groups, or individuals to assume an ongoing responsibility for serving the individual. This is especially important for clients who participate in long-term homework programs.

7) When counseling is provided in a client's residence, it should be recognized that the type of counseling offered will be influenced by the nature of the home environment. Thus, individual counseling may be difficult to arrange in a home where privacy is rare. More often than not, the home ecology necessitates counselor informality and, in many instances, family group rather than individual counseling. Whereas the counselor who works in his office has access to a variety of counseling aids—occupational information files, procedural manuals, immediate recourse to supervision, and instant consultation of case records—these are out of his reach when he works in the client's home.

8) In counseling, it should be kept in mind that the parameters of a homebound client's decisions differ from those of other clients. If he is restricted to his home and neighborhood, and is dependent upon others, the client may, indeed, be unable to control large segments of his life. Counseling in such instances may have to focus upon an acceptance, rather than a modification, of this reality. For example, clients who rely upon others for physical care cannot readily decide to disengage themselves from these individuals, however strong the need to do so may be. Therefore, counseling help is needed to explore areas even in such a constricted situation in which client decision-making is possible and, through exploiting these areas fully, the counselor can help the homebound person to retain, and even to enhance, his sense of self-worth.

ECOLOGICAL   CONSIDERATIONS

Counseling the homebound client also concerns human ecology, an emphasis that has important implications for rehabilitation workers. Although the limitations possessed by homebound clients usually receive the rehabilitation spotlight, it is the environment which really defines the nature and extent of homeboundedness. In the most obvious terms, the architectural barriers in clients' homes and communities really set the limits of most homeboundedness. Beyond architectural barriers, however, community and family attitudes, the unavailability of comprehensive rehabilitation services, the lack of suitable rehabilitation residences, and the apathy of some rehabilitation workers—all contribute a physical and human ecology that promotes unnecessary dependence and impoverishment among homebound persons. Any positive alteration of this ecology can redefine a homebound person's status to such an extent that, in some cases, he ceases to be homebound.

Looking at the problem from a related point of view, the Programmatic Research Project noted that only a small proportion of homeboundedness in the samples studied was attributable solely to the extreme nature of the disability. On the contrary, most of the homeboundedness observed was sustained and exacerbated by social factors. The nondisabled world seems to draw a line demarcating the adjustments it will make for atypical people, determining whether it will or will not make its buildings accessible to people in wheelchairs, provide free or low-cost special transportation to severely disabled persons, offer decentralized rehabilitation and employment facilities in local neighborhoods, and supply comprehensive services designed to reduce or eliminate homeboundedness. Such decisions are often made against the homebound usually not through malice or hostility, but through omission and default.

At this point in time, nondisabled society seems little disposed to initiate a major effort to restructure the environment so that it will become more hospitable to homebound persons. Simultaneously, however, society is to some degree currently doing just this for other minority groups. Rusalem (1970), in an analysis of obvious social bias against homebound persons, concluded that the environment continues to be unfavorable for the homebound person because homebound people lack the power needed to pressure society into effectuating change. Minorities that are able to mobilize group strength, call upon powerful advocate organizations and individuals, arouse public anxiety, issue threats, conduct demonstrations, challenge existing ideas in the mass media of communication, and even resort to violence have had some success in breaking down public resistance to environmental restructuring. The homebound group, however, lacks all of these instruments and, as a consequence, is one of the most impotent of all American minorities. Lacking organizational potential and sources of influence, the homebound are powerless in a power-sensitive rehabilitation establishment.

Rehabilitation counselors who serve the homebound cannot counsel in a social vacuum. If American society is so denying to homebound individuals that it blocks their access to fundamental human rights and prerogatives, counseling alone will not enable them to function adequately. Yet, this is precisely the situation of the homebound person today. Community apathy, employer resistance, denial of service, and absence of opportunities all combine to create an environment that defies ready human adaptation, an environment which creates unnecessary homeboundedness, prolongs dependency and poverty, and prevents the homebound individual from achieving appropriate social, personal, and economic self-fulfillment. Counseling the homebound to accept such conditions is not only unthinkable for rehabilitation workers but impractical as well.

Despite their legal right to rehabilitation services, hundreds of thousands of homebound persons each year are systematically denied this right by arbitrary agency policies and procedures, administrative decisions, and counselor indifference. Those who would serve the homebound cannot discharge their responsibilities to homebound persons by being oblivious to these conditions nor by accepting them as inevitable. In this light, the counseling of homebound rehabilitation clients imposes nothing less than a special advocacy role upon the counselor. In these terms the thrust in counseling should not be merely upon changing the client so that he will adapt more readily to a world that was not made for him but also to have counselors move out into that world and to take leadership in changing it.

All too often in the past, the rehabilitation counselor has functioned as a representative of currently constituted society. If an employer has

made a dubious demand that handicapped workers behave in some stip-
ulated but not wholly rational fashion, such as accepting more modest
remuneration than other workers, some counselors would hasten to
comply, attempting to convert the client into the type of working unit
desired by the employer. In view of the fact that unreasonable demands
should be made upon the homebound no more than upon other groups
in society, the counselor is no longer justified in passively accepting the
world as it is. In the case of the homebound, at least, this is not usually
a suitable world, and only by counselor participation in changing that
world will the client be able to live as rich and full a life as he merits.

TRENDS, ISSUES, AND RESEARCH

Stronger support for rehabilitation programs for homebound persons
has been accompanied by a trend toward a broader advocacy for this
group. In an address before the National Conference on the Rehabilitation of Homebound Persons in February, 1971, Edward Newman,
Commissioner of the Rehabilitation Services Administration, called for
a higher rehabilitation priority for the homebound. His view reflects the
positive action taken both by the Social and Rehabilitation Service and
the Rehabilitation Services Administration to stimulate the development
of broader services for the homebound. In the wake of this dynamic
leadership, state and voluntary rehabilitation agencies are launching
programs for the homebound in unprecedented numbers.

As part of this effort, the Programmatic Research Project has translated this improved climate into action by promoting the rehabilitation
of homebound persons in all sections of the United States. Despite this
commendable effort, however, the rehabilitation of the homebound remains in an early stage of development. Even today, fewer than 10 per
cent of all homebound persons who could benefit from rehabilitation
services are receiving such services. Among the steps that remain to
be taken are:

1) The designation within each state rehabilitation agency of a
special division, group, or person to assume the major responsibility
in that state for developing rehabilitation services for the homebound.

2) The allocation of special funds to assist rehabilitation agencies

that serve the homebound to meet some of the additional costs of working with this population.

3) The establishment of at least one National Research and Demonstration Center for the Rehabilitation of Homebound Persons to serve as the fulcrum for nationwide efforts in this field.

4) The creation of regional rehabilitation centers for the homebound which may work with homebound persons who cannot benefit from local programs.

5) The development of an advocacy organization of rehabilitation workers and homebound persons to provide leadership in the battle to reorient public behaviors toward this disability group.

6) The creation of rehabilitation residences which would permit homebound persons to live with their peers in a rehabilitation-oriented ecology.

7) The redesign of institutions housing homebound persons so that those who reside in them would be enabled to develop their potential and enjoy opportunities to work, achieve optimum independence, and acquire a sense of autonomy and self-worth.

8) The redesign of existing state and local legislation that limits industrial homework so that such legislation will be more responsive to the rehabilitation needs of homebound persons.

9) The inclusion of materials and experiences relating to the homebound in training programs for rehabilitation workers in the various disciplines.

10) The assignment of a high priority to research and demonstration projects concerning the homebound.

REFERENCES

Cohen, M. October, 1956. What can be done for the homebound child? Recreation 49:8:375–77.

——Autumn, 1956. Expanded work for the homebound. Vocational Guidance Quarterly 5:1:13–15.

Federation of the Handicapped. 1968, 1969, 1970, 1971. Programmatic Research Project on the Rehabilitation of Homebound Persons: Progress Reports. Unpublished.

Gersten, J. 1968. Comparison of home and clinic rehabilitation for chronically ill and physically disabled persons. Archives of Physical Medicine and Rehabilitation 49:615–42.

Katz, H. 1961. Program for the homebound in New York City of the New York State Division of Vocational Rehabilitation, in R. Tickton, ed., A guide to comprehensive rehabilitation services to the homebound disabled. Washington, D.C., National Association of Sheltered Workshops and Homebound Programs.

McKenna, N. A. M. et al. 1967. Attitudes of homebound patients toward eleven home employment opportunities. Perceptual and Motor Skills 25:776.

Rusalem, H. 1967. Penetrating the narrowing circle. Rehabilitation Literature 28:7:202–17.

——1970. Powerless in a power-sensitive rehabilitation establishment. Journal of Rehabilitation 10:19–21.

——1971. Exploring the widening circle. Rehabilitation Literature 32:8.

——Papers from the National Conference on the Rehabilitation of Homebound Persons. In press.

Rusalem, H., R. Baxt, and I. Barshop. 1967. Rehabilitation of the neighborhood-bound older disabled person. New York, Federation Employment and Guidance Service.

U.S. Congress. 1954. Vocational Rehabilitation Act Amendments. 83d Cong., 2d sess., S Doc. No. 2759, Public Law No. 565. Washington, D.C., U.S. Government Printing Office.

U.S. Office of Vocational Rehabilitation. 1955. Study of programs for homebound individuals. House Doc. No. 98, 84th Cong., 1st sess. Washington, D.C., U.S. Government Printing Office.

FRANKLIN C. SHONTZ

SEVERE CHRONIC ILLNESS

A DISCUSSION OF REHABILITATION PRACTICES with the severely chronically ill must deal with a problem of considerable magnitude and complexity. The severely disabled comprise a heterogeneous population. They come from all age groups and socioeconomic backgrounds; they cannot be identified by any specific illness or bodily condition. Few rehabilitation programs are specifically designed for persons with severe chronic disabilities. Consequently, there is no common body of knowledge gained from shared professional experience. Furthermore, much of what is now being done for the chronically ill is, in the opinion of the writer, probably misguided and unproductive.

Subsequent sections of this chapter therefore do not attempt to describe current rehabilitation practices. Despite this restriction, a consideration of the principles of rehabilitation practice with the severely chronically ill can be rewarding. Recent theory and research provide leads and suggestions which have important implications. A number of these will now be examined.

DEFINITION

The problem of defining severe chronic illness has been discussed elsewhere (Shontz, 1962) and need only be summarized. Briefly, medical definitions are useful for describing characteristics of diseases; but, be-

FRANKLIN C. SHONTZ, Ph.D., is Professor and Director of Training and Research in Somatopsychology-Rehabilitation, University of Kansas, Lawrence, Kansas.

cause of the dynamic nature of the human organism and the complexity of individual diagnoses, medical definitions cannot be used to identify a homogeneous group of persons as the chronically ill. Person-oriented definitions label as "chronically ill" those people who are cared for in rehabilitation settings or hospitals for chronic diseases. These definitions, although often operationally convenient, ignore the fact that many persons in institutions suffer rejection only. They are disabled by social problems rather than by medical conditions.

For present purposes, the writer finds that the most useful definition of severe chronic illness or disability incorporates both medical and social considerations in a rehabilitation context as follows: A severe chronic illness is *a combination of medical and social limitations that drastically restricts long-range rehabilitation goals.* Because rehabilitation practices generally stress vocational activities, the severely chronically ill may be identified by rule-of-thumb as persons with long-term diseases or disabilities and for whom economic independence is improbable.

This definition also has its weaknesses. First, it does not explicitly recognize important differences between the types of problems presented by the chronically ill whose disabilities are primarily medical (for example, persons with debilitating, progressive physical conditions such as muscular dystrophy or multiple sclerosis) and the chronically ill whose disabilities are strongly psychosocially determined (for example, the amputee who is physically capable of vocational rehabilitation but cannot successfully achieve it because he is too old, has a drinking or drug problem, is severely disturbed behaviorally or seriously retarded intellectually).

Second, like many definitions that apply to people, it can acquire a static quality; it may suggest that specific persons can be labeled "severely disabled" and that this label will apply forever. Such is clearly not the case. On the medical side, advances in treatment methods and the development of sophisticated devices for improving patients' abilities to communicate, ambulate, and care for themselves constantly reduce handicaps and make economic rehabilitation possible for many who could not expect it in the past. On the social side, any positive change in attitudes or practices affecting the employment of persons with disabilities could quickly alter the status of many severely disabled persons.

For example, general removal of architectural barriers would markedly reduce the number of persons with disabilities who must currently be regarded as severely handicapped.

The rehabilitation worker who deals with the severely chronically ill must be prepared to alter his conception of what constitutes severe disability at a moment's notice. This caution applies not only to his conception of chronic illness in general, but also to his assessment of individual clients.

INCIDENCE

An appreciation of the magnitude of the social problem of severe chronic illness and disability may be gained from U. S. Department of Labor statistics (cited by Usdane, 1970). According to these statistics, at least 22.6 million Americans (more than one in ten) have physical disabilities; nearly half the men and women over sixty-five years of age have handicaps.

Racially and ethnically, persons with handicaps represent a cross-section of America, although a somewhat greater proportion of the working-age, nonwhite population (24 per cent) is handicapped than of the working-age white population (16 per cent). Slightly more than half the population of persons with disabilities live in cities; about one-third live in the South. The major handicapping disabilities are heart conditions, arthritis and rheumatism, mental and nervous conditions, hypertension (without heart involvement), impairments of the lower extremities or hips, and visual impairments.

Eighteen million persons with disabilities (more than three-fourths) are of working age, but 48 per cent of this working-age group (about 8.6 million) are not in the labor force. Only 36 per cent of the working-age handicapped are employed full time. The 8.6 million persons with handicaps who are of working age but are not in the labor force and the 4.6 million persons with handicaps who are not of working age comprise a total of 13.2 million people with disabilities who are not gainfully employed. This figure is undoubtedly too high to be an estimate of the number of persons with severe physical disabilities. But, even if it were in error by as much as 50 per cent, the scope of the problem it represents for society would still be very great.

INITIAL EVALUATION AND
ASSESSMENT OF CLIENT POTENTIAL

Two independently conducted programs of research provide insights and suggestions about client assessment in relation to rehabilitation outcome. These results are impressive because the studies were conducted by different investigators at separate institutions and used entirely different types of subjects. Yet, both produced similar conclusions, some of which were unanticipated.

WORK INHIBITION: THE ICS (INSTITUTE FOR COMMUNITY STUDIES) PROJECT

Although research on the concept of Work Inhibition was carried on for several years at the Institute for Community Studies in Kansas City, Missouri (Tiffany, Cowan, and Tiffany, 1970), only one part of the over-all investigation is of concern here (Tiffany, Cowan, and Shontz, 1969). This research attempted by experimental means to alter subjects' tendencies to produce statements reflecting self-initiated efforts to obtain employment.

None of the forty-three subjects in the project was institutionalized. All were men twenty to sixty years of age, not physically disabled to the extent of hindering employability, and showing no evidence of brain damage, alcohol or drug addiction, or of incapacitating psychiatric disorder. However, all subjects had unstable work histories: long periods of unemployment and substantial amounts of job hopping and vocational impermanence.

Subjects came from two sources: (a) local offices of state employment agencies, which referred clients with long histories of repeated short-term job placement; and (b) respondents to a newspaper advertisement offering a day's work to people who had trouble holding jobs. This difference in subject source is critical, for subjects from each source differed markedly not only in responsiveness to the experimental procedure but also in psychological characteristics measured before and after experimental treatment.

During initial evaluation, subjects who answered the newspaper advertisement presented themselves as independent and self-directed. They strengthened this stance in response to experimental efforts to increase their expression of self-direction through differential social reinforcement of verbal behavior. By contrast, subjects referred by placement agencies showed little initial tendency to describe their job-seeking activities as self-initiated and were less responsive to selective reinforcement of statements expressing self-direction of behavior.

Given the general cultural tendency to view self-directedness (independence) as desirable, the "advertisement" subjects gave the appearance of being better candidates for counseling and placement than did the agency referrals. However, close examination of intensive interview data and of personality test scores obtained before and after experimental treatment suggested that this appearance was deceptive.

For the self-directed, advertisement-answering subject, work instability proved to be a record of repeated frustration. These people shared the conventional American dream for success but they repeatedly failed to achieve it because they lacked tolerance for frustration, could not sustain long-term interpersonal relationships, denied their weaknesses, were prone to impulsivity, and solved problems only by running away from them.

For the non-self-directed, agency-frequenting subject, work instability often appeared to be an appropriate adaptation to problems posed by recognized general interpersonal ineptitude. These people accepted their dependence on others for help in finding work. The jobs available to them through the placement agencies were neither offered nor accepted as permanent, and all parties understood that no deep or long-range commitment was being made. This type of unstable worker is accepted for what he is, and no one (including himself) expects more of him than he is capable of giving.

Marked changes on personality tests were not expected from a single experimental procedure; nevertheless, some statistically significant changes did occur. Of the two sources from which the subjects came, only those referred from agencies showed improvement on before-and-after measures of self-concept and of experienced control over the self.

The investigators concluded that the chronically unemployed client who looks best in an evaluation interview, who seems to show the most spontaneous initiative, and who seems most sensitive and responsive to the counselor's suggestions may be the poorest prospect for long-term counseling. Changes of verbal behavior in these clients are probably superficial and not indicative of real change in personality structure. The work-inhibited client who seems most resigned to his fate, who is most dependent, and who is least obviously changed by the counselor's actions actually seems the better prospect for beneficial influence from counseling. Changes produced in him are more likely to be deep and long-lasting, even if not immediately evident in surface behavior.

THE WADSWORTH V.A. PROJECT

The Wadsworth V.A. Center Project (Armatas, Hewitt, Lohrenz, and Remple, 1970) subjected sixty-four institutionalized adult men to an intensive program of milieu therapy and vocational training. The program for each participant lasted approximately one year and consisted of counseling, human relations training, special living arrangements which encouraged independent, responsible behavior, and vocational training at appropriate schools. The subjects were from a population of chronically institutionalized, emotionally disabled individuals.

As might be expected, rehabilitation success rates were not high. Fifty per cent did not complete the program. Of the remaining thirty-two subjects, only fifteen were clearly successful. Success for twelve more was judged to be questionable; five subjects who completed the program were judged to have failed in rehabilitation. Obviously, level of achievement varied widely within the sample, but this variability enabled the investigators to relate outcome to measures of subject characteristics taken before the program was begun.

Men who clearly failed had described themselves at the start of the program as dominant, assertive, self-confident, and free of personal problems, other than those related to physical health. The investigators noted that these subjects had professed eager interest in the project and were initially regarded by staff members as promising candidates for rehabilitation.

Unexpectedly, the individuals who proved to be most successful in the program described themselves initially as weak, dependent, submissive, and conforming. As the project progressed, these subjects continued to perceive themselves as weak and dependent, but they gradually assumed a somewhat more aggressive and even rebellious stance.

Subjects who completed the project but were judged to be unsuccessful showed a change toward increased recognition of the reality of personal problems and appeared, at the end of the project, to have reached about the same psychological state as successful subjects presented initially.

The investigators noted that they had learned three valuable lessons from their results: (a) clinical judgments concerning individuals who initially look like "good" prospects can be quite erroneous, and individuals who look "normal" are most likely to be those who deny problems and cannot tolerate the admission of weakness or defeat; (b) very dependent, unassuming individuals with long patterns of dependency, particularly if such individuals acknowledge interpersonal problems and weaknesses, are surprisingly good candidates; and (c) candidates who successfully complete rehabilitation do not show dramatic personal changes, but success can probably best be measured in terms of a dependent individual learning to transfer his dependency from an institution to an outside environment (Armatas, et al., 1970, p. vii).

COMMON FINDINGS AND IMPLICATIONS

Both studies show that common-sense notions of what constitutes desirable psychological prognostic signs may be grossly in error. In both investigations, one group of subjects looked "good." They were classic "self-starters," showed ambition, desire, and initiative; in short, they appeared well-motivated for rehabilitation. Yet, both studies concluded that these subjects are poor candidates. The ICS project found them to be only superficially influenced by attempts to alter their underlying conflictual states; the investigators predicted that such persons would fail to complete successfully any program that threatened to touch upon deeper psychological processes. The Wadsworth project showed that these predictions are correct.

In both investigations, a second group of subjects looked "poor." They seemed weak, dependent, timid, and ineffectual. Yet, both studies concluded that such persons are better candidates for rehabilitation. The ICS project found that these persons showed slight but significant positive gains on tests of personality following manipulation of their verbal behavior. The Wadsworth project found that these clients stayed with and completed the program and were successfully and relatively permanently placed into the community.

There is a truism in rehabilitation that the best predictor of future behavior is past behavior: clients who did well before disability are most likely to do well later; clients who achieved little in their predisability days are likely to achieve little as a result of rehabilitation. This doctrine is probably reasonably correct (although it has rarely been subjected to rigorous statistical evaluation). According to this dictum, virtually none of the subjects in the studies summarized here qualifies as a candidate for rehabilitation—all are at the low end of the continuum of life accomplishment. Both investigations studied persons for whom prospects were poor. Yet, both investigations suggest that favorable change is possible for at least some of these persons; and because this chapter concerns rehabilitation with those for whom rehabilitation is least feasible, the findings can be integrated into important practical recommendations.

SEVERE DISABILITY AND THE WISH
FOR INDEPENDENCE

Obviously, when a person is prevented by medical and social factors from realistically anticipating a return to economic independence, he gains little from dreaming about and working toward future independent accomplishment. Cases exist in which overwhelming medical and social incapacitations are brilliantly overcome, but they are rare, and they may serve only to make life more difficult for the ambitious client without great talent who suffers by comparing himself with those who achieve exceptional success. For the most part, persons with no prospects for future economic independence, who show "healthy" signs of desirable motivation for independent vocational activity, should probably not be regarded as the best candidates for programs that emphasize other types of life goals. Such clients are likely to be counterdependent, defensive, rebellious, and prone to denial. Attempts to persuade them to accept what they regard as lesser goals are likely to provoke reactions which will disturb both client and therapist and which may exaggerate disruptive psychological processes.

Persons who are more passive, dependent, timid, and conforming are probably better candidates for programs of rehabilitation that aim at goals other than those defined in vocational terms. With such clients, dependency provides the lever by which greater independence of behavior may be produced. The commonly cited similarity between the situations of the severely disabled person who requires expert assistance and of the child in relation to his parents should not be over-stressed, but it is more than sheer coincidence. The person with a severe disability who is dependent on agencies and professional personnel is somewhat like the child who continually relies upon his parents for guidance and direction. The wise parent knows when to provide what the child asks for and when to insist that he seek it for himself. The client with a severe disability but who insists on "making it on his own" behaves somewhat like a child who tries to grow up too soon. Rebelling against authority which he feels cannot be trusted, he thrusts himself, unprepared, into situations which make demands upon him that he does not know how to meet.

SOME PROBLEMS OF MANAGEMENT

HOPE AND THE AMBITIOUS CLIENT

The above might suggest that the severely disabled client who tries for more than seems reasonable is to be abandoned, and that programs should be instituted only for easy-going, passive, dependent, conforming clients, while those who are most strongly motivated for conventional success are left to bloody their heads against the stern walls of reality.

In some cases, planned nonintervention against unrealistic ambition is best. Consider a person with a rapidly progressing terminal illness who insists that if it were not for the incompetence of the hospital personnel he would be on his feet and back at work. Little is gained by demanding that such a person "face up to facts." Clearly, in this and similar instances, ambition serves a useful self-protective purpose. So long as the patient continues to accept care, and so long as affairs in his life situation are in order, there is no reason for breaking down his hopeful retreat from reality. Benign acceptance of abuse from the patient by the hospital staff is part of the course of his treatment.

In other cases, planned nonintervention is necessary, although undesirable. When resources are limited, there may be no alternative to providing services only to those most likely to benefit from them.

Ideally, assistance is given even to those who stand relatively little chance of benefiting from it. What kind of program might be best for those who do not accept the limitations and necessary dependencies of their life situations? The question cannot be easily answered.

Wright (1960) has pointed out that *hope* serves vital psychological purposes. The functions of hoping in parents of children with disabilities has been studied in detail by Wright and Shontz (1968). Unfortunately, rehabilitation personnel frequently act as though hope and "reality" are mutually contradictory. Wright (1968) found that college students endorsed the idea that it is good to be "realistic" and bad to be "unrealistic"; most also believed that being unrealistic means having aspirations that are too high.

Wright pointed out how these attitudes can influence rehabilitation practices. When a therapist or counselor feels that a client aspires to more than he can attain, he is likely to regard the client as unrealistic. Since being unrealistic is bad, the worker communicates disapproval of the client's aspirations. This is done in the name of good psychology, since therapists are taught that adjustment to reality is the prime requirement of mental health. However, the result is likely to be that the client refuses to accept the communication, becomes angry with the communicator, strengthens his own beliefs, and perhaps rejects rehabilitation altogether.

Mistaken Assumptions. One common fallacy in this form of rehabilitation practice stems from the assumption that encounters with reality are always beneficial to psychological well-being. The invalidity of this notion is obvious when one considers that ghetto environments are real, but few would maintain that it is psychologically healthy for people to be forced to encounter them.

Beneficial encounters with reality possess two characteristics. First, the individual accepts his own behavior. He may be encouraged, supported, coaxed, cajoled, or shamed by others into finally making the encounter, but he ultimately acknowledges it as his own act. Second, despite his anxieties and fears, he emerges from a beneficial encounter with a greater sense of mastery, accomplishment, or self-worth than he had before. To force a client to face reality by undermining his hopes accomplishes neither purpose effectively and is, in fact, likely to make future encounter more difficult.

Another fallacy in an approach that stresses the hopelessness of reality for people with severe disabilities stems from the supposition that rehabilitation workers know more about the client than he does himself. Rehabilitation workers must remind themselves again and again that their prognoses are judgments and guesses, and that these are often wrong. Regrettably, few rehabilitation specialists fully appreciate the importance of the total life situation in the client's over-all adjustment, and almost no effort is made to keep rehabilitation workers informed of their clients' fates (see subsequent section, *Monitoring the Rehabilitation Process*). Lack of feedback and critical assessment of the predictive validity of clinical prognoses encourages stereotypes that prevent the specialist from appreciating the limitations of his ability to anticipate what is in store for many individuals.

Recommended Practices. Prevalent practices are easily criticized; recommendations for improvement are more difficult to specify. When a client expresses unrealistic hopes for the future, perhaps initially the most important question to be asked is: how harmful are these hopes in the immediate present? When independence, initiative, and self-confidence provide the motivation for active participation in beneficial therapeutic programs, the immediate benefits of unrealistic expectations are often great enough to justify supporting (or, at least not attacking) the client's hopes.

The decision to attack a client's defensive retreat into unrealistic hope must be made with caution. Because defensive retreat is a normal, and probably necessary, stage in the course of adaptation (see subsequent section, *Satisfactions and Dissatisfactions in Disability*), it should be actively opposed only when it has become so pervasive and permanent that spontaneous recovery is highly improbable and when there is greater danger in allowing it to continue than in ignoring it. This last state of affairs might occur when a patient with grossly unrealistic hopes approaches discharge. If such a person has suicidal tendencies which will be activated by later disappointment, it is less dangerous to attack his defenses while he is still in the agency, where depressive responses can be managed and worked through, than to force him to deal with them later on his own.

These cautions are complicated by the consideration that long-lasting defenses to which a client has a high level of personal commitment are extremely difficult to disrupt. Furthermore, successful disruption of such defenses is almost certain to provoke profound and intense responses. Consequently, anyone who decides to attack a defensive retreat of this type must be prepared for a struggle. The client's most likely initial response will be to resist and reject the attacker. If the attack is eventually successful, the attacker must then be willing to assume responsibility for picking up the pieces when the client's hopes collapse.

Prevention. The best approach to unrealistic defenses is to prevent them from reaching the point where massive intervention is required. Careful consideration of the needs of the newly disabled client suggests how this may be done. The first basic need of such a person is to assure himself that he is being competently cared for and that those he loves are minimally threatened by his personal crisis. Constant reassurance on these matters is essential as preparation for the client's ultimate acceptance of his condition. Such assurance is conveyed, in part, by specific things that are said directly. More important, it is conveyed by the general atmosphere of the agency. Clients experience fewer disruptive defenses in a setting where staff and patient morale is high and outlooks are genuinely optimistic than in a setting characterized by dissension among staff and depreciation of client worth.

The second basic need of many newly disabled persons is to mourn their losses (cf. Wright, 1960). Rehabilitation personnel focus so strongly on future possibilities that they tend to forget that the client himself is for some time far more concerned about what he no longer has than with what he may get later. To talk with the client about his loss seems cruel, and indeed it is, when such talk serves no useful purpose. But it is by no means cruel to remind the patient who deteriorates physically because he resists treatment that he has, in fact, suffered loss and that the purpose of prescribed therapies is to help him overcome the effects of that loss as much as possible. Such an approach is certainly kinder than one which says "you're getting treatment because your doctor says you're supposed to get it" or one that leads the patient to believe that he'll be as good as new in no time if only he cooperates. Treatment is, of necessity, a reminder of loss; it is likely to provoke a degree of mourning and depression. The therapist who accepts and understands his patient's need to work through this encounter in his own way, and who is not tempted into providing unnecessary support for maladaptive defenses, gives more than physical help.

SATISFACTIONS AND DISSATISFACTIONS
IN DISABILITY

RESEARCH SUMMARY

Reports of personal experiences, written by persons with disabilities, provide valuable information about the psychological aspects of chronic illness. *Experiments in Survival* (Henrich and Kriegel, 1961) contains thirty-one first-person reports describing virtually all aspects of life with a handicapping condition. The present author has conducted a study of this volume, the procedures and results of which are partly summarized below.

Procedure. Each report was evaluated on a variety of measures dealing with subject characteristics, psychological content of reports, and formal structure of reports. One psychological variable was satisfaction-dissatisfaction. The measures derived from this variable were similar to measures devised originally by Dollard and Mowrer (1947). A sentence was tabulated as reflecting satisfaction (s) if it communicated pleasure, hope, success, comfort, relief from distress, or a similar experiential state. A sentence was tabulated as reflecting dissatisfaction (D) if it communicated discomfort, pain, distress, anxiety, fear, displeasure, or a similar experiential state.

A second psychological variable was achievement-frustration. A positive score (A) was assigned to each sentence that communicated past, present, or anticipated efforts to achieve some socially or medically desirable goal. A negative score (F) was assigned to each sentence that communicated either failure or rejection of opportunities to achieve.

Appropriate statistical tests were used to determine relationships among pairs of variables. Only findings of major importance are summarized below.

Quantitative Results. Of primary concern is the fact that severity of disability correlated significantly with only one other measure: medical diagnosis. In this particular sample of persons with disabilities, those with polio were relatively severely incapacitated by their conditions, while those with cerebral palsy were relatively mildly disabled.

The lack of correlation between severity of disability and all other measures indicates that, contrary to what might be expected on a common-sense basis, the severely disabled reported as much satisfaction and interest in achievement as did the mildly disabled. The close similarity of findings on psychological measures for the total group and for the subgroup of persons with severe disabilities is evident in the table.

SELECTED QUANTITATIVE RESULTS FROM
THE STUDY OF FIRST-PERSON ACCOUNTS
OF DISABILITY EXPERIENCES

Measures	Total Group (N=31)		Severely Disabled (N=7)	
	Mean	S. D.	Mean	S. D.
Sum S	34 *	11.0	36	11.0
Sum D	30	8.9	27	8.5
Sum A	38	14.2	36	16.2
Sum F	10	6.4	8	5.6

* Entries indicate percentage of sentences expressing the psychological state described.

In general, expressions of satisfaction slightly exceeded expressions of dissatisfaction. (Types of satisfactions and dissatisfactions are described in the next section.) Positively oriented interests in achievement exceeded expressions of frustration by almost four to one in the total group (more than four to one among the severely disabled). As might be expected, high levels of achievement orientation were closely associated with high levels of satisfaction.

Qualitative Considerations. The following paragraphs briefly summarize the types of satisfactions and dissatisfactions described in reports written by persons so disabled that full economic independence is either doubtful or clearly impossible:

N. D. described her fears and discomfort at the onset of disability; but she counteracted these by noting that she had complete confidence in the competence of her physicians. She described benefits gained from the community of patients in the hospital and told how she had established lasting friendships and learned the importance of living harmoniously with others. Now her main dissatisfactions are with people who try to force their wills upon her—the "helpers" who pretend to know more about what is good for her than she does herself.

D. W. expressed primary concern over loss of his role as husband, father, and provider for his family. He is eager to participate in all forms of rehabilitation and is pleased at the gradual improvement he experiences. After four years in rehabilitation, he continues to hope for eventual return to independent employment, but, as he says, "I have learned patience and tolerance."

D. L., who is virtually confined to her bed, stated that, "The severely handicapped person knows with passionate certainty that the wish to be part of life is the only ambition that makes any sense." She defined her task as that of finding her way back into living. That she has done by writing, tutoring in English, by aiding in church projects, and by assisting in registration for local adult education courses. Primarily, however, she emphasized her increased appreciation of generally unnoticed events. "There are more discoveries to be made than the imagination can foretell. Each day has its precious, expectant quality, is potentially a birthday. "

L. G. is a young man with Bechet's syndrome. He has been to several hospitals and has experienced frequent setbacks in rehabilitation, but he finds comfort in religion and in socializing with others in the hospital; he has long talks with a fellow patient, for whom he has developed an attachment. L. G. is often discouraged, but he continues with his exercises and clings to the hope that if he really tries he can help himself get well.

D. P. noted that after seven years of struggle with her medical condition, she decided there were too many interesting things to do to justify expending all her effort on the task of getting well. With very considerable mechanical assistance from others she has collaborated in writing books about nature. She requires constant physical care, but to her "Life is so wonderful . . . that I have no wish to complain of having less of it than someone else. If a great deal of it is desirable, then even a small amount is something to be prized."

COPING WITH DISABILITY

Understanding of these cases is increased by considering them in the light of psychological constructs that describe and explain reactions to stress and crisis. In his theory of stress, Lazarus (1966) identified three forms of response to stressful situations. One form is *direct action*: behavior designed to overcome or escape physically from the stress agent. In disability, active coping directed toward overcoming the stress agent is seen in patients' efforts to get well through vigorous activity or to defeat their conditions by hard work. D. W. represents the clearest example of well-organized activity of this sort.

Active coping directed toward escape from the stress agent is less possible in cases of disability, for the disability is an everpresent fact of life. No cases of active escape are represented in the preceding reports, since the only completely effective direct escape action against permanent, pervasive disability is probably suicide.

Another form of response to stress is cognitive; it involves *reappraisal* of the meaning and significance of the stress agent. Although Lazarus refers to this form of response as "defensive," that term is misleading, since cognitive restructuring may also enhance self-worth. The case of D. P. illustrates the point; after seven years of active coping, she completely reinterpreted her situation. Perhaps it was defensive to decide that the struggle to get well was not worth the gains it produced, but it was hardly defensive to decide that writing books about nature is more gratifying and worthy of attention and energy. Restructuring is implied as well in the cases of N. D., D. L., and L. G., all of whom indicate that they have found sources of satisfaction that are not blocked or threatened by their disabilities; they have managed the stress of disability by turning their attentions elsewhere.

Purely defensive reappraisal is not represented in the cases summarized here, but its general characteristics are easily specified; it consists of denial of the reality of disability. Except in persons with brain damage, cases of pure denial are rare. At the same time, elements of some form of denial are probably present in every struggle to adjust to severe physical disability.

The third form of response to stress occurs when the other two fail; it is *anxiety*. Like denial, anxiety rarely constitutes the whole of a patient's permanent adjustment to his condition, but it is doubtless present to some degree in every case where illness or disability seriously interferes with normal life processes. Because anxiety is commonly regarded as a symptom of neurotic disturbance, a reminder is in order. Anxiety is also a precursor and accompaniment to personality growth. As such, its presence may indicate that a client has given up unproductive defenses and is preparing for movement toward psychological maturity.

The implications for rehabilitation practice are clear. When anxiety is neurotic, that is, when it represents defensive retreat from constructive behavior (as, for example, when it is used to manipulate others for selfish purposes), little can be done within the ordinary rehabilitation setting, unless one is prepared to undertake the complex and difficult task of personality reorganization through intensive psychological counseling or a relatively complete program of systematic behavior modification. However, when anxiety represents either normal distress at facing unknown situations or the residual discomfort that occurs when ineffective modes of behavior are abandoned, support, guidance, and encouragement are obviously called for and can produce important positive personality growth.

The three forms of response to stress are to some extent interchangeable. For example, a client actively engaged in rehabilitation may experience so little success for his effort that (like D. P.) he decides to direct his energies elsewhere. The decision is likely to take place by way of cognitive reappraisal, and the period of transition is likely to be associated with anxiety.

Furthermore, the three types of response often work together in the adjustment process. A person with a disability of sudden onset may experience severe anxiety when previous behavior mechanisms fail to produce essential psychological satisfactions. Anxiety may then serve as a drive to seek new interpretations of the situation. If the new interpretation is hopeful, it supports direct action through cooperative participation in rehabilitation.

Defensive and Growth Functions. All three forms of response to stress (direct action, cognitive reappraisal, and anxiety) are two-sided. On the one hand, each serves the psychological function of defense against threat. On the other, each prepares for and promotes genuine personality growth. In an earlier discussion of the psychological aspects of severe chronic illness, Shontz (1962) pointed out that persons with disabilities face two general types of coping problems. The first type is negative and requires behavior that neutralizes the threat of loss. The second type is positive and requires the discovery of new values to take the place of those no longer available.

Lazarus' theory of response to stress makes a related distinction between *primary and secondary* processes of threat appraisal. Primary threat appraisal is the individual's judgment of the danger that a stress agent will thwart personal motives. The stronger the motives endangered, the greater the threat. Accordingly, the greater the threat, the greater the need for neutralizing behavior. Secondary threat appraisal is a judgment of the probable effectiveness of coping actions in restoring motive gratification or in removing the stress-producing stimulus.

Through primary threat appraisal a client in rehabilitation decides whether he needs assistance; on the basis of primary appraisal, he evaluates the negative character of his disability, the degree of threat it imposes. Through secondary appraisal the client judges whether assistance received is sufficiently beneficial to justify continued cooperation; successful secondary appraisal provides the basis for the discovery of positive possibilities in life.

Transactions in Rehabilitation. Lazarus makes a special point of the fact that, while threat appraisal is a psychological process, its form and intensity are not entirely determined by the personality of the threatened individual. Threat appraisal is a *transaction* to which both organism and environment contribute.

Rehabilitation has long followed the practice of assigning responsibility for failure to patients' personal characteristics (for example, lack of motivation). Sometimes the assignment is correct. However, awareness of the transactive nature of the behavior-determining process reveals that the environmental setting of the agency is often as responsible for rehabilitation failure as are the personality dynamics of the clients. More is said of the influence of the environment on behavior in rehabilitation in a subsequent section of this discussion.

The Course of Events During Coping. Fink (1967) and Shontz (1965) described the process of adjustment to crisis as a series of recurrent approach-avoidance cycles, in which the person successively copes with and retreats from the problems he has to face. The cycles tend to diminish in both frequency and force with time. In the earliest stages of adaptation, emotional involvement is strong, and a complete cycle may take place in a matter of minutes or hours. In later stages, the cyclical process may be so weak and slow as to be unnoticeable.

Fink divided the course of adaptation into four stages: shock, defensive retreat, acknowledgment, and adaptation. Shock is a relatively quickly passing period of intense encounter with the crisis and its dangers (primary threat appraisal). Defensive retreat is a neutralizing response which involves cognitive restructuring so that the situation appears to be less dangerous or threatening than it actually is (denial). Acknowledgment is a prolonged series of re-encounters with the crisis in which each new coping effort produces both an increment of ability to cope with threat and a corresponding tendency to retreat temporarily into the defensive belief that "now everything will go along smoothly." Acknowledgment fades gradually into adaptation, or stabilized adjustment. The over-all level of psychological maturity following adaptation may exceed that which existed when the crisis was first encountered.

Fink argues that adaptation is not complete until all four stages have been passed through. He also stresses that the victim's psychological needs during the first two stages differ from his needs during acknowledgment. While in shock or defensive retreat, the victim is primarily concerned with lower-level needs for physiological integrity, freedom from pain and his safety and security. While in the stage of acknowledgment, his needs become growth-oriented; he seeks love, esteem, and self-actualization (Maslow, 1970).

Crisis and Satisfaction. By definition, the essential difference between the severely disabled and the rest of the population of persons with physical disabilities is that the former group has little or no opportunity to seek growth-oriented satisfactions in independent vocational activity. Although this is a serious loss in a society that equates independence with self-worth, first-person accounts show that persons with severe disabilities do not necessarily lead lives of despair. They report the same general levels of satisfaction and dissatisfaction as do persons with less severely disabling conditions; furthermore, the over-all balance of their reports slightly favors the expression of satisfaction. Also, persons with severe disabilities describe far more interest in achievement than concern over frustration. In this they do not differ from persons with less handicapping physical conditions.

Of course, the types of satisfactions and achievements experienced by persons with severe disabilities are not always identical to those experienced by persons with less severe disabilities—but the differences are less important than might be expected. The lives of persons who have successfully adapted to their conditions reveal that psychological well-being is less dependent upon freedom from the need for care by others than is generally supposed. Persons with severe disabilities often report that they have gained remarkably in their appreciation of themselves and others, of life itself, of religious beliefs, of nature, of small improvements in their somatic state, and of "ordinary" things like rain, birds, and trees. Such sensitivity is not unique to persons with severe disabilities; it is available to anyone willing to take the time to develop it.

This discussion has emphasized the potentiality for severe physical disability to stimulate psychological growth and development. Indeed, a fundamental assumption has been that the human organism in crisis cannot remain static. The rehabilitation worker provides vital services when he is aware of the stage of reaction through which his client is passing, when he provides satisfactions appropriate to the client's needs, and when he guides the client through the process of crisis resolution to a higher level of personal maturity.

MONITORING THE REHABILITATION PROCESS

ASSESSMENT IN INDUSTRY

The process of rehabilitation is sometimes analogized to industrial operations in which raw materials (clients) enter a processing plant (rehabilitation setting) and are discharged, sometime later, in an improved state. People are by no means equivalent to sheets of steel or bales of cotton, but some instructive things can be learned from industrial practices. Perhaps the most important of these is the necessity for continuous monitoring of the effectiveness of procedures.

The unlikely analogy of a phosphate mine illustrates the point quite clearly. Although the machinery used is technically complex, the basic problem of phosphate mining is simple; it is to remove and refine ore-bearing earth. Gigantic shovels extract the raw material from deep pits. This material is transported to the refining plant, where it undergoes a series of sieving operations and chemical processes, each successive stage producing a finer and more concentrated grade of ore. The various grades of ore are dried and shipped to factories for conversion into directly usable products, primarily fertilizers. Aside from the sheer power and magnitude of the operation, the most striking feature of the mining process is the care and expense devoted to continuous assessment of its effectiveness. Samples of raw earth are evaluated before it is dug. During each successive treatment of the ore, samples are taken for chemical analysis. Residual waste is tested daily to see whether useful substances are being discarded. After the processed ore has been dried, it is tested once again. Before it is shipped, samples are taken from every railroad car and given final analyses; these are sent to the receiver of the shipment to guarantee that the material meets specifications. A crew of chemists, working with complex, sophisticated scientific instruments, is occupied full-time performing these analyses. They are expensive, but management realizes that to be uninformed of the effectiveness of their operations and of the quality of their products is far more expensive in the long run.

ASSESSMENT IN REHABILITATION

The temptation to say that we are more concerned about the quality of our fertilizer than about the quality of our people is too great to be resisted. Virtually no continuing program of rehabilitation assesses its clients, its processes, and its results often enough, or uses the assessments it does possess adequately. Judgments that should be made from a firm data base are typically made on the spur of the moment and are as likely to be wrong as to be right. The wasted expense of misapplied professional time is incalculable.

These remarks do not imply that large batteries of tests should be administered helter-skelter to every client in a rehabilitation agency. Assessments must be relevant to purposes. Chemists in a phosphate mine do not test for maple sugar content in the ore. Neither should rehabilitation agencies administer tests that are inappropriate to their purposes.

Many agencies use complex tests of personality. The well-known Minnesota Multiphasic Personality Inventory and such time-consuming individual tests of intelligence as the Wechsler Scales are examples. Most of the sophisticated information that can be derived from these instruments is neither used nor needed. Much briefer instruments, administered by technicians, would probably serve assessment purposes reasonably well, except in cases where special problems present themselves.

Neither do these remarks constitute endorsement of the quality-control analogy from industry. Rehabilitation agencies are not factories, and rehabilitants are not "products." The ore from a phosphate mine can be evaluated by a single, uniform standard: phosphate content. People cannot be evaluated in the same way. A distinction between two types of criteria will help to specify needs of rehabilitation.

Output Criteria. An output criterion leads us to judge a process by evaluating the finished product. An output criterion for industry might be "number of units of production per man-hour of work." An output criterion for rehabilitation might be "number of clients successfully placed on jobs each month."

An output criterion need not deal with large numbers of outcomes. A surgeon who is dissatisfied with the results of an operation applies an outcome criterion to his work, even though he deals with a single case. The important thing about an outcome criterion is that it is directed only at the result of a process and not at the process itself.

Access Criteria. An access criterion leads us to judge a process by evaluating the properties of the process itself. For example, if an engineer knows that mechanical techniques are more effective than chemical means, he can say immediately that a plant that uses mechanical techniques is "better" than one that uses chemical techniques. In rehabilitation, if a counselor knows that there is no market for watch repairmen but a demand for machinists, he can judge that a training program in watch repair is not as feasible as a training program in machine operation, although both may be capable of turning out equally high numbers of well-qualified workers. Physicians realize that medical treatments are not uniformly successful. They also realize that, regardless of success rates (output criterion), a hospital in which they have access to highly versatile treatment facilities is "better" than a hospital in which possibilities for performing complex procedures are minimal.

Consider the situation of a person with severe multiple sclerosis, for whom recovery is highly unlikely. If success were judged by outcome alone, such a patient might be refused physical therapy because it could produce no improvement (such as increased strength or coordination of muscles) and is therefore unjustified. However, if rehabilitation success were determined by criteria of accessibility, the same patient could be admitted to therapy, on the grounds that, even without significant physical improvement, he will gain support for hope by continued participation in a therapeutic program.

A Logical Objection. The objection may be raised that the concept of access criteria is superfluous. In the case just cited, an outcome criterion is implied; the hoped for outcome is psychological instead of physical.

This argument has merit, but it ignores two important points. First, it ignores the fact that, in rehabilitation, goals for different individuals are typically so complex and varied that the attempt to establish outcome criteria for individual clients results in different outcome measures for every patient. Such a procedure would destroy the main advantage of the outcome-oriented approach: the use of a single uniform standard for assessing effectiveness.

Second, the argument ignores the more subtle fact that the philosophical bases of the outcome-oriented and the access-oriented approaches differ. In its extreme form, the outcome approach focuses on ends. It says, in effect: how you produce what we want is irrelevant; all that matters is that it be produced as quickly and as efficiently as possible. The access approach focuses on means. In its extreme form, it says: success or failure is irrelevant; what matters is whether all that could be done was done as well as possible. In the example cited above, the access approach disregards whether muscle strength and coordination (the standard output criteria) improve; it asserts that making physical therapy accessible to physically ill patients is beneficial, regardless of outcome.

EVALUATION OF REHABILITATION PROGRAMS

In actual practice, rehabilitation cannot be realistically assessed by a single type of criterion. A "good" rehabilitation program provides high-quality services to all clients. The problem of evaluation is to discover and apply assessments that permit accurate description of the operation of the program as a whole. Both outcome and access criteria are required.

Outcomes in Rehabilitation. Outcomes should be assessed in three ways. First, evaluations must take into account the uniform goals of the program. For example, if the purpose of an occupational therapy program is to teach activities of daily living, appropriate measures of outcome could include the length of time it takes clients to dress themselves before and after treatment, or more simply the number of clients who do, in fact, routinely perform specified activities for themselves before and after treatment.

Second, outcome evaluations must take into account goals of the program that vary from client to client. They should recognize that improvement in speech therapy is more important for client A than for client B, while elimination of contractures is more important for client B than for client A. The use of individualized goals is complicated by the fact that goals often change during the course of rehabilitation. Once client B's contractures have been relieved, speech therapy and activities of daily living take on an importance they did not previously possess. Ideally, each client's rehabilitation course should be recorded on an individualized chart which identifies specific goals and defines objective criteria for determining when each has been reached. (If necessary, goals may be weighted by priority.) This chart should be kept up to date, not only through routine assessments of the client's level of achievement but also through the addition of new goals, as these become relevant; previous goals or priorities should be revised as new insights are gained into the client's needs; long-range follow-up should be routine. The client himself must participate as fully as possible in establishing these goals.

Third, outcome evaluation must take into account clients' assessments of over-all effectiveness of operation. Periodic surveys of client attitudes and opinions, during and after rehabilitation, provide valuable information and suggestions about how program operations may be improved or made more relevant to clients' needs.

Access to Rehabilitation Facilities. Effectiveness of access must be assessed both quantitatively and qualitatively. Quantitatively, access is assessed by counting the number of hours of client and staff time devoted to various rehabilitation activities.

The value of a program does not bear a simple positive relationship to the number of patient-treatment hours it provides. A program that makes excessive demands on its staff and facilities is no better than one that allows professional staff to sit around with nothing to do. Each setting has an optimal capacity, and effectiveness is best evaluated by the degree to which operations are kept within specified limits of variation from the optimum.

Qualitatively, a program must be judged according to the suitability of its staff and facilities for performing services the agency was designed to provide and meeting the needs of the clients it serves. These two aspects of the problem are not necessarily correlated. A hospital may be well equipped to deal with physical problems but inept at handling psychosocial needs. If rehabilitation is to meet its obligations to the whole client it must evaluate itself not only in terms of its capacity to achieve goals defined by specialized professional personnel but also in terms of its ability to provide facilities and services valued by the clients themselves.

In the final analysis, an evaluation of the effectiveness of a rehabilitation program can never be expressed numerically. Relevant quantitative data are useful and should, by all means, be collected. But assessment of the value of a rehabilitation program is a decision for which human beings ultimately bear responsibility. Means, standard deviations, ratios, and correlation coefficients summarize and make explicit the facts upon which judgments are based, but here their utility ceases. Only a qualified person, whose judgment must be trusted, can decide what the figures mean.

EFFECTS OF THE ENVIRONMENT

From an administrative point of view, a rehabilitation agency is organized to provide specific types of services to specific types of people. From an economic standpoint, the organization functions best when services are delivered uniformly and with maximum efficiency to all who require them.

The standard of *uniformity* is intended to assure that no clients are given special treatment; all are treated equitably. The standard of *effi-*

ciency is intended to assure that agency funds are spent wisely and for intended purposes. Unfortunately, in actual practice, these admirable intentions are often distorted. In the face of overwhelming pressure to provide more services to more clients than an agency is capable of handling, the demand for uniformity becomes an implement for authoritarian control; client individuality is ignored, and the agency places pressure on inmates to conform and become behaviorally passive. In the face of budgetary inadequacies and cutbacks, efficiency comes to mean simple cheapness. "Expensive frills," such as research, assessment programs, group therapy, modern diagnostic or therapeutic equipment, adequately trained staff, and opportunities for client self-determination, are eliminated. The agency becomes a place that provides only the bare necessities. It sometimes defends its position by asserting that "if we make life too comfortable for clients, they will never want to leave."

A SOCIOLOGICAL STUDY

The worst features of rehabilitation for the severely chronically ill are documented by Roth and Eddy (1967) in *Rehabilitation for the Unwanted,* a study of rehabilitation in a hospital for chronic illness. Significantly, the fictitious name given to this institution is Farewell Hospital, a name that is probably appropriate to a large proportion of agencies for the severely disabled.

At Farewell Hospital, selection for rehabilitation typically takes place at a weekly line-up, where a physician evaluates candidates (who usually do not realize that they are candidates) by skimming over medical records and examining patients briefly. A strong bias exists in favor of younger patients with "appropriate" disabilities, such as hemiplegia, amputation, spinal cord injury, multiple sclerosis, arthritis, muscular dystrophy, and improperly healed fractures. Patients rarely take part in selection decisions; many do not know about rehabilitation and are not aware that a decision is being made about them.

Direct patient care is typically the responsibility of nonprofessional "caretaker" personnel, who are poorly paid, receive little recognition for their work, have no important decision-making powers, and have poor or virtually nonexistent relations with specialized professionals. Ward personnel do not want "helpless" patients and try to have them transferred elsewhere.

Administrative requirements of the institution take precedence over personal preferences of the inmates. Privacy is impossible; the patient is under constant surveillance, and anything he does (as well as anything he has done in the past) may be used against him. His needs are defined by others; he keeps few personal possessions; he exerts no control over planning his own treatment or discharge, when the time comes. The pace of life is so slow that it makes his time and effort seem worthless.

Roth and Eddy also stress the point that success in rehabilitation is transactionally determined (cf. preceding discussions of stress and crisis). It is not attributable to either patient or environment, but is the product of the relationship between patients' personal characteristics and the responses they elicit from their environment. Whether a given personality trait leads to success or failure depends upon whether it causes the staff to do things that improve or diminish the patient's chances of receiving the treatments and services he needs.

To be successful, an inmate need not be pleasant. A demanding and unpleasant patient may be disliked, but his chances are good if he is persistent and demands the right things. At the same time, the demanding inmate runs the risk of having his transaction with the environment go wrong. He may be labeled "crazy"—in which case his aggressive traits may lead to rejection on psychiatric grounds and to ultimate failure.

WHAT CAN BE DONE?

Few rehabilitation agencies have the staff and facilities to undertake massive programs for altering the basic personality traits of their inmates. Even if they did, no reputable psychologist could maintain that such programs would have a high probability of success. Nevertheless, adjustments of environmental characteristics do lie within the realm of possibility, and improvement of rehabilitation settings can greatly increase their efficacy as devices for improving client welfare.

Most obvious is the need for agencies serving the severely chronically ill to take the real needs of clients more seriously. For a large proportion of such patients, the most important contributions rehabilitation can make are to reduce physical discomfort and to provide meaningful (or, at least, enjoyable) activities for taking up time.

The typical emphasis of modern rehabilitation on the positive value of economic activity, medical improvement, steadily increasing independence, and quick discharge is congenial to the view that clients in rehabilitation should not be too comfortable or settings too pleasant. This doctrine assumes that progress is achieved through use of the carrot (discharge, which is desirable) and the stick (continued treatment, which is painful and unpleasant), and that, left to his own devices, the human being (or, at least, the rehabilitation client) prefers inactivity to action. With regard to the first assumption, it is doubtful that discharge is in fact desirable to many severely chronically ill patients. Making such a patient miserable in the rehabilitation institution may induce him to seek escape from it at all cost, but it will not transform the prospect of life in a nursing home into a plan about which he will possess any positive enthusiasm.

As for the second assumption, there is no evidence that indolence is a fundamental trait of the normal human organism. Indeed, all data indicate that enforced inactivity is psychologically and physiologically intolerable. The so-called unmotivated client is rarely inactive, except when in a state of depression, schizoid withdrawal, physical paralysis, or coma. The most bothersome of the presumedly unmotivated clients are not those who are forced by their medical conditions to be helpless but those who are physically capable of assuming responsibility for themselves yet who seem to choose not to do so, in defiance of medical opinion and administrative doctrine. Of course, such persons are motivated; their motives are merely deviant. They choose safety and security to the risk and anxiety of independence. The fact that some persons make this choice is annoying. It is also inconsiderate, since use of limited facilities to care for these individuals prevents the use of these facilities for others in more desperate need. But it by no means proves, nor does it even remotely suggest, that human beings are basically lazy.

Such careful observers of human behavior as Goldstein (1939, 1940, 1942), Rogers (1942, 1951, 1961), and Maslow (1970) have asserted that the human organism is fundamentally growth-oriented and self-actualizing. Given proper conditions, the human being is naturally motivated toward fullest possible development of his potentialities. When such development does not occur, it is not due to inherent weakness of the organism but because the environment fails to provide conditions essential for growth. In actual practice, rehabilitation workers can do a great deal to alter faulty conditions existing in rehabilitation settings. However, a philosophy that teaches the desirability of discomfort does not achieve that end.

One solution to the problem of institutionalization is to arouse clients' interests in activities that can be most successfully engaged in outside the agency setting. To achieve this, the agency must provide interest-stimulating activities; it must activate and care for its clients' growth needs. These are precisely the needs many agencies currently regard as dangerous because of the mistaken fear that satisfied clients will resist discharge.

Assume that a patient with a severe disability is dependent, likes the hospital setting, and does not wish to leave. When economics dictate that he be transferred to a less expensive place where care is inadequate, and where the environment is depressing or hostile, is there any justification for describing this patient's resistance as "hospitalitis" or for believing that the source of the problem lies within him? A more realistic and reasonable course of action would be to agree with him that he is right in feeling as he does and to work toward improving the types of institutions to which such unwanted people are typically sent.

There are those within society for whom economic independence is not feasible. The rehabilitation movement has largely ignored these individuals because they are poor investments, burdens on the economy. It will be a sign of maturity when we regard improvement of the human condition of those who can never be expected to pay their own way as a worthy enterprise.

REFERENCES

Armatas, J. P., J. L. Hewitt, L. J. Lohrenz, and H. D. Remple. 1970. Rehabilitation of the chronically institutionalized. Wadsworth, Kans., Wadsworth Veterans Administration Center.

Dollard, J. and O. H. Mowrer. January, 1947. A method of measuring tension in written documents. Journal of Abnormal and Social Psychology 42:3–32.

Fink, S. L. 1967. Crisis and motivation: A theoretical model. Archives of Physical Medicine and Rehabilitation 48: 592–97.

Goldstein, K. 1939. The organism: A holistic approach to biology derived from pathological data in men. New York, American Book.

——1940. Human nature in the light of psychopathology. Cambridge, Harvard University Press.

——1942. After-effects of brain injuries in war. New York, Grune and Stratton.

Henrich, E. and L. Kriegel, eds. 1961. Experiments in survival. New York, Association for Crippled Children.

Lazarus, R. S. 1966. Psychological stress and the coping process. New York, McGraw-Hill.

Maslow, A. H. 1970. Motivation and personality. 2d ed. New York, Harper & Row.

Rogers, C. R. 1942. Counseling and psychotherapy. Boston, Houghton Mifflin.

——1951. Client-centered therapy: Its current practice, implications and theory. Boston, Houghton Mifflin.

——1961. On becoming a person: A therapist's view of psychotherapy. Boston, Houghton Mifflin.

Roth, J. A. and E. M. Eddy. 1967. Rehabilitation for the unwanted. New York, Atherton.

Shontz, F. C. 1962. Severe chronic illness, in J. F. Garrett and E. S. Levine, eds., Psychological practices with the physically disabled. New York, Columbia University Press, pp. 410–45.

——May, 1965. Reactions to crisis. Volta Review 67:364–370.

Tiffany, D. W., J. R. Cowan, and F. C. Shontz. 1969. Work inhibition and rehabilitation. Part II: Psychosocial correlates of work inhibition. Part III: Experimental treatment of self-direction in work-inhibited clients. Kansas City, Mo., Institute for Community Studies.

Tiffany, D. W., J. R. Cowan, and P. M. Tiffany. 1970. The unemployed. Englewood Cliffs, N.J., Prentice-Hall.

Usdane, W. A. 1970. Opening remarks, Conference on Psychology and Rehabilitation, Asilomar, California, October 26–28.

Wright, B. A. 1960. Physical disability—a psychological approach. New York, Harper & Row.

——June, 1968. The question stands: Should a person be realistic? Rehabilitation Counseling Bulletin 11:291–96.

Wright, B. A. and F. C. Shontz. November, 1968. Process and tasks in hoping. Rehabilitation Literature 29:322–31.

J. HERBERT DIETZ, JR.

CANCER: MEDICAL FACTORS*

CANCER CAN BE THOUGHT OF as a variety of nearly two hundred different diseases, but with one general characteristic: that of the multiplication of a disorganized and diseased group of cells within the body which grow and spread either locally or by transportation to other areas of the body. Cancer is a disease which can arise in any tissue of the body, although some tissues are more prone to its development than others. No type of body tissue is spared and no age group is totally exempted from the development of cancer, but the risk is greater by or after middle age. (Shimkin, 1964).

NATURE OF THE DISEASE

Cancer cells undergo changes in their size and shape and in the pattern of their nucleus. The changes apparently occur over a period of many years, being a gradual and continuous process rather than one which is sudden. In many forms of tumor, the transformation begins in a single area, but in others it may begin in multiple areas simultaneously.

Once the changes have occurred, the small initial group of cells begins to invade its surrounding area. Abnormal multiplication of the in-

J. HERBERT DIETZ, JR., M.D., F.A.C.S., is Associate Professor of Rehabilitation Medicine, Institute of Rehabilitation Medicine, New York University, and Consultant in Rehabilitation, Department of Surgery, Memorial Hospital for Cancer and Allied Diseases, New York, N.Y.
    * A glossary of medical terms is given on pp. 171–74.

dividual tissue cells beyond the limits followed by normal cells results in an abnormal growth, often with disorderly cellular structure and tissue architecture. This process can destroy areas of normal tissue which are neighbor to the cancerous process. Multiplication of the cancer cells will proceed indefinitely unless treatment retards this process or stops it.

Cancer, by growth, can not only invade normal tissue, but it can also spread to other areas in the body by both lymphatic and blood channels.

The spread of cancer from a localized origin is by several different routes:

1) The tumor may spread by direct extension into neighboring tissues.

2) It may advance along channels of lymphatic drainage.

3) It may be carried in the blood stream as a free floating cell and be stopped in the capillary system of any organ of the body. This happens most frequently in the lungs, bones, and the liver. The cancer cell has a particular characteristic in that it can live and reproduce itself in an area of the body other than its site of origin.

4) It may spread by diffusion into a body cavity after direct invasion. This spread is found in the peritoneal or pleural cavities.

The spread to a new site, whether by lymphatic channels, by veins, or by diffusion in body cavities, is called a metastasis. Such secondary growths tend to duplicate the original growth, and in their new location they may develop without check in similar fashion to the original tumor.

Different types of cancer tend to undergo different modes of spread and location of their metastasis. For example, cancer of the bone, such as an osteogenic sarcoma, may first appear in the lungs as a metastatic deposit, while a prostate cancer usually first metastasizes to bone.

CLASSIFICATION

Cancer is usually classified in three main categories: carcinoma, which develops from epithelial tissue; sarcoma, which arises in connective tissue; and lymphoma and leukemia, which develop in lymphatic and blood-forming tissues respectively. This latter group of malignant diseases usually first appears in already generalized form. However there are unicentric forms of both lymphosarcoma and Hodgkin's Disease.

Occasionally separate cancers arise in several different organs, or in separate sites in the same organ, at the same time, which suggests that there may be a common cause. (American Cancer Society, 1970).

INCIDENCE AND DISTRIBUTION

As has been said previously, there are approximately two hundred different forms of cancer, but there is much greater incidence in some sites of origin than in others. The principal current primary sites of cancer in women are in the breast (23 per cent), intestines (13 per cent), uterus (13 per cent), skin (13 per cent), ovary (4.5 per cent), lung (4 per cent), and the lymphomas (3.5 per cent), in that order. In men the order of incidence is in the skin (23 per cent), the lung (18 per cent), the intestines (10.9 per cent), the prostate (10.6 per cent), urinary bladder (4.5 per cent), and the lymphomas (4 per cent). For the adult American the over-all most frequent site of internal cancer is colon and rectum. Almost half of the cancers of childhood are a form of leukemia.

Cancer is second only to heart disease as a cause of death in the United States. There has been a general increase in the incidence of cancer, which is contributed to by several factors including population growth, longer life expectancy, in general as a result of control of other diseases, better methods of diagnosis and treatment of first cancers, and a better-informed public which seeks earlier medical care. The present annual incidence of new cancer in the United States is 635,000. Adding the current new cases of cancer to those still being treated from previous calendar years, it can be estimated that about 975,000 Americans will be under treatment for cancer during a given year. More than 52 million Americans now living will have cancer, and at present four out of every ten new cases will be cured.

The ecology of cancer is such that there is a difference in the incidence of cancer in various parts of the world from the standpoint of sites of origin in the body. In Africa, Asia, and Indonesia primary liver cancer is common, but it is rare in other areas of the world. Iceland, Scandinavia, and Japan show a higher rate of cancer of the stomach than the United States, while breast cancer in the United States and western Europe is more frequent than it is in Japan. Areas of the world where cigarette smoking is practiced widely show a higher incidence of cancer of the lungs than where cigarette smoking is not common habit. (Pack and Ariel, 1968; Healey, 1970).

CAUSE OR PREDISPOSITION

Research over the years has accumulated a great deal of data covering the different varieties of cancer, factors which promote or decrease the ability of cancer to reproduce and invade, and also some of the predisposing factors and internal and external influences which favor cancer development. Hereditary elements, immunity factors, internal and external effects of irritants and chemicals, cellular reaction and transformation, viral agent effects—all are felt to have a bearing on development of the changes called cancer.

Predisposing causes of cancer include conditions which produce long-standing irritation. The hot pipestem of a pipe smoker can lead to cancer of the lip. Exposure to sunlight in farmers and sailors results in heightened frequency of cancer of the skin and also the lower lip. A habit of betel-nut chewing in large population areas of the world couples with a high incidence of cancer of the cheek. Friction from a belt or clothing may cause a malignant melanoma to arise in a pigmented mole. Specific chemical agents have been found to be associated with the development of cancer, and in this area the most important finding is that of the association of cigarette smoking with cancer of both the lung and larynx. Aniline dyes can cause cancer of the urinary bladder in workers handling the dyes. Radium paints have caused cancer of the bone in workers handling these paints to paint numerals on clock dials.

There are many cancers which develop without any yet-known external predisposing conditions or factors. In these instances it may be considered that the factors which ultimately cause the change into cancer are forces which are operative within the body, or in other words endogenous to the individual. An example would be hormones. Some cancers, such as cancer of the breast and prostate, are considered to be hormone dependent, and can often be controlled by changing the patient's hormone balance. This is a form of chemotherapy. There is also a group of benign conditions or lesions which can undergo change into a cancer. These include polyps in the colon and rectum, which may become adenocarcinoma; cystadenoma of the ovary, which may become a cystadenocarcinoma; von Recklinghausen's disease, which may change from a neurofibromatosis to malignant schwannoma; senile keratosis, which may become a skin carcinoma; and leukoplakia of the mucous membranes of the mouth, which may become squamous carcinoma. The benign conditions are frequently termed precancerous, and as such they are not considered trivial, but are treated with intent to remove or prevent the possibility of malignant change. (Mozden, 1965; American Cancer Society, 1970).

DIAGNOSIS OF CANCER

The diagnosis of the presence of cancer in the patient with symptoms depends first on the patient's history and then on a careful physical examination with attention to all accessible regions of the body and finally on the performance of special diagnostic procedures. These special procedures include biopsy, which means the surgical excision of an entire small neoplasm, or a portion of a larger tumor, or the removal by aspiration through a large bore needle of a core of tissue. Microscopic examination of the specimen then allows identification of presence or type of cancer. This microscopic examination permits the pathologist to evaluate and study the characteristics and the arrangements of the tissue cells in comparison to the regional normal tissue. From this study he can make a diagnosis of the type and the grade of malignancy of the cancer being investigated. (Committee on Guidelines for Cancer Care, 1970).

Cells which have broken away from their tumor area in exfoliation and have become dispersed in the various body secretions can also be studied in a smear preparation. This is a technique which was developed by Dr. George Papanicolaou and is termed a "Pap smear." Characteristic changes in the cells recognized by the pathologist will determine his opinion as to the possible presence of malignancy in these exfoliated cells. When he is suspicious of cancer, then a surgical biopsy is also done in order to confirm the diagnosis as correct.

X-ray examinations of the patient by check of the lungs and gastrointestinal tract, bones, and kidney-bladder system are methods of detection of the presence of cancer as shown by changes in the x-ray patterns and shadows. Metastatic disease in the lungs and the bones can also be detected by this method, and scans made of uptake of radioactive material will show the presence of tumor or metastases in the thyroid, liver, bones, or brain.

The background of the patient's general health also must be considered when making a cancer diagnosis, in the effort to provide comprehensive care for the patient. Therefore, additional laboratory examinations are made, including blood sugar and blood urea nitrogen as well as urinalysis and hemogram. Special tests of liver, lung, kidney, and heart function are made according to indications from the history and examination findings. A test for blood in both the urine and stool will give a lead as to the possible presence of a malignancy in the related systems. If x-rays show a questionable stomach lesion, the absence of free acid in the stomach will suggest the possibility of a cancer rather than a benign ulcer, as cancer of the stomach is more frequently associated with the absence of free hydrocloric acid and benign ulcer with a high free acid. Special blood tests are now being studied which will show serological indications of the possibility of cancer, particularly in the gastrointestinal tract.

TREATMENT

Treatment of cancer follows three basic directions: surgery; radiation therapy; and chemotherapy. These may be used alone or in combination, depending upon the type and status of the tumor. Increasing knowledge is being developed as to which combinations are most effective in particular circumstances. All methods have been curative of specific types of cancer both alone and in combination, and to date only these methods have resulted in valid cases of cancer cure. (Pack and Ariel, 1968).

In the surgical approach to the treatment of cancer, excision of the primary tumor mass is performed, including a wide margin of adjacent normal tissue surrounding the tumor and including the regional lymph nodes. This method is a typical one for breast cancer, when a radical mastectomy is performed, for cancer of the colon and rectum treated by abdominal perineal resection, and for the radical neck dissections performed for cancer of the head and neck. Cancer in these areas has a known tendency to metastasize to regional nodes. Under these circumstances, the cure rate is apparently better than when only local excision is performed without removal of the regional lymph nodes.

If a cancer is localized in a spot which is both solitary and can be removed by appropriate surgery, this type of cancer can be considered curable. If, on the other hand, the cancer has metastasized to the regional lymph nodes, this reduces the chances of cure and increases the radical nature of the surgery which has to be done, and which has to encompass not only the area of the lesion but also all of the lymph nodes draining the site of that cancer's origin. When this situation is encountered, x-ray treatment is often combined with surgery to attempt to insure for the patient control of the disease process. (Pack and Ariel, 1968).

When cancers grow in size, additional problems may be created. There may be interference by pressure with the function of another organ. An example of this would be partial obstruction of the bowel, preventing normal passage of bowel content, with alternating constipation and diarrhea and eventual complete obstruction. A tumor in the brain can obstruct the normal drainage of cerebrospinal fluid, with the resulting increased pressure within the skull causing headache, nausea, and projectile vomiting. Cancer of a vocal cord will interfere with its function and cause hoarseness as a symptom. Cancer which spreads to a bone may erode the supporting structure of the bone and result in a fracture of the bone. This is termed a pathological fracture to differentiate it from a fracture resulting solely from injury. Pressure of a growth upon a nerve or nerve root may create pain or increasing weakness of the muscles supplied by the nerve. Treatment of these problems may be by surgery for removal or bypass, or by radiation therapy or chemotherapy to shrink the tumor and reduce the pressure or obstruction (Dietz, 1969; 1971).

At times, the surgery may require sacrifice of important structures in order to make a cure possible. These operative procedures include the performance of colostomies, alteration of facial structures, and the various amputations. There is an increase in the patient's ultimate disability and particular efforts are required toward his rehabilitation in the effort to improve the quality of his survival. The rehabilitation includes the performance of such plastic and reconstructive surgery as will increase the cosmetic effectiveness of the end result and the provision of such orthotic or prosthetic devices as will increase the functional end results. (Synderman, 1970). Current improvements in understanding of human physiology and in improved modalities of therapy have increased the rate of cure and permitted the performance of operative procedures previously not considered feasible.

In the event of distant metastases being found, such as by bone cancer to lung, either cure can be effected or life remarkably prolonged by the procedure of surgical resection of the pulmonary metastases. This is due to the fact that such may be the only area to which metastasis has occurred, and is solitary in that sense. Similarly, metastatic disease in the liver can be removed by resection or lobectomy, and the patient's life appreciably prolonged in a state of appropriate disease control.

Combination of treatment by giving x-ray therapy before surgery may render a tumor more suited for appropriate removal and may assist in the control of spread. Radiation therapy may also be given postoperatively to control any residual tumor cells. Radioactive materials may also be implanted during surgery into inoperable tumors to control their growth and spread for at least temporary periods. (Ariel, 1968; Raventos, 1968).

Drugs used as chemotherapeutic agents may also be used before, during, or after a surgical procedure to assist in the destruction of the cancer cell (Karnofsky, 1968).

When the patient has developed prolonged and intractible pain as a result of the effects of the incurable cancer, he may be subjected to measures of pain control which involve neurosurgery. These include division of a nerve supplying the area which is painful, division of nerve roots at the spinal cord level for the same reason, and division of the pain-carrying nerve tract in the spinal cord. This is called a chordotomy, which may be done with or without the exposure of the spinal cord by surgical procedure. An occasional patient may need to be subjected to brain surgery in the form of a thalamotomy or lobotomy to alter perception and recognition of pain.

Radiation therapy as a method of cancer treatment is based on the fact that the cancer cell is more sensitive to x-rays than is the cell of normal tissue. X-ray machines, radio-isotopes, and radium, (infrequently at present) are the sources of radiation therapy used for patient treatment. Treatment may be given by use of an electric or radioactive element beam source, from the standpoint of the source being entirely outside the body and directed at the patient. This form of irradiation can be focused for a maximum effect at a given tissue level by the use of modern equipment with high-voltage sources. Treatment may also be given internally from the standpoint of placement of the sources of radiation within a body cavity, and implants of radioactive material can be placed within tumor tissue. Radioactive isotopes, which are radioactive chemicals prepared in the presence of the atomic reactor, can be injected or instilled into body cavities in fluid form to control cancer in these regions and to reduce the production of fluid by the lining membranes. Radioactive drugs given intravenously course through the body and are selectively picked up by the malignant tissue causing the effect of the radiation to be maximal in the tumor area. These materials can also be placed in containers such as gold seeds and implanted in tumors otherwise not removable by surgery. Some forms, such as radioactive iodine and phosphorus, can be given by mouth (Ariel, 1968; American Cancer Society, Inc., 1970).

Radioactive isotopes used for treatment have a short half-life, and their duration of effect is, therefore, limited. The half-life of each is known. That of radioactive gold, for example, is approximately three days. At the end of that period the radioactive gold is half as active as it was at the beginning of the treatment, at the end of six days it is one-fourth as active, and so on, progressively.

Radiation therapy, when it is applied externally, is given by several different types of machine. They are called "bombs" if they contain such radioactive material as the radioisotope Cobalt 60, the gamma rays from which have a penetrating power in tissue roughly comparable to the beam from a three-million-volt x-ray machine. Similar machines can be built using other radionuclides such as Cesium or Iridium. There are also the betatrons and linear accelerators and other super-voltage machines which produce a focusable beam of radiation. These high-voltage machines, in comparison to the old low-voltage units, tend to spare the patient's skin from the effects of the radiation and concentrate on the deeper tissues. Their effectiveness is much greater for deep-seated tumors than were the older type of low-voltage units.

Specific drugs can be used to both destroy cancer cells and suppress their capacity for reproduction, while sparing the normal tissue. These drugs include hormones, steriod compounds and ACTH, antimetabolites, polyfunctional alkylating agents, and the previously described radioactive isotopes. There are also miscellaneous drugs which are useful in their direct effects on the cancer cell. All agents are often used in combination, as well as with other treatment approaches. Depending upon their nature, these drugs produce their effects by reacting with genetically important material within the nucleus of the cell to produce changes in the mutation characteristics of the cell and death of the cell. They also interfere with metabolic pathways which the cells use in production of various substances essential to their cellular health.

The chemotherapeutic agents have most marked side effects on those cells of the normal tissues of the body which are undergoing rapid multiplication or the production of certain substances. Accordingly, they affect the cells of the lining of the gastrointestinal tract, creating nausea and vomiting. Loss of hair is frequent. The cells of the bone marrow, which are actively reproducing in order to form new blood component units, are affected and the patient will develop anemia and low white cell counts. Adequate white cells are necessary to protect the patient against infection. Careful monitoring of these side effects is necessary in order to determine the dosage level at which the drug should be continued, or whether it should be stopped, at least temporarily, for the patient to regain a satisfactory ongoing status. (Karnofsky, 1968).

An occasional approach in the treatment of cancer by drugs is that of localized perfusion of tumor tissue areas by injection of a chemotherapeutic agent directly into blood vessels supplying the tumor region. The remainder of the body is clamped off from approach by the drugs during the treatment. This is done to direct a higher concentration of drug to tumor tissue with less effect upon the body in general and better control, it is hoped, of the cancer area.

Cancer which involves the lining of the chest or the abdomen frequently produces excessive fluid secretion which results in fluid accumulating in the chest or the abdomen. Compression of lungs or abdominal órgans causes interference with normal function. Relief is necessary by the procedure of tapping to remove the fluid from within whichever cavity it may be found and by the instillation of radioactive isotopes, as described above. In the chest it is occasionally necessary to surgically remove the pleura by the procedure of a pleurectomy in order to remove the malignant tissue which secretes the fluid and to eliminate the space in which fluid can accumulate by promoting adhesion of lung to chest wall.

Pain, when it develops, is a result of obstruction by the tumor of a normal organ passage, of direct pressure by a tumor on a nerve pathway, or the presence of infection. Pain does not arise because of tumor presence only.

The management of pain is accomplished by different methods. Search for infection must be made. Control of infection will usually relieve related pain. For the initial relief of pain symptoms use of medications is attempted. Such medication is kept as uncomplicated and as low in narcotic content as possible. Addiction is something to be avoided, in view of the fact that in an unfortunately short time narcotics can cause addiction and at the same time their effect upon pain control is reduced. The patient then becomes dependent upon the drug and still suffers pain. If moderate amounts of drugs cannot control the pain, radiation therapy may be tried for radiosensitive tumors in an attempt to shrink the tumor and relieve pressure or obstruction. Hormone therapy may be attempted, if the tumor may be hormone dependent. Chemotherapy also may be tried to effect control of the tumor, reducing both size and pressure. Surgery is frequently needed to either remove or bypass the area of obstruction or relieve pressure-caused pain. Occasionally, interruption of nerve pathways for pain transmission is necessary. As previously stated, the peripheral nerve itself may be blocked or sectioned. A nerve root section may be performed, or a chordotomy may be done by a percutaneous or by an open surgical approach. Sensory nerve sectioning has been found to be most useful in head and neck areas but less useful elsewhere. Chordotomy and nerve block are of relatively temporary effect and are used primarily in patients with advanced cancer. Chordotomy usefulness is greatest in pain which originates at or below the chest level.

The patient with advanced cancer may develop a state of malnutrition resulting from poor caloric and protein intake. He will need supplemental feeding both orally and by vein, and occasionally by tube feeding when there is difficulty in swallowing.

Increased efforts are currently being directed toward identification of the problems and the approaches for a concerted effort to control cancer. Determination of specific causes and possible immunity factors and the prevention of body changes will lead to either control or prevention of the majority of cancers. Principal research objectives at the present time are: to reduce the effectiveness of external agents which may increase the probability of cancer development in existing individuals and future populations; to modify individuals, by vaccination, for example, which would decrease the likelihood of their developing cancer; to prevent the conversion of the normal cell to one capable of forming a cancer by blocking or interfering with steps involved with the conversion of the cells capable of forming a cancer; to prevent tumor establishment in those cells already capable of forming cancer, such as cells of precancerous tissue, as previously described; to achieve accurate assessment of the presence and the extent and the probable cause of cancer risks in both population groups and individuals as an aid in prevention, in cure, and in prognosis; to cure as many patients as possible and maintain maximum control of disease continuing in patients who are not cured; and lastly, to restore patients with residual deficits as consequence to their disease or treatment to as nearly a normal functioning state as possible (National Cancer Plan, 1972).

REHABILITATION

Current statistics reveal that each year more than 600,000 new cases of cancer will develop in the United States. Over 250,000 of these patients will be cured of and will have survived their first bout with cancer. The rest will eventually develop recurrent or metastatic cancer and will require additional treatment. Each of these patients will have possibly undergone radical treatment, as previously stated, either in the form of surgery, chemotherapy, radiation therapy, or a combination of these approaches. The radical nature of the treatment often leaves extensive physical deficits to which both the patient and his family must make adjustment. The time of survival for the patient who has not been cured by his initial treatment is lengthening because of increase in the control of disease. Both cured and controlled patients have frequent needs for rehabilitation care in order to improve the quality of their survival (Dietz, 1969).

The disabilities presented by the cancer patient represent a general category of all disabilities and do not differ essentially from those arising from other diagnostic backgrounds. There are, in addition, disabilities particularly related to the effects of cancer or its treatment, such as neuropathies secondary to the remote effects of cancer on the nervous system, the secondary effects of treatment agents used, and such focal problems as pathological fractures. Older cancer patients in particular may also be victims of additional forms of chronic disabilities, the result of other diseases prevalent in this age group, and adding to the need for care. (Mozden, 1965). Provision of appropriate rehabilitation care is a challenge which is in proportion to the extent and variety of the disabilities encountered. Each patient must be taught by the members of the treatment team how to circumvent and also to compensate as much as possible for whatever disability occurs.

The first step in the program of rehabilitation care is prompt recognition by the treating physician of the presence of existing disability and, ideally, the recognition of potential disability, such as may follow scheduled treatment. Initial examination and evaluation of the patient and the provision of the first orders for care can be made at the patient's bedside, without waiting for him to reach a status of readiness for being removed to a specialized rehabilitation service area. (Dietz, 1969).

The disability encountered may be either acute or chronic. Acute disability is found in the immediate postoperative period, when there may be enforced immobilization, pain, fear, and confusion. Chronic disability is found when there is long-standing handicap. Prompt attention to the patient in the form of preventive as well as definitive rehabilitation therapy can reduce both the degree of disability and the time needed for recovery. For surgical cases, preoperative as well as postoperative training and counsel are of benefit. Dependent upon each patient's needs and findings, there should be an individually prescribed care program made for physical and occupational therapy, training in the activities of daily living, psychosocial evaluation and counseling, as well as the supply of such orthotic or prosthetic devices as may be required.

Realistic goals should be considered in programming rehabilitation of the cancer patient. There is an undeniable element of unpredictability. However, in instances where life expectancy is limited, efforts toward keeping the patient functioning at maximal potential may produce results that transcend any economic return. The housewife, who can be trained to carry on her role as mother and homemaker for any appropriate time, is a worthwhile candidate for rehabilitation effort.

In the past, eligibility rulings for rehabilitation programs excluded many patients with residual disease, overlooking the special human needs of patients with an uncertain future.

Early in the course of examination and care a goal for the patient should be established. Suggested are the following categories: "restorative," if the patient can be expected to be without remarkable residual handicap; "supportive," if ongoing disease or handicap must persist, but the disability can be lessened; and "palliative," if there is increasing disability to be expected and the patient has progressed to an advanced stage of disease. Regardless of the classification of the type of disability or the goal, early availability of care is important. Rehabilitation should not be delayed until completion of definitive treatment, but should start with onset or recognition of disability.

Rehabilitation should be concerned not only with the physical adjustment to the loss of an organ, but also with changes in the social and vocational status of the patient after he has been discharged from the hospital, and with the emotional, psychological, social, familial, and personal aspects of life after treatment. This program should be the responsibility of every member of the medical team which takes care of the patient, including his personal physician and other members of the medical staff and the hospital personnel. Help should be obtained from the various community organizations which are available for assistance.

Rehabilitation benefits should be made available to the widest possible population of cancer patients. In the past, such efforts were usually started only after completion of all other treatment. They were concentrated on those patients in which the disease or handicap had become stabilized and where it could be anticipated with security that the financial investment would be justified by future productivity. Unfortunately, cancer patients do not fall into this mold until much valuable time has been lost waiting to rule out possible recurrence of disease.

The extent of rehabilitation provided to a cancer patient depends on the needs of the individual patient. Some patients can accept their diagnosis and status more readily than others. Many (perhaps the majority) feel that they have been threatened by the diagnosis, badly maimed by surgery, or have lost vital structure function from which they can never recover. They may feel that they are unable to resume a normal existence in a job, at home, or in the community. Rehabilitation should be planned to involve the patient from a point prior to his surgery throughout his stay in the hospital and continuing after his discharge to the point where he can live with his family and in his community with the maximum degree of efficiency (Dietz, 1969; 1971).

The psychological problems of the patient are sometimes as devastating as the physical consequences of the disease. Therefore, attention should be paid to the psychological as well as the physical and vocational rehabilitation needs of each patient. The severe psychological effects of the diagnosis of cancer and the presence of the patient with cancer in the family unit also require consideration and extensive assistance in order to provide the patient with the appropriate amount of familial background support which he desperately needs throughout the course of illness. Reaction to a diagnosis of cancer or to the shock of a sudden disability can take the form of fear and anxiety, withdrawal, depression, or emotional breakdown. There is disruption of social and vocational setup as a result of the presence of disease. The effect upon the family unit of the cancer diagnosis and the illness of the family member all create complex and varied reactions, many of which are never to the patient's advantage (American Cancer Society, Inc., 1970; Healey, 1970).

The psychologist and the vocational councelor can provide valuable assistance to the patient with emotional upset or who needs to make plans for his occupational future. These members of the rehabilitation team should be called for guidance and instruction whenever indicated. The social service worker can provide detailed inquiry into the family structure and can develop intimate knowledge of the living and possible working conditions to be faced by the patient after discharge from the hospital.

Job placement for the disabled patient with a cancer diagnosis is often difficult. Positive understanding is needed by the employer to modify problems of acceptance of the employee's cancer diagnosis. Planning helps circumvent limited ability for the patient in the use of public transportation and aids in the facing of competition in the labor market and the possible need for specialized job placement within the limitation of residual disabilities. A great proportion of the patients are in the employable age group, and the average patient of forty-nine may have as many as sixteen years of employability left, figuring on retirement age of sixty-five (Dietz, 1969). The impact of these psychosocial problems is discussed in the following chapter.

Disabilities encountered in the cancer patient depend upon both the anatomical region or organ system affected by the cancer and upon given treatment. Rehabilitation care is varied according to individual case findings and needs and can best be discussed under headings of disease region and cancer treatment procedure.

AMPUTATION AND DISARTICULATION FOR
BONE AND SOFT TISSUE MALIGNANCY

Preoperative training in ambulation with crutches is of great value to the lower extremity amputee, who has not yet been weakened by a period of immobilization, has no wound discomfort, is not affected by medication, and has not developed fear. Postoperatively, the patient can be instructed in strengthening exercises to the residual normal extremities and his ambulation training can be continued (Dietz, 1969).

Consideration of the provision of any prosthesis for the patient should begin preoperatively, if possible. The consideration of "cure" should not restrict the rehabilitation program or planning for a prosthesis. Amputation because of a malignant tumor does not constitute an a priori contraindication to a prosthetic fitting. If there is no evidence of metastasis and the stump is suitable for fitting, a limb should be fitted at the earliest possible time for both adult and child (Research Division, 1965).

The approach of fitting a prosthesis either immediately after surgery or early in the postoperative period is of particular value for the cancer patient. In both instances there is immediate postoperative application of a snug plaster of Paris cast over a light, thin, wound dressing. This cast creates sufficient support to prevent edema and swelling of the stump and appreciably lessens pain and discomfort. In the case of immediate fitting, a pylon or coupled articulated prosthesis is added by the surgeon and the prosthetist while the patient is still on the operating table. In the case of early fitting, the pylon-coupled prosthesis is fitted ten or twelve days after surgery, when the operative dressing is first changed, the skin sutures removed, and the wound found to be in satisfactory condition.

Use of an early total-contact prosthesis creates an increased proprioceptive sense and utilizes the phantom sensations present. Success in early prosthesis application depends upon the amputation surgery technique, including proper and secure attachment of the muscle and fascia to or over the bone end, so as to afford good stump control (Burgess, Romano, Zettl, 1969).

As with lower extremity amputation, upper extremity loss needs to be treated with a positive approach, including the provision of an appropriate prosthesis and training, with special attention paid to one-handed activity proficiency.

Children who are amputees should be considered promptly for the provision of a prosthesis. Child amputees with malignancies survive in significant percentage for one to five years and wear their prostheses successfully for a year or longer, the majority of them full time (Research Division, 1965).

The earliest and most useful prosthesis for the interscapulothoracic amputation is a shoulder-cap cosmetic prosthesis. Little can be said for any form of functional prosthesis after this type of operative procedure. A shoulder disarticulation does not disturb stability so radically, and in such cases a functional prosthesis can be prescribed.

For those rare instances where there is an appreciable residual stump length of the upper extremity, progressively better prostheses can be made.

Immediately after the operation, the upper extremity amputee should begin occupational therapy for training and dexterity, have strengthening exercises for any residual stump, and learn techniques of one-handed activities. The training should continue after fitting for the prosthesis, with emphasis on the use of the new replacement appliance.

CANCER OF THE BREAST

Rehabilitation following radical mastectomy has three main goals: restoration of external appearance; maintenance of range of motion and function in the operated arm and shoulder; and aid in psychological adjustment. The patient's severe psychological and emotional reactions require support, reassurance, and encouragement from the surgeon, the rehabilitation team, and the family. The patient must be instructed in the performance of early routine exercises to preserve and restore function, and should be given an appropriate prosthesis for early restoration of symmetry in appearance. She should have a prosthesis as immediately after surgery as possible. This would include the light-weight dacron fluff filled prosthesis which is supplied by the "Reach to Recovery" program of the American Cancer Society, where available.

Approximately 50 per cent of mastectomy patients experience some degree of postoperative lymphedema. Lymphedema disability is proportional to the extent and disfigurement the edema creates. Treatment has been varied. Salt-free diets, diuretics, mechanical aids for massage with intermittent compression, elastic sleeves, and surgical procedures have all been tried. Intermittent compression must be repeated daily and throughout the day.

In the care of both early postoperative and long-standing lymphedema, preventive measures are of great value. Infection must be meticulously avoided and antibiotics used liberally if there is a suggestion of infection. Mastectomy patients should never be given any form of injections or vaccinations or have venupuncture performed in the arm on the operated side, and they should be warned about the danger of infections in the fingers and hand, trauma or sunburn, for which they should seek immediate care. Use of the American Cancer Society's "Reach to Recovery" pamphlet is recommended. An occasional patient may require psychiatric advice and therapy.

CANCER OF THE BOWELS

There is great importance in the surgeon's effort in placement, construction, initial care, and training of the colostomy for the patient. This is the surgeon's responsibility, and it will not be discussed in detail in this chapter (Committee on Guidelines for Cancer Care, 1970).

The presence of a colostomy may develop great adjustment problems for the patient (Druss, O'Connor, Stern, 1969). There may be leakage, odor, and noisy expulsion of gas, causing anxiety and embarrassment. Loss of sexual function occurs in about 50 per cent of male patients. Travel, especially by air, becomes more difficult, as changes in air pressure are sufficient to increase gas expulsion and bowel activity.

Rehabilitation should start, whenever possible, during the preoperative stage with advice and possibly a visit from another colostomy patient. Postoperative continuity of care should be provided daily by the same nurse, trained especially in colostomy handling. Management is generally better by irrigation technique. The first irrigation, because of its great impact, should be done under the best circumstances by an expert. In planning for the patient consideration should be taken of the patient's preoperative bowel habits to set up his individual routine. Variations in equipment and technique of care should be permitted according to the individual patient's needs (Turnbull, 1961; Datona, 1967; Postel, Grier, Localio, 1965).

Prior to discharge from the hospital the surgeon should discuss home plans with the family to insure adequate preparations and obtaining of needed equipment. A nurse may give a helping hand during the first few days at home. Further assistance may be obtained from another patient who has successfully lived with a colostomy and also from "ostomy" clubs. Regular follow-up facilities should be provided for all patients (Turnbull, 1961; 1966).

CANCER OF THE FACE AND MOUTH

Radical surgery leaves severe cosmetic problems as well as functional defects in speech, mastication, swallowing, and salivary control. With head and neck cancer, there is a special terror coefficient. It is extremely difficult for the patient to mask or hide his problem, which can create severe psychological reactions. Rehabilitative care should start in the preoperative period with purposeful information and support, and oral hygiene instruction. During and after surgery the surgical and dental team can supply either a temporary or a permanent prosthesis— functional if possible. Reconstructive plastic surgery requires patience and understanding on the part of the patient and may involve repeated procedures over a long period of time (Synderman, 1970).

Social Service should work extensively with these patients and their families. Speech therapy may be able to assist and vocational counseling should be obtained (Dietz, 1969).

CANCER OF THE LARYNX

After laryngectomy, speech training becomes the most pressing need in rehabilitation. Esophageal speech is the preferred method. To avoid development of bad communication habits in the immediate postoperative period, and until he has learned to talk, the patient should communicate only by writing and signs. Only a trained speech therapist or another laryngectomee, a successful speaker, should undertake speech training. Learning time varies. Return of smell and taste may take several months after loss of function. At the time of discharge each patient should be provided with a post-laryngectomy kit, containing the main essentials required for good care. Social service and vocational training play large ongoing rehabilitation roles. There may be a laryngectomy club in the patient's community, and he also may obtain help from the International Association of Laryngectomies and through the American Cancer Society (Diedrich and Youngstrom, 1966; Lauder, 1969).

RADICAL NECK DISSECTION

Radical neck dissection results in varying degrees of trapezius muscle paralysis, secondary to section of the accessory nerve. Treatment requires initial support of the arm and shoulder with a sling to prevent overstretching of the trapezius, and patients should be taught to support their arm and shoulder when seated. An exercise program is needed for training and movement to facilitate abduction of the arm at the shoulder. During the healing following this procedure, trapezius muscle electrical stimulation may be beneficial.

CANCER OF THE LUNGS

Rehabilitative measures for patients with the cancer of the lung should include preoperative training in breathing control and proper coughing technique. Postoperatively effective coughing is taught by correct control of respiration rather than by force or volume of expelled air. Activity of accessory musculature is reduced to minimize discomfort. Moistened air helps prevent the drying of bronchial secretions which makes it very difficult for the patient to cough and properly eliminate these secretions. Intermittent positive pressure breathing apparatus, the use of sustained maximal inspiration, and the "yawn" maneuver help to provide the patient with proper pulmonary ventilation and in the prevention of problems of respiratory insufficiency.

Manual splinting of the chest helps to reduce both discomfort and apprehension. If postural drainage is ordered, it should be continued until coughing is nonproductive and the patient ambulatory (Dietz, 1969, 1971; Brompton Hospital Physiotherapy Department, 1967).

CENTRAL AND PERIPHERAL NERVOUS SYSTEM INVOLVEMENT

Malignancies, whether primary or metastatic, involving the brain, spinal cord, or peripheral nerves create motor and sensory deficits and affect coordination. Treatment for the patient should begin as soon as the disability is diagnosed or the surgery completed. The entire spectrum of plegias and peripheral neuropathies may be encountered. The general treatment is the same as the standard recognized care program for such disabilities unrelated to cancer.

Control of persistent pain may require a neurosurgical approach. Causalgia and paraesthesia are occasionally helped by the application of hot packs or cold packs or by gentle massage. Sensory losses can be assisted by training and by substitution of other sensory modalities.

REMOTE EFFECTS OF CANCER OF THE NERVOUS SYSTEM

Remote effects of cancer on the neuromuscular system and the similar effects of steroid medication and cancer chemotherapeutic agents may result in muscular weakness and wasting, most frequently involving the limb girdle and proximal muscles. It is important to teach the patient exercises as preventive measures against the effects of disuse and lack of range of motion (Brain, Forbes, 1965).

PATHOLOGICAL FRACTURES

Pathological fractures may occur as a result of primary or metastatic bone involvement. Depending on the individual disability and the procedure performed in treatment of the fracture, rehabilitation begins with appropriate motion and exercises, and later, according to needs and ability, training and assistance in ambulation with suitable supports. Otherwise, a goal of wheelchair mobilization should be sought.

PSYCHOSOCIAL AND VOCATIONAL PROBLEMS

The patient with cancer may develop great psychological problems. These are discussed in the next chapter. Effort must be made to gain support of the family and help from religious advisors and mutual assistance groups. Social service personnel can direct in assisting and understanding patients' needs. Community resources should be fully utilized. The vocational counselor can aid in motivation of the patient toward rehabilitation and work. Solution is urgently needed of problems of employer acceptance for work of the applicant who has a record of treatment for cancer (Dietz, 1969).

CONCLUSION

Early recognition of patient disability and of rehabilitation potential should be made by the medical staff attending the patient, and rehabilitation therapy should be started as early as possible to reduce disability and hopelessness, frustration and despair on the part of the patient. Training and counsel preoperatively for the patient about to undergo surgery will increase the psychological and the physiological benefits. The same criteria should be used in the consideration of disability from cancer or its treatments as are used for disabilities not connected with any cancer. There is need for rehabilitation care in goals of restorative and supportive nature as well as for palliation for the patient with advanced and incurable cancer.

It is considered unrealistic and contrary to good rehabilitation practice to defer provision of rehabilitation services for a waiting period in order to determine the status of a patient's disease or the question of disease spread. It is not possible to make an accurate judgement of life expectancy or length of time for engaging in useful activities for a patient with cancer, in spite of the general tables available.

It would be a great service to the cancer patient if the physician would change his basic appraisals and concepts of results of cancer treatments from those of possible "cured" to those of "controlled." This type of consideration would eliminate the unfortunate problems which are created by arbitrary time limits of two to five years before consideration of eligibility of the cancer patient for a positive rehabilitation program or for vocational rehabilitation services.

Consideration should be given to each patient on an individual basis with evaluation of all medical findings, the prognosis and the maximal eventual gain to the patient, his family, and the community. By so doing, comprehensive medical care would be provided for the patient to effect improvement in his quality of survival.

GLOSSARY

ABDOMINOPERINEAL RESECTION—Excision of the rectum by combined abdominal and perineal (space between anus and genitalia) approach.

ACTH—ADRENOCORTICOTROPHIC HORMONE—Hormone produced in the pituitary gland which stimulates activity of the cortex of the adrenal gland.

ADENOCARCINOMA—Malignant tumor composed of glandular tissue.

ALKYLATING AGENT—A highly reactive chemical compound which causes damage to DNA and so interferes with cell reproduction.

ANTIMETABOLITE—Chemical which interferes with or prevents processes of normal cell life.

BIOPSY—Removal by surgical excision of a small part or the whole of a (small) mass for identification by microscopic examination.

CANCER—A malignant new growth.

CAPILLARY—Any one of the minute branch vessels which connect the smallest arteries and veins forming a network in nearly all parts of the body.

CARCINOMA—A malignant new growth made up of cells originating in the coverings of the external and internal surfaces of the body, including the lining of the blood vessels, stomach and intestines, and other small organs.

CARDIOVASCULAR—Pertaining to the heart and blood vessels.

CAUSALGIA—Persistent burning pain usually following peripheral nerve injury.

CEREBROSPINAL FLUID—Fluid forming in the brain and bathing brain and spinal cord.

CHEMOTHERAPY—Treatment by use of appropriate chemical substances, including hormones.

CHORDOTOMY—(or cordotomy) Interruption of the nerve tracts carrying pain in the spinal cord.

COLOSTOMY—Surgical opening to the outside from the large bowel.

CONNECTIVE TISSUE—The tissue which binds together and is the basis for the various parts and organs of the body, including bone.

CONVERSION—Process of the change into another state or form.

CYSTADENOCARCINOMA—Malignant tumor arising from epithelial cells and forming cystic spaces of variable size.

CYSTADENOMA—A tumor developing from a cyst or its lining cells, benign but possibly precancerous.

DIURETIC—A medicine which stimulates the flow of urine and thereby eliminates body fluid.

DNA—DEOXYRIBONUCLEIC ACID—A nucleic acid found in cell nuclei and which sets the pattern for cell reproduction.

ECOLOGY—Study or state of the environment and life history of an organism or situation.

ENDOGENOUS—Originating within the organism.

EPITHELIAL TISSUE—Cells growing mostly in sheets and adapted for covering or lining of body tissues or organs. Skin itself is the most obvious form.

EXFOLIATION—Separation of cells as free units.

HEMOGRAM—A tabulated representation of the differential blood count.

HODGKIN'S DISEASE—A form of cancer which arises particularly in lymph nodes and also in spleen, liver, or bone marrow.

HORMONE—A chemical substance produced in an organ, which when carried to another associated organ, excites in the latter a functional activity.

ISOTOPE—See Radioactive isotope.

KERATOSIS—Thickening, piling up, of skin.

LARYNGECTOMY—The surgical removal of the larynx (or voice box).

LESION—A spot or site of change in body tissue due to disease or cancer.

LEUKEMIA—Cancer of the bone marrow involving white blood cell elements.

LEUKOPLAKIA—Formation of white thickened patches on mucous membranes of mouth, cheeks and tongue. May be precancerous.

LOBECTOMY—Surgical removal of a lobe, such as lung, liver, etc.

LOBOTOMY—Surgical division of nerve pathways in the frontal lobe of the brain to interrupt (change) response to pain.

LYMPH—A body fluid which bathes and nourishes the cells of the body and flows through spaces between cells and in channels called lymphatics.

LYMPH NODE—Nodules of specialized nature occurring along the course of lymphatic vessels and channels usually occurring in groups and tending to strain out of the lymph such foreign substances as bacteria and cancer cells.

LYMPHATIC—Pertaining to lymph, as the spaces and channels in the tissues through which lymph flows.

LYMPHEDEMA—Swelling of a limb or body part due to a blockade of lymph fluid drainage.

LYMPHOMA—Malignant tumor of lymphoid tissue origin.

MASTECTOMY—Surgical removal of the breast, male or female. Radical mastectomy includes wide surgical removal of the muscles of the anterior chest and the lymph nodes and fat of the armpit.

METABOLISM—The sum of all the physical and chemical processes by which living organized substance is maintained, including those transformations which make energy available for use by the organism.

METASTASIS—Transfer of disease or cancer from a site or origin in one organ or tissue to another at a distance.

MODALITY—Employment of a treatment agent, usually a physical agent.

MUTATION—Change to assume one or more new characteristics.

NEUROFIBROMATOSIS—(Von Recklinghausen's disease) Hundreds of small nodular growths originating from the sheaths of nerves, scattered throughout the body. Basically a benign disease, but cancer may develop in any one or several of the growths.

NEUROPATHY—Disease or loss of function of a nerve.

NUCLEUS—The core or center of a cell, contains special protein and DNA.

OMENTUM—The apron-like fatty folds of peritoneum which attach from stomach and large bowel.

ORTHOTIC—Pertaining to a brace or splint.

OSTEOGENIC—Having origin from bone.

PARESIS—Weakness or partial paralysis.

PATHOLOGIST—A physician specializing in the diagnosis and study of changes caused by disease in the tissues of the body, and in abnormal chemical and metabolic body changes.

PERFUSION—To run a drug or chemical through the blood vessel system of an organ or body part.

PERIPHERAL—At a distance from the center or source.

PERITONEAL—Pertaining to the lining of the abdominal cavity and covering of the abdominal organs.

PLEGIA—Total paralysis.

PLEURAL—Pertaining to the lining of the chest cavity and covering of the lungs.

POLYP—Pedunculated (having a wide or narrow-footed base) growth from a mucous surface. May be benign, precancerous, or malignant.

POSTURAL DRAINAGE—Procedure of positioning and tipping a patient to improve drainage, especially from the lungs.

PRECANCEROUS—Pertaining to a state or condition which could eventually become a cancer.

PROPRIOCEPTIVE—Pertaining to perception or sense of body (or body part) position in space.

PROSTHETIC—Pertaining to a replacement of a lost limb or body part.

PROXIMAL—Close or closer to the center or source.

PSYCHOSOCIAL—Pertaining to psychological and social background, situation or reaction.

PULMONARY—Pertaining to the lungs.

RADIATION THERAPY—Treatment of a disease or cancer by exposure to x-ray from any active source.

RADICAL MASTECTOMY—*See* Mastectomy.

RADICAL NECK DISSECTION—Surgical removal of all lymph nodes of the neck (on one side or both) to eliminate local cancer spread.

RADIOACTIVE ISOTOPE—Chemical substances made radioactive by exposure to an atomic reactor.

RADIOSENSITIVE—Sensitive to exposure to radiation therapy.

RESECTION—To surgically remove part or all of an organ or tissue mass.

SARCOMA—Malignant tumor arising from connective tissue.

SCAN—A study of the patterns created by the radioactivity of special medicines given to the patient. Used to locate presence or spread of certain tumors.

SEROLOGICAL—As found by tests of the blood serum.

STEROID—A term applied to any one of a group of substances, especially as related to the hormones produced by the adrenal gland cortex.

THALAMOTOMY—Surgical, electrical, or chemical destruction of local nerve tracts in the thalamus of the brain to alter reaction to pain.

TISSUE—Body cell group and type classified by function into epithelia tissue, connective tissue, muscular tissue, nervous tissue, and blood.

TRANSPOSITION—Placement in a different position.

TRAPEZIUS MUSCLE—The large muscle of the top of the shoulder (slope from neck base) and upper back which shrugs the shoulder.

VENUPUNCTURE—The procedure of insertion of a hollow needle into a vein for withdrawal of blood or injection of material.

REFERENCES

American Cancer Society. 1970. A cancer source book for nurses. New York, American Cancer Society, p. 120.

Ariel, Irving M. 1968. Radioactive isotopes in the treatment of cancer, in Cancer management. Philadelphia, Lippincott, pp. 181–95.

Brain, Lord and N. Forbes, Jr. 1965. The remote effects of cancer on the nervous system. Contemporary neurology symposia 1. New York, Grune and Stratton.

Brompton Hospital Physiotherapy Department. 1967. Physiotherapy for medical and surgical thoracic conditions. 3d rev. London, Brompton Hospital, p. 32.

Burgess, Ernest M., R. L. Romano, and J. H. Zettl. 1969. The management of lower extremity amputation (TR 10-6, Superintendent of Documents). Washington, D.C. U.S. Government Printing Office, p. 122.

Committee on Guidelines for Cancer Care, Commission on Cancer, American College of Surgeons. 1970. Guidelines for cancer care. Chicago, American College of Surgeons, p. 208.

Datona, Elizabeth A. 1967. Learning colostomy control. American Journal of Nursing 67:3:534–41.

Diedrich, William M. and K. A. Youngstrom. 1966. Alaryngeal speech. Springfield, Ill., Charles C. Thomas, p. 220.

Dietz, J. Herbert, Jr. May 1, 1969. Rehabilitation of the cancer patient. Medical clinics of North America 53:3:607–24.

—— 1971. Rehabilitation of the cancer patient, Howard A. Rusk, ed., Rehabilitation medicine. 3d ed. New York, Mosby, pp. 634–56.

—— 1969. Cancer rehabilitation in the work force. Transactions Bulletin No. 43, Industrial Hygiene Foundation of America, pp. 61–65.

Druss, R. G., J. F. O'Connor and L. O. Stern. 1969. Psychologic response to colectomy. Arch. Gen. Psychiatry 20:419.

Healey, John E., ed. 1970. Ecology of the cancer patient. Interdisciplinary Communications Program, The Smithsonian Institution, Washington, D.C., p. 184.

Karnofsky, David A. 1968. Clinical application of chemotherapy, in Cancer Management. Philadelphia, Lippincott, pp. 214–20.

Lauder, Edmund. 1969. Self-help for the laryngectomee. 2d ed. San Antonio, Texas, Lauder.

Mozden, Peter J. 1965. Neoplasms, in S. J. Myers, ed., An orientation to chronic disease and disability. New York, Macmillan, pp. 323–61.

National Cancer Plan. 1972. U.S. Department of Health, Education and Welfare National Cancer Institute, 1972.

Pack, G. T. and I. M. Ariel. 1968. The history of cancer therapy, in Cancer management. Philadelphia, Lippincott, pp. 2–27.

Postel, A. H., W. R. N. Grier, and S. A. Localio. 1965. A simplified method of irrigation of the colonic stoma. Surgery, Gynecology and Obstetrics 121:595.

Raventos, A. 1968. Radionuclide beam units, in Cancer management. Philadelphia, Lippincott, pp. 151–54.

Research Division, School of Engineering and Science, New York University. 1965. Prosthetic fitting of children amputated for malignancy. New York.

Shimkin, M. B. 1964. Science and cancer. Public Health Service Publ. No. 1162. Washington, D.C., U.S. Department of Health, Education and Welfare, p. 137.

Synderman, R. K. 1970. Cancer, a chronic disease. Plastic and Reconstructive Surgery 45:5:502.

Turnbull, R. P. 1961. Instructions to the colostomy patient. Cleveland Clinic Quarterly 28:134.

———— 1966. Construction and care of the ileostomy. Hospital Medicine 2:145:38.

CANCER: PSYCHOSOCIAL FACTORS

CANCER. The word strikes terror in the hearts of all who hear that dread diagnosis. Despite brilliant medical advances toward control of the disease and increasing extension of survival time in the past quarter of a century, cancer continues to be shrouded by attitudes of defeatism (Healey, 1970). Fear, real and fantasized, becomes the constant companion of those who seek treatment for cancer, and of the ones who love them. Fear of death, fear of separation, fear of disability, helplessness, pain, and disfigurement are all realistic anxieties that must be faced. Small wonder that a pall of pessimism hangs over the diagnosis and that the challenging medical decisions are further complicated by severe psychosocial problems impinging upon the patient and his family.

It was in the early 1950s that Doctor S. J. Kowal (1955), after the death of his wife from cancer, became interested in psychological factors surrounding early diagnosis, or recognition, of the preneoplastic state. He made an intensive review of the literature and found that the role of the emotions in cancer had been subject to avid interest and concern by physicians of the eighteenth and nineteenth centuries. At that time, three outstanding physicians committed themselves to the theory that there are indeed implications of psychological stress in cancer. Parker (Kowal, 1955) expressed his deep conviction that depression, appearing as grief, induced a predisposition to the disease. In 1846 Walshe

BEATRIX COBB, PH.D., is Distinguished Horn Professor, Texas Tech University, Lubbock, Texas.

(Kowal, 1955) said, "It would be vain to deny that facts of a very convincing character, in respect to the agency of the mind in the production of the disease, are frequently observed." Sir James Paget (Kowal, 1955) states "We can hardly doubt that mental depression is a weighty addition to the other influences that favor the development of the condition." In the nineteenth century, Herbert Snow (Kowal, 1955), surgeon to the Cancer Hospital in London, tried to interest the medical profession in emotional influences in cancer through the publication of several books and articles, but was forced to conclude that the time was not ripe for its adoption.

And then Freud hove into view and reinforced psychosomatic concepts to medical thinking. The concept was first applied by such leaders as Alexander (1950), Dunbar (1955), and others to the etiology of such diseases as ulcers, asthma, and the like. However, it was not until around the 1950s that serious consideration was given the idea of emotions in cancer.

Around this time, four groups widely divergent as to geographical location but intent upon similar ideas became interested in systematic research in the area. Perhaps the first group formed was that in Chicago, led by Doctors Finesinger and Abrams (1953). Almost simultaneously groups began work at Memorial Hospital in New York (Sutherland, 1952), Texas M. D. Anderson Hospital in Houston (Cobb, 1952), and in the Veterans' Administration Hospital in California (West, 1954). These efforts began with high enthusiasm and deep dedication on the part of the participants, but one by one these groups disbanded in the middle and late 1950s. The psychological dynamics surrounding the discontinuation of programs contains a common element reiterating Doctor Snow's experience a century earlier. Medical thought continued to remain not only untouched, but often actually scathingly rejecting of data and concepts reported. With no reinforcement from the field, the researchers then turned one by one to less controversial and more rewarding areas of endeavor. Only one group remains active in the field, the New York team.

Whether the late twentieth century shall prove different from the period of Doctor Snow's discouragement is something the future holds hidden. It is with some encouragement that we do note the turning in the past decade of the investigative curiosity of the modern physician toward some interest in psychosocial factors in cancer, as evidenced in the reports of three interdisciplinary conferences on cancer, *Ecology of the Cancer Patient* (Healey, 1970).

Two comprehensive areas of investigation growing out of the formulation of early findings in psychological studies and observations have to do with a constellation of psychological factors revolving around the social-cultural background of the cancer patient, and a second galaxy focuses upon the implications of psychological stress in the course of the disease. The first constellation would seek to delineate possible psychological patterns that might be instrumental in predisposing an individual to cancer, or that might act as a precipitating mechanism initiating the cancerous growth. The second galaxy would explore the possibilities of a psychological resistance to the onslaught of the disease, psychophysiological interaction in the course of the disease, and the psychological role of the physician and its impact on the course of the cancer. Each of these areas will be reviewed briefly.

PSYCHOLOGICAL PATTERNS IN
PREDISPOSITION TO CANCER

Grinker (1956) tells us that the hereditary factor in cancer implies that some genic predisposition to the formation of new growths is inherited in some fashion. Hereditary predisposition, however, does not mean that there is a cancerous potential within a structure, or a somatic system, which slowly unfolds or blossoms like a seed endowed with self-action. In hereditary predisposition, rather, there is required an adequate stimulus from the environment of the organism, the organ, or the cell, to bring the predisposition into action. "What is this stimulus? Must it be physiological, or might it not be psychological in nature? Is it possible that the hereditary factor, even though it is not proven, may be a potent psychological weight on the individual with a cancerous ancestry that swings the balance in the favor of the initiation of the disease?" (Cobb, 1960).

The point here is that it is difficult to separate a hereditary process from a familial repetition of the disease augmented by psychological influences. The psychiatrists speak of such incidents as "anniversary syndromes." Whatever this may be, whether predisposition or anniversary syndrome, it is of concern to the practicing physician when it intrudes between him and the successful control of malignancy when working with a patient.

In the area of predisposition also lies the moot question of organ selection in cancer. We have no right to assert at this time that psychological factors are significant in locating the site of cancer. We do have unexplained incidents that make us wonder.

Adler (1963) pointed out, in his theory of organ inferiority, that each individual inherits an organ that is "inferior," that under stress this is the organ most likely to succeed in becoming impaired, and that the personality of the individual is molded in the process of compensating for and adapting to this inferiority. Is it possible that the woman who acquires cancer of the breast may be so predisposed by the conscious, or unconscious, knowledge of this flaw in her body? Is it probable that psychological factors, involving the symbolic meaning of the organ to that individual, may be impinging upon the physiological defect in such a way as to become instrumental in the onset of the disease?

Alexander (1950) would question also if specific chronic emotional states bring about certain disturbances of body function, ultimately resulting in cancer; and is a specific organ involvement selected because of stress made to bear upon it through endocrine imbalance and concomitant shifts in body function? Or, putting it another way, we might ask: is the hormonal imbalance a contributing factor to the psychological stress? The possibilities are not mutually exclusive.

Dr. Grinker (1956) has another way of questioning. He asks if the selection of organ is a secondary process dependent upon the availability of a location and the processes that made that location suitable in the presence of a generalized tendency.

In this area of predisposition to cancer, very few social scientists have reported studies. Perhaps the study "Relationship of Body Image to Site of Cancer" by Fisher and Cleveland (1956) of the Veterans' Administration Hospital in Houston has some bearing on the subject. The authors conclude that personality variables may play a significant role in the total complex of factors that determine the site of development of cancer. Fisher and Cleveland themselves label these results as tenuous, and emphasize the need for much further study in the area.

Doctor Wolfgang Luthe (1956) of the University of Montreal proposed two hypotheses pertinent to the subject, and indicated that he was involved in research in the area.

First, he presented the hypothesis that,

malignant processes are due to weakness, or defect, or genetic growth, control or timing and that the site and type of tumor is determined by particularities of the functional pattern of an individual's genetic constellation. In this case, the involvement of psychological factors would be, if involved at all, of secondary nature.

Second, he proposed the hypothesis that,

the developmental possibility of malignant growth exists in every human person, and that specific consequences of deficiencies in the organism's homeostatic and adaptational mechanisms are responsible for the onset and course of neoplastic processes. Here, the psychological variables may be decisively involved by modulating functional dynamics in certain parts of the neurohumoral axis.

If definitive research has been accomplished in either of these two proposals, no report is available to the writer. Certainly, there is need for elaboration of these topics. Research in this complex physiological area, however, must be led by the expert medical investigator who is in command of all the knowledge available in the area of endocrinology as well as cancer. The social scientist's role would be that of adjunct, assisting in collecting pertinent social-cultural data and interpreting it to the principal researcher, who would then integrate its substance into the total complicated picture under scrutiny.

PRECIPITATING PSYCHOLOGICAL FACTORS

There are many known causes of cancer, but so far no single common factor has been designated. Among the intrinsic factors of proved importance, in addition to the inherited biological determinents discussed above, are such variables as age, sex, and hormonal influences. If we grant that certain biochemical, metabolical, and hormonal activities are significant for the development of cancer, and recognize the influence of mental process on some of the hormonal steroids as taking place through the intermediation of the hypothalamus, it is not unreasonable to conjecture that psychological factors may effect cancer through the elaboration or suppression of certain hormones through this pathway. When we ask what the factors are which trigger the change from cellular order to cellular chaos, could we not question further, is an emotional force the finger on the trigger at times?

If long-continued anxiety can produce a premature aging syndrome with its alterations in adrenal, gonadal, and hepatic function, (and this has been demonstrated by researchers, one instance of which is reported in *Anxiety and Stress* by Grinker *et al.* (1956)), it might be presumed that certain chronic emotional changes may be significant in the development of carcinoma. Basic emotional states, such as anxiety, anger, or depression, would seem worthy of study; the effect of these states on metabolism and endocrine function would seem a fruitful focus of elaboration.

Inhibition of an organ or system activity might well be as involved as hyperactivity. What happens to the metabolism in structures thus inhibited, and how this influences the change in growth, or maintenance of growth, of its component parts, is of interest in this study of precipitating factors.

From 1952 to 1956 numerous researchers from New York to California started reporting results of individual investigations having to do with personality and/or psychological factors as precipitating events leading to cancer. Renneker and Cutler (1952), in Chicago, led the field by reporting in 1952 their observations that women with cancer of the breast are masochistic, sexually inhibited, deficient in motherliness, and incapable of discharging hostility felt toward their own mothers, covering over instead with a pleasant facade. During 1954, 1955, and 1956, a rapid succession of replications or similar studies were reported from Greene in the East (1954 and 1956), Wheeler and Caldwell in St. Louis and Houston (1955), and LeShan and Worthington in New York City (1955 and 1956). Four consistent findings were common to all this work done independently in all parts of the country. The patients studied have in common:

1) Loss of an important relationship prior to the development of the tumor;
2) inability to express hostile feelings and emotions;

3) unresolved tension concerning parental figures;

4) disturbance in the sexual area.

This background of psychological stress, however, was not demonstrated as unique to any particular cancer site. Renneker and Cutler concentrated on cancer of the breast, with Wheeler and Caldwell adding cancer of the cervix and noncancer control patients. Greene reported on both males and females; his patients, however, were suffering from the pymphomas and leukemias for the most part. LeShan and Worthington also studied patients with various cancerous sites.

Psychological trait specificity to cancer was not demonstrated by any of these researchers, nor were they actually attempting to do so. These were really exploratory studies. Grinker (1956) points out that similar personality descriptions might be made of patients suffering from multiple sclerosis and thyrotoxicosis.

The implication might be that sufficient study has not been made of either the psychological dynamics of the so-called normal individual or of the other disease entities to warrant a claim that these personality traits are in any specific way conducive to the onset of cancer. They could be coexisting and unrelated. The fact, however, that a state of depression seems almost a universal precursor of the cancerous state would seem to be worthy of intensive investigation, whatever the cause.

Greene (1954 and 1956) highlighted other areas indicative to fruitful study. He stated that his patients had first recognized symptoms of the disease while having to adjust to stresses arising from multiple sources. Symptoms leading up to the recognition often included anorexia, nausea, vomiting, pain, anxiety, and depression. These symptoms could frequently not be correlated with extent or degree of neoplastic activity, but could be understood on a psychological basis.

Greene further reported that the majority of patients studied showed an affect of sadness or hopelessness for weeks, or months, prior to the apparent onset. He again highlighted the idea of separation from a key person or goal, with the ensuing depression, as a possible precipitating factor to cancer.

S. J. Kowal (1955 and 1956) of Boston, made an exhaustive eight-year study of this type of depression, attempting to differentiate it from the psychoneurotic and psychotic depressions of the psychiatric literature.

He found that loss of a vital figure or goal, eventual dissipation of resistance, and final collapse or hopelessness simulating a depression was constant in his population.

In attempting to differentiate this depression, Kowal explained that the neoplastic state is a constitutional one characterized by a general retardation of normal growth, or some equivalent state. When the neoplasm begins to develop it is found that the body separates functionally into two portions, the non-neoplastic portion and the neoplastic one. From the point of view of mass, at that time the non-neoplastic portion is much larger than the other. If these two portions are visualized as in actual conflict for nutritional supplies, the growth of the neoplasm might be explained, not on the basis of aggressiveness, which is the customary explanation, but on the basis of the failure of the non-neoplastic portion to accept, or utilize nutritional materials. In the depression preceding the cancerous state, then, he suggests that there is struggle between two active forces of aggression and restraint, resulting in a shifting equilibrium between the two forces, and if the malignant growth is victorious, an exhaustive state of depleted energy is observed. A Greek word signifying "emptying out or collapse" was remodeled to "catarosis," so that this exhaustive state could be described as a catarotic depression as distinguished from the usual psychoneurotic or psychotic depressions that emphasize the element of restrained aggression or blocked goal.

From a therapeutic viewpoint, this conception implies that any agent applied so as to stimulate normal growth again in the non-neoplastic portions of the body might result in regression of the neoplasm and restoration of the normal status. From the point of view of emotional influences on cancer, then, the salutory effect of stimulating hope could become equivalent to restoring normal growth activity. According to this theory, massive supportive therapy, with the aim of restoring the will to live by supplying actual aid in all the needed areas and slowly creating new goals for living, could become a vital aid in cancer therapy.

At this point, the efforts to elucidate precipitating factors merge with those involved with psychological resistance to the onslaught of the malignant state. Before we turn to this second galaxy of psychological factors with implications toward host resistance tending to control the disease, we should reiterate that there is much to be done in this intriguing area of precipitating factors in cancer. Intensive study of the role of emotional pressures in cancer could produce added insights to bear upon the problem.

PSYCHOLOGICAL HOST RESISTANCE IN CANCER

In 1953 a symposium was held at the Veterans' Administration Hospital in Long Beach, California, that touched off an avid interest in a phenomenon labeled by the participants as "host resistance" to cancer. The exciting question under discussion was, "Is there such a thing as psychological resistance to cancer which might result in control or regression of the malignant growth?" This idea was so unique that even Doctor P. M. West (1954), one of the leaders in the investigation, confessed,

Ten years ago I would have been quite shocked at the idea of emotional factors ever invading the field of neoplasia. True to my conservative and revered teachings, my attitude even five years ago was . . . let the psychosomaticists play around with peptic ulcer, mucous colitis, asthma, and hypertension, but cancer . . . never! This is one disease that is purely organic and belongs forever and exclusively in the realm of the surgeon, the radiologist, the pathologist and the autopsy room (page 306).

In 1948, when Doctor West started his intensive study of cancer patients, the autonomous nature of cancer had been successfully challenged by Huggins (Huggins and Hodges, 1941) as far as prostatic carcinoma was concerned. Mere alteration of the endocrine balance of the host sufficed in many cases to arrest or produce regression of this disease. At this time also, the reversal by nitrogen mustard of the progressive course of other types of neoplastic disease had become an accepted fact. Perhaps it was because of the use of these drugs that attention was focused on the degree and duration of clinical responses obtained, and the side effects that might occur.

Anyway, it was only a short time until Doctor West and his coworker, Doctor Ellis, found themselves involved in a grim game. They found, for example, that the same dose of nitrogen mustard that might put one man with Hodgkin's Disease back on his feet for months or years in apparent perfect health, would in another patient in a comparable stage of the same disease do nothing at all, and the patient would fail and die. Very shortly they realized that they could predict upon first contact with the patient whether or not he would be one who would respond or fail. The success of their predictions was so great that they examined the clues by which they were making the prediction and realized that they were mostly psychological. They then called in psychiatrists and psychologists from the University of California at Los Angeles and started a full-scale search to pin down these nebulous but potent clues.

Eugene M. Blumberg (1954) reported on the results of psychological testing of fifty patients with cancer in which it was attempted to elucidate the psychological differences evident in the patient who did resist the onslaught of the disease and returned to normal living and the patient who rapidly succumbed to the malignancy. The individuals with fast-growing cancer were described by Dr. Blumberg as having more defensiveness, a higher anxiety level, and less ability to reduce tension through motor discharge than the group surviving longer.

The population for this study consisted of fifty individuals, all males, with many types of carcinoma. Would this hold true in a population of females? And since cancer is known to be many diseases, would the findings be repeated in a sample consisting of a single type of cancer? Alan Krasnoff (1959) did a replication study of the procedures explained by Blumberg, utilizing only patients with melanoma, but including both males and females. He was unable to replicate the results. This is not to say there is no evidence of psychological resistance to the disease involved. It does, however, indicate that proving the point and identifying the ingredients is not a simple matter.

PSYCHOLOGICAL IMPLICATIONS
IN THE TREATMENT OF CANCER

As has been seen in the review of the series of conferences on cancer as late as 1967, 1968, and 1969, a great deal of patient fear and depression is observed by physicians during the treatment phase of cancer. Material has been presented in the literature which indicates that three important psychological factors should be understood to meet the emotional needs of the cancer patient. First, the treatment team should be aware of the intimate meaning of the psychological impact of a cancer diagnosis to the patient and his family. Second, the anxiety aroused by the unknowns surrounding treatment in cancer as well as the fear of mutilation should be well understood by those in close contact with the patient and his family. Finally, the physician must be aware of the significance of the doctor-patient relationship in the course of cancer. Each of these psychological variables is summarized below.

PSYCHOLOGICAL IMPACT OF CANCER

Inasmuch as cancer seems to be synonymous with the concepts of pain, mutilation, and death, the diagnosis evokes psychological responses in keeping with the intimate meaning of the disease to the patient, and in keeping with his realistic knowledge of the disease and its process. It is, however, vital that the physician be aware of the possible range of meaning that the diagnosis of cancer may have for the patient in order that he may work effectively with the patient and his family. Renneker (1957) classified these emotional responses to the impact of the diagnosis of cancer into three phases:

1) Emergency, shock reaction to the suspicion or fact of cancer and its consequences.
2) (a) early, usually short-term adaptive measures for dealing with the trauma, and (b) beginning means of coping psychologically with the basic threat to life.
3) Long-term adaptive patterns of dealing with the basic threat to life.

As a physician works with his cancer patient, he usually finds him in the first phase—that is, in shock and disbelief, often accompanied by strong feelings of depersonalization. These feelings are sometimes expressed in such statements as, "This can't be happening to me," or, "They made a mistake, it is just a tumor." Often the feeling is not expressed verbally at all, but its psychological and physiological signs are present. If the doctor is alert to this fact, he will remember that the patient may not be absorbing the instructions he is given or the gravity of the situation.

As the shock wears off, the second phase sets in, and the counselor, nurse, and/or physician may observe early adaptive measures employed by the patient to cope with the treatment. Often the patient uses psychological defenses, such as denial or projection, in coping with this threat. Denial seems to be a common maneuver. It may be used for only a short period of time and then brushed away by reality. Or it may become a lingering retreat into which the patient withdraws until treatment or the growth of the cancer itself forces reality upon him. Often this patient will lose himself in hypomanic activities which exhaust his energies to the point that he cannot think of the reality of the diagnosis. One patient, facing the threat of an adrenalectomy in connection with prostatic cancer, concentrated upon the fact that he would have to take an adrenalin substitute each day and worried for fear he would forget to take his pill. He worked on ways and means of remembering this for ten days. When he solved the problem by deciding to place the number of pills representing the number of days in each month in a bottle the first of each month so he could count each day to be sure he had taken the pill, he fell into depression and then really faced the operation for the first time.

Depressive reactions are also common to the patient with cancer. This depression may serve the useful function of allowing the patient to mourn for his impending loss in terms of a changed body image or a threat to his well-being. Once the mourning period has run its course, he seems able to move forward to adaptation to the new body image and new goals. There are times, however, when the patient seems unable to work through this depression and achieve acceptance by himself. This patient needs referral to a therapist (be it a social worker, psychologist, or a psychiatrist) who may spend the time necessary in order to assist this patient who feels alone, unloved, and without hope to a hopeful acceptance of his disease.

The psychological impact of the diagnosis of cancer, then, is not a simple emotional stress. It is complex and it is deep. We should also remember that not all cancer patients go through the process described above. In fact, it has been observed clinically that some patients labeled as hypochondriacal at onset of cancer suddenly become more adjusted than they have ever been and relax with almost an unsaid "I have tried all these years to make you realize that I am sick, and now I have proof."

PSYCHOLOGICAL REACTIONS TO TREATMENT OF CANCER

Cancer often necessitates radical or mutilative treatment, either surgery or radiation. Emotional reaction to the threat of the treatment itself is often present. Ian MacDonald (1957) recognized the extreme of this reaction as the "Psychologically Inoperable Group." He explains:

It should be recognized that there are certain patients with lesions which are technically and biologically operable, but whose psyche is such that severe mutilative or exenterative surgery is so distasteful that death from disease is preferable to the prospect of continuing life with the intolerable sequelae of the contemplated procedure. Such patients constitute a small minority, but they should be recognized by the surgeon as a "Psychologically" inoperable group (MacDonald, pp. 555–56).

The unknowns surrounding the use of radiation create undue anxiety in the minds of many patients and their families. Careful preoperative instructions from the physician, nurses, or social workers may help avoid many of these reactions. The fact that radiation is harmful is difficult to conceal in assisting the patient to understand how he can be radiated and not harmed. The fact that the treatment machines are housed in shielded enclosures and that the patient is left alone while the radiologist observes through a small window is frightening. Often the room "feels" strange to the patient because it is soundproofed from the shielding structure. Even small clicking sounds made by the machines may become unbearable if the patient does not hear them as an expected occurrence. Radioactive iodine is surrounded with an aura of mystery and fear because when given it tastes like a glass of water. But the precautions surrounding the giving of it are frightening to the patient. Cobb (1958) told of a patient whose family had visualized her unattended in a room with radioactive beams shooting all around her after she had taken radioactive iodine. This anxiety was produced because the doctor had told them not to go into her room to visit for a certain number of hours after she had had the radioactive cocktail. These fears are intensified by lay articles reported in newspapers and magazines. MacDonald (1957) recommends a period of psychological conditioning for the patient and his family to offset these fears.

This psychological conditioning according to MacDonald should include three phases. First, the physician should carefully outline the type of treatment to be employed and the resultant "deformity or physiological disruptions" the patient should expect. Second, an individual who has undergone the contemplated procedure may be introduced to the patient. This becomes a reassuring factor, and the patient may ask questions he hesitates to ask the physician. Third, family members should be briefed separately from the patient in order to assist them to become a bulwark of emotional support for the patient. Each of these factors will be briefly discussed.

The briefing on the treatment schedule should be reassuring but accurate. Cobb (1960) reports a case where such careful briefing resulted in early recuperation from radical surgery. A fifteen-year-old girl was faced with the trauma of hemipelvectomy. Her concern was focused more on her horror of becoming limited to a wheelchair than on the loss of the limb. She was first carefully instructed as to the need for the surgery and the relief from the pain she had endured that it would bring. She was then told that she could be walking on crutches as soon as she felt ready to learn to manipulate them. As soon as the wound healed, she was assured, she would have an artificial limb tailored just for her. Her acceptance of the operation and the challenge to walk again were gratifying to the physician and psychologist and reassuring to the family members. Within fifteen days after the operation, she was manipulating the crutches and walking quite well. Although a limb was made for her, it was seldom used. She lived naturally and richly for the some eighteen months after surviving the operation, continuing school activities on her crutches.

Another patient, a man faced with a surgical procedure for prostatic cancer, was briefed by his physician as to the nature of the operation. He did not ask questions, but did not understand how the procedure could possibly be accomplished; so he withdrew from medical treatment and went to a quack practitioner, who promised him instant healing. Some six months later, when no miracle had occurred and his condition was growing more critical, he again presented himself for medical aid. By that time the disease process had spread to the point that surgery was no longer feasible.

The confidence the patient has in his physician and the care with which he is briefed on the treatment to be employed play an important role in the recovery of the patient. This explanation is the foundation of psychological conditioning.

Bringing an individual who has undergone the procedure to be employed to speak with the patient is often reassuring. Sometimes, however, it can result in augmented anxiety. One beautiful young woman (Cobb, 1958), who was told she must have her voice-box removed, panicked. In good faith, a man who had learned esophageal speech following such an operation was sent to visit with her. His restored voice was raspy and reminded her of Donald Duck's. She was so repulsed that she retreated into a transient neurotic conversion which had to be treated for several months before the cancer could be excised.

More often, however, the cancer patient can reassure the individual recently diagnosed more effectively than anyone else. In fact, the organization of "Cancer Anonymous" has been suggested by a number of patients and physicians as having a strong potential in the psychological conditioning of the cancer victim and his family.

The third item conducive to psychological conditioning of the patient for radical treatment procedures in cancer is the careful briefing of family members. Not only does the family need to know the extent of the deformity and the resulting physiological and psychological disruptions, but they also need to be aware of a frank prognosis for the patient. By preparing the family members and giving them an opportunity to express their shock and grief, the physician, or the psychologist, may be able to guide them toward the role of emotional support the patient will surely need.

Unassisted, a family member may become a most important element in sustaining the emotional strength of the patient, or he may become a detrimental influence.

A husband whose wife was dying of cancer visited her each day with cheerful stories and, at great emotional expense to himself, a smile on his face. One day the wife lashed out at him, accusing him of not caring if she died since he was always happy. Stunned and anguished, he stumbled into the office of the psychologist, and after a time blurted out his story. After thinking through his actions and gaining insight as to how his behavior might affect his wife, he decided the thing to do was to level with her as to how much it hurt to see her suffer, and then help her to think of other things. He did this. She relaxed in the knowledge of his love, and together they shared the sorrow of impending separation. When "acting out" his "feeling" that he must be cheerful at any cost, the husband was actually adding to the anguish of his dying wife. When he could share her sorrow, he gave her the emotional support she sought.

All of the fears just reviewed have to do with the extensive treatment involved. This phase also carries with it the anxiety provoked by loss or damage to parts of the body. The woman with cancer of the breast or cancer of the cervix undergoes psychological stress revolving around the symbolic meaning of this loss to her "womanhood." To lose a breast is for many women loss of sexual attractiveness. The husband of one patient reported to Cobb (1959) his reaction of repulsion to the scar following surgery, which led to his rejection of his wife and a divorce. This man fought the feeling, but simply could not love a woman he felt to be disfigured. This may be an extreme example, but it may also be repeated many times. A woman needs reassurance of love when faced with a loss such as this. Another patient reported by Cobb (1959) spent her last night, before the operation for cancer of the cervix, in her wedding gown. Her quiet statement, "I feel this is the last night I will be a whole woman" belied the turbulence of her grief.

This emotional impact of the loss of an organ is not limited to women. It is a traumatic experience for men to have prostatic surgery when there is a threat of loss of sexual activity. There is mourning of the loss of a limb. Certainly there is psychological distress when there is facial disfigurement, as in cancer of the neck or face. The loss of a voice and the resulting discordance of esophageal speech is mourned by the patient. All of these traumas must be considered in the treatment of the whole person.

The treatment phase is an anxiety-producing experience for a cancer patient. The treatment team should be aware of the misinformation he may have, the psychological meaning of the treatment prescribed, emotional meaning surrounding the organ involved, and include information and reassurance as a part of the treatment plan.

THE SIGNIFICANT ROLE OF THE DOCTOR-
PATIENT RELATIONSHIP IN CANCER

The relationship with the doctor is probably more important to the cancer patient than in most illnesses. Often the physician is perceived by the patient as literally standing between him and a certain death. Fear of death, of severe and mutilating treatment and combat with all the unknowns surrounding cancer, can be debilitating physically as well as psychologically.

It is to the doctor that patients turn for information and reassurance. Usually, they want to know what can be done for them, and how and when it will be done (Cobb, 1952). Uncertainty only adds to the anxiety.

Controversy continues among physicians as to whether a patient should be told he has cancer, or not told. Many doctors do not want their patients told because they fear it will be detrimental to their responses to treatment. Others say that the patient should be told the truth.

MacDonald (1957) states that the discerning physician can soon separate his patients into three general groups: the "emotional cripples," who may need some shielding from the truth of their condition; the "tough guys," who demand the "undiluted truth" or will not cooperate in treatment; and the "intermediate majority," who have received some factual information and had their questions answered.

While we consider the urgent need of the patient for a genuine relationship with his doctor, the physician himself and his emotional response to the patient and to the disease must not be forgotten. Cancer is a baffling disease. Its cause eludes scientific understanding. Because he cannot "cure" the disease, the physician may have a depressive reaction to the diagnosis, a reaction that may be misinterpreted by the patient as disinterest or lack of hope.

The physician's response to the patient and his needs is draining, both physically and psychologically. A close working relationship with deeply troubled, frightened, and life-threatened patients demands a strong yet loving ego. It also demands a great deal of time. Under these circumstances it is truly understandable when the physician seeks to remain professionally distant from the patient. But the patient suffers from this psychological avoidance.

If the doctor-patient relationship is important to the individual with a cancer diagnosis, how much more urgent is the relationship when that patient enters the terminal stages. There are times when the physician seems to forget how great the need for emotional support grows as death approaches. As long as the doctor calls, shows interest, and seems to care, the patient feels he is not fighting alone. He draws hope and comfort from the presence of "his" doctor. If the physician is traumatized by the downward course of the patient, and his own inability to change this course, the patient can accept the fact. If the doctor stays away, or rushes in and out of the room, the patient feels rejected. As long as the physician shows he cares and is there to help in any way possible, the patient hopes and grows to accept death.

This emotional responsibility must also be shared by the family and close friends. The clergy can possibly be of great assistance. Sutherland (1957) said, "The patient's attitude toward his own death must be fortified by religion or other philosophies." With the medical care and emotional support of "his" doctor, family, friends, and minister, the patient can face death, and may even welcome it as a peaceful release from pain.

The consensus of opinion seems to be that in cancer, probably more than in any other disease, the doctor's psychological role is an extremely important one. It is also agreed that this role is emotionally laden and time consuming. It is a role that each physician must recognize, in accordance with his professional image and his interactions with his patients.

REHABILITATION OF THE CANCER PATIENT

Rehabilitation begins with the medical diagnosis and definitive treatment of the cancer patient, but complex psychosocial and vocational problems brought about by the ravages of the disease and radical treatment are not transient. They are permanent. The ultimate goal of return to optimal functioning—physical, mental, and social—may often be blocked by residual psychosocial and vocational factors.

Pursuing this thought, in order to build effective rehabilitation programs in cancer, four urgent areas of need were highlighted in the previously mentioned National Interdisciplinary Conference (Healey, 1971). First, an overwhelming need for education of physicians, nurses, and paramedical members of the treatment team was stressed, as well as family and community instruction. Second, dissemination of knowledge was identified as a major problem in rehabilitation. Third, specific research needs dealing directly with cancer in this interface area of medicine, psychology, and rehabilitation counseling were enumerated. Fourth, it was pointed out that to meet all these needs extensive financial support was mandatory.

EDUCATION FOR EFFECTIVE REHABILITATION

Members of the Conference (Healey, 1971) pointed out several times that perhaps the greatest stumbling block in the rehabilitation of the cancer patient is educational in nature. They not only called for added stress on cancer in the education of medical students but also pointed out that education of the physicians in the field was a paramount need. This educational urgency also extends to the allied groups. The average nurse, psychiatrist, psychologist, dentist, physical therapist, etc., does not know enough about this complex disease to feel comfortable, professionally or personally. Certainly, the vocational rehabilitation counselor (the latest member of this team) needs intensive and extensive instruction in the medical and psychosocial aspects of cancer.

Beyond this team educational need looms the dearth of accurate information for the family members of the patient and the members of the community in which he must live out his span of life.

Some effort has been expended in the education of the team members. At the University of Texas M. D. Anderson Hospital, Houston, and in other cancer research hospitals throughout the country, short-term courses for nurses, physicians, volunteers, and just recently for rehabilitation counselors, have been held. These courses have been well attended and enthusiastically received, but the need for additional training is still massive.

Public education has been the goal of the American Cancer Society for a number of years. Much has been accomplished. Much remains to be done.

DISSEMINATION OF CANCER KNOWLEDGE

Lack of communication and dissemination of knowledge is a major deterrent to rehabilitation. A pertinent question is—how can knowledge about cancer best be disseminated to treatment team members and to the public?

In the Cancer Conference (Healey, 1971) it was pointed out that the busy physician is difficult to reach, and the logical solution would be to give him information when he needs it. A Fact Bank where stored information could be secured by dialing a phone was suggested as a possible means of reaching the doctor.

An alternative approach could be direct public education through the lay press. For such a program, professionals in the field of public relations, promotion, and communication should be utilized.

Interinstitutional cooperation could also improve dissemination of knowledge through joint sharing. This method should extend to intrahospital as well as interinstitutional instruction.

PSYCHOSOCIAL RESEARCH TOPICS

That basic research on the cause and treatment of cancer should continue full speed was understood by all participants in the Conference. But a number of pertinent research topics were discussed at length that might well bring into the team approach the research skills of the psychologist, sociologist, and epidemiologist, and other professionals.

Research on attitudes, the quality of success, the team approach and specific roles of its members, and goals of rehabilitation were enumerated as pertinent investigations. Each will be summed up briefly below.

Research on attitudes. In cancer this is a provocative topic. The prevailing pessimistic and defeatist attitude toward cancer held by physicians and patients alike is one of the greatest deterrents to successful rehabilitation. Attitudes are nebulous though powerful. Careful investigation should be initiated to elucidate the effects of such attitudes, how they came into being, and how they may be counteracted.

What happens when the patient is released from treatment and returns to his home community? Does he pick up life and move forward to productive endeavors? Or, does he find rejection and disillusionment awaiting him? Although the treatment hospitals usually keep contact with a patient over a five-year period, the focus seems to be on the physical condition of the patient and the control of the cancer, rather than the status of the total person.

This area of research in *quality of success* might well be a cooperative effort between the physicians and the rehabilitation counselors. The counselor will be in the district to which the patient returns. He can play an important role in assisting the patient back into the stream of productive living. And, he will know the community and have opportunity to enhance the understanding of potential employers, co-workers and family members "back home."

Research on effective team approach. Here the well-trained psychologist or sociologist can make a valuable contribution. The focus of the research might well be to clarify the functions and roles of the various members of a multidisciplinary team approach to total rehabilitation of the cancer patient.

An important fringe benefit of such research would be the education of the various members of the team as to the skills, techniques and approaches of all the disciplines involved. From this experience could then come accurate educational efforts in the dissemination of knowledge gleaned.

Certainly, the role of the rehabilitation counselor should be studied carefully in such an investigation. This knowledge could then be applied in the development of the rehabilitation counselor as a valuable member of the cancer treatment team.

Although efforts directed toward the total rehabilitation of the cancer patient are at present woefully inadequate, a start has been made. It is a new endeavor for the rehabilitation agencies; it is a new experience for the physicians. To be successful it calls for concerted teamwork. Miller (Healey, 1971) points out that perhaps the key to total rehabilitation of the patient is the awareness by the physicians that emotional and vocational blocks are present in the lives of their patients. Added to this must be their awareness of the contributions the psychologist, medical social worker, and rehabilitation counselor can make toward the total rehabilitation of their patients as well as of the importance of these 'new' disciplines as professional members of the team. When the physician can accept this fact, the patient's emotional problems can be worked through, the rehabilitation counselor can work with the positive assets of the individual, the patient can set up realistic goals, and the employer and co-workers can receive information and support essential to successful job performance of the rehabilitated cancer patient.

THE COUNSELING ROLE

Work with the cancer patient involves a strange dual role for a counselor. The first, adjustment counseling, is concerned with such factors as control of anxiety, acceptance of the diagnosis and treatment, and knowledge and emotional support to cope with the physiological limitations and/or disfigurement that are so often permanent residuals in cancer. In the second, counseling for death, the acceptance becomes adjustment to the inevitability of death, and emotional support as the individual faces the realistic agony of stark separation trauma.

ADJUSTMENT COUNSELING

The role of the adjustment counselor in cancer is more complex than with the usual emotionally disturbed patient. First, in cancer the counselor must have a depth knowledge of the disease itself. Cancer is not a simple entity. It is many diseases in that its diagnosis, course, and prognosis varies with the organ or system involved. Treatment is complex and tends to change rapidly with new research findings. The physician on the case must be well-known to the counselor and his philosophy and treatment plan respected at all times. Actually, the counselor becomes an extension of the physician. He assumes the role of interpreter, in the course of which he often finds he needs to interpret the doctor and his treatment prescriptions to the patient and vice versa to communicate the patient and his needs to the physician. All of these factors must be considered prior to and during the regular assignment of exploring and lessening the anxieties of the patient.

If the concept of psychological resistance to cancer discussed above is accepted, the counselor's challenge is to combat anxiety in order to free the energies of the patient to fight the onslaught of the disease. The antidote seems to be "hope through intelligent coping with facts can conquer fear" (Cobb, 1953).

The new counselor questions, how may one build this hope under the dire threat of cancer? Cobb (1952) reported pertinent guidelines for the counselor to explore with the patient in order to set up a plan of action. First, before misconceptions and false fears may be corrected, the counselor must learn the intimate meaning of cancer to the individual with whom he is working. Second, the psychological meaning of the organ invaded must be explored before the debilitating anxieties can be understood. Third, often the counselor will find that the threat of the strange, new horizontal world of the hospital is as anxiety producing as the diagnosis. With these emotionally laden feelings from his patient and the medical facts from the physician on the case at hand, the counselor may turn to his major task of replacing "feelings" with facts and lending emotional support during treatment and convalescence or until death, as the case may be.

INTIMATE MEANING OF CANCER

Before the counselor can understand the anxiety he senses in the patient and initiate hope as a foundation for acceptance, he must know the personal meaning that cancer holds for that individual. Research (Cobb, 1959) has disclosed that cancer means many things to diverse people. Approximately 12 per cent of a group of patients studied seemed not really able to comprehend the diagnosis. To them they had a "bad disease." Twenty-six per cent held a vague, diffused fear of cancer, and their anxiety seemed free-floating rather than focused on the disease per se. Ten per cent verbalized an intelligent, knowledgeable fear because they knew about cancer, its treatment, and realistic chances for survival or demise. To the remaining 52 per cent of the sample studied, cancer meant simply death.

One young man of some twenty-one years had been in treatment for a number of months, but had not been told specifically that he had a form of cancer. After one period of hospitalization his insurance slip was returned to his address indicating the amount paid on the hospital expense. He glanced at the slip and a word jumped up at him, "Hodgkin's Disease." He pulled down a medical dictionary and looked for the definition of the term. It was there, "cancer" . . . "prognosis: probably two to five years." He recalled blacking out at the impact. As he returned to consciousness, a thought would come to mind—he would remember—then "gone—all gone" would chase the bright spot away and dark, threatening, imminent death took its place. After some time, he thought of his doctor and actually started running toward the hospital. Fortunately, he did not live too far from the hospital. He burst breathless and almost incoherent into the doctor's office and demanded to know the truth.

To this patient cancer meant "death." Had he been conditioned psychologically at the outset of treatment, the shock would not have been so great. His confidence in the physician and the staff was badly shaken by this incident. It took several months of hard work and much unnecessary anguish to work through his chaotic feelings and arrive at acceptance, faith, and hope.

Sometimes the anxiety experienced by the patient is based on fantasy, and is hence unnecessary. One young woman undergoing radiation therapy as part of the treatment schedule for cancer of the cervix suddenly became hysterical. Upon referral, the psychologist learned she had half overheard members of the staff talking and thought they had said she was pregnant but that the treatment would kill the baby. When she was reassured, the hysteria was no longer present.

A number of patients became nauseated when radiation therapy was administered. The number suffering from nausea greatly decreased when careful explanation of the machine and the soundproof room in which it was housed was made. Again, psychological conditioning for treatment was effective.

THE ORGAN INVOLVED

As was indicated earlier, the organ involved by the cancerous growth may pose a severe emotional problem to the patient. The loss of a breast is always a deep ego blow to a woman. She needs extra support from her counselor, but even more so from her husband. Here the psychologist must work through this trauma with both. Not only does the husband need to express and work through his fears and feelings, but he also needs help in learning to assume the supportive role for his wife. A number of couples are not able to cope with this problem, and a divorce ensues. Many, however, with insight and real desire, live through the crisis together and emerge with a deeper relationship than ever before.

Men also experience deep anxiety when the mutilation of the organ involved threatens their manhood. Cancer of the prostate poses such a problem to some individuals. Again with the help of an informed counselor, or physician, and the loving support of an insightful wife, this problem can be faced successfully.

Facial disfigurement, a scar on the neck from a radical thyroidectomy, the loss of a limb, obesity caused by chemotherapeutic agents used, all these and countless other individualized traumas need to be known to the counselor, aired for catharsis, and replaced by acceptance and hope.

The basic emotion with which the counselor must come to grips is anxiety. In the cancer patient, anxiety may be based on realistic fears with which the patient must learn to cope. It may also be based on misinformation or fantasy. In either case, the counselor must work in the light of knowledge of the depth feelings of his client and the possession of correct information to supplant the erroneous before he can build the foundations of hope, faith, and acceptance.

THE HORIZONTAL WORLD

The new counselors may be amazed to find that even well-educated and highly intelligent adults often find the horizontal world of the hospital baffling and anxiety provoking. Several factors are at work here. First, the adult is precipitated into enforced dependency. Often this arouses fear that comes out as hostility, uncooperative behavior, and varied management problems on one end of a continuum, and whining, wheedling dependency on the other. It is not easy for an independent, self-sufficient man or woman to shift gears to dependency and uncertainty in a strange new hospital world. The indignity they feel perpetrated upon them by many of the medical procedures is a great psychological stress. The unknowns surrounding what the medical staff may consider routine procedures add much to the emotional discomfort of the patient.

Once again, the psychological conditioning of the patient can add much to the comfort and adaptation of the patient, as well as to the smoothness of the physician's schedule.

COUNSELING FOR DEATH

If the counselor has come to terms with death himself, he can be more comfortable working with the acute anxieties impending demise activates in the client. This is not to say that he is to impose his own philosophy, or truce with death, on the patient. It does prevent much uneasiness within the counselor as he allows the individual to come to his own terms with extinction.

To counsel for acceptance of death is at once devastating and richly rewarding. No sensitive, empathic counselor can work with the deep emotional concerns of an individual facing certain death without reeling at times under the impact of the unyielding bludgeon of time running out. It is fulfilling because at no other time in the life of man is the need for emotional support, for understanding, even for moments of diversion, more urgent, than when an individual comes to the "bend in the road" beyond which inevitable death awaits.

When a counselor first meets face to face the challenge, and the urgent need, to work with a patient preparing to die, his inclination is to bolt. He tends to rationalize, "I don't know what to say," or "I might say the wrong thing." Far too often the physician, the family, and even close friends of the patient utilize this same defense. The patient, then, is left to face the traumatic experience alone. So, the counselor gathers his courage around him and listens, and grows emotionally himself as he does so. He learns that it is not so much *what* he says, as it is *caring* for the patient, and by *being there,* giving the emotional support the dying person so desperately needs.

The goal in this counseling for death is still to give emotional support to the point that the patient can gain insights, face his problem, and work through it to some semblance of peace within and without. Each individual must work out his own reconciliation with the "grim reaper" just as he had to resolve his life problems in his own characteristic way.

If the patient has always met his life problems head on and fought fiercely to overcome them, he is likely to meet death in the same way. Cobb (1962) speaks of a man who in his terminal days kept quoting the following lines from Browning's "Prospice":

> I was ever a fighter so—one fight more,
> The best and the last!

And he died fighting, asking no quarter, and never verbally admitting the possibility that he might die.

A gentle, wonderful old gentleman, on the other hand, looked upon death as a door of release through which he would walk to a richer life without pain or heartache. When his time came he went as William Cullen Bryant's line in "Thanatopsis" reads,

> Like one who wraps the drapery of his couch
> About him and lies down to pleasant dreams.

Often, the patient is preoccupied with unfinished business. Meeting financial obligations, planning for the future of loved ones, making their "going" easier on their families—all these are often concerns that need to be shared with someone. Sometimes, the dying individual hesitates to discuss these problems with those close to him because it hurts both the patient and the family member so very much. Often, the patient will even ask the counselor's help in ways and means of making the departure easier for the family.

There are those who have a need to deny the approach of death. Certainly, the counselor respects that need, and lets the patient lead. If the patient seems to feel an urgency to explore the possibilities of his death, he should be allowed to do so without the counselor attempting to reassure him falsely that he will live. Neither should the counselor present a hopeless picture; hope is always present. Realistic hope can be offered based upon persistent efforts to treat the disease and the possible cure based on research always under way.

Each individual must be considered as a separate entity when he is preparing for death, but Cobb (1962) suggested three general rules applicable to "a successful interpersonal relation with the person facing death."

First, to listen is the cardinal rule. A warm, emphatic listener is often all the patient needs to start his journey through his fears, his treatment, his family, and finally the courage to look at death.

One patient experienced a terrible recurrent nightmare for weeks. In this nightmare, it was dark, and she sensed an awesome presence behind her. Terrified, she would start running. The faster she ran, the closer the presence seemed to get, and finally a calm voice would say, "You can't escape me—turn around." At this point her horror would wake her. She reported this nightmare consistently several times to her counselor, with no seeming insight as to its meaning. She was young, beautiful, and just beginning to live. To admit that death was near was too traumatic to verbalize. Finally, the counselor asked her once more "What do you think the meaning of this dream could be?" She thought for a moment, drew herself up with quiet dignity, and said, "I know what it means. It's death hovering over me, and I can't outrun it." She then started making peace with death, "got her house in order" she said, and never had the nightmare again. The counselor did not interpret the dream. The patient did the interpretation when she was ready.

Second, correct information can be supplied by the counselor. Sometimes the dying patient wants to know more about additional treatment. Sometimes he wants to know about side-effects of the medication. Quite often, the patient reaches a point where he wishes to speak with a clergyman. When the patient so indicates, the counselor can arrange such a visit.

At times the dying man wishes to talk about death itself. Cobb (1962) reports an incident where a man, who had endured lingering pain for eight years, asked "What do you have to do to die? I've been so near to it and pulled out, and the pain was so terrific, that it scares me. I just don't believe I can stand to die" (Cobb, p. 255). This patient was reassured when told that death does not always mean a painful struggle, that it could be a gentle release from pain. The counselor was grateful that when death came to this patient, it was as gentle as going to sleep.

Third, the counselor can "stand by" emotionally and physically. This is no "rose garden" for the counselor, for the individual preparing for that long journey is probably the loneliest person in the world. The counselor becomes a warm human contact with life. Often a touch on the shoulder, or hand, soothes the "weary wanderer between two worlds" (Cobb, 1962).

The psychologist, or counselor, might well ask "What kind of behavior can be expected as the patient waits for death?" In cancer this is an extremely pertinent question. With constant research, new drugs and treatments are initiated from time to time. At times, these new techniques seem literally to "drag one back from the brink of the grave" (Cobb, 1962). For a few days, or weeks, even months, the patient can live an almost normal life. This rejuvenation brings on episodes of false hope. Eventually, the disease takes over again and rebellion, bitterness, and despair seem dominant. After this fleeting miracle has happened a time or two, the mature person, who is working toward psychological conditioning for death, learns to accept the joy of the reprieve, and to bow to the inevitable, when their Indian summer is over. These fortunate individuals go to meet death with dignity and humility. "As they meet life, each individual must also face death in his own way" (Cobb, 1962, p. 257).

A most important facet of counseling for death is the preparation of the family for this tragic separation. It is in these long hours of "waiting for the call" (Cobb, 1958) that the patient desperately needs the support of family. Too often, the family member is so distraught that he cannot contain his own sorrow let alone absorb the mourning of the dying.

One instance, reported by Cobb (1959), told of a young mother of four who was told by her husband (a former mental patient) that he wished she would hurry up and die, that he couldn't stand the drawn-out ordeal of her getting better, then worse—still knowing she could not survive. The only other member of her family to whom the counselor seeking emotional comfort for the patient could turn was her mother. In fifteen minutes of conversation with the mother, the counselor perceived that she was an alcoholic.

A concerned minister who had known the patient for several years, and in whom she had great faith, became her "support" along with the counselor. When the day of her death arrived, and the physician told the counselor, the husband and mother (who had not visited the patient for over a month) were called and urged to come. After protests of "I can't stand it!" they were persuaded to come. The counselor will always remember the happiness mirrored on the patient's face when she exclaimed "Just look who came to see me—my little mother and my husband!" Two hours later she was gone.

In most families, however, there is at least one member strong enough to stand by with comfort and love. Often the total family, even the children rise to the occasion, and give splendid support to the patient. In such cases, the desire to help, to give of themselves, brings the family circle closer as the members face a common threat. This "giving" to one they love serves as a psychological conditioning for the impending separation, and when death comes acceptance is already near.

Counseling for death, then, is listening and giving unselfish support and warm understanding to the patient and his family. It is permeated by shared sorrows and sparked by unforgettable moments of splendor when a patient, or family member, rises to peaks of selfless love in attempts to shield the other. It is a depth experience which lends comfort and eases anxiety in the hearts of the patient and those who love him, and to the counselor it adds a depth of humility, and realization of the courage and dignity of all mankind.

REFERENCES

Abrams, R. D. and J. R. Finesinger. 1953. Guilt reactions in patients with cancer. Cancer 6:474–84.

Adler, Alfred. 1963. Individual psychology. Paterson, N.J., Littlefield, Adams.

Alexander, Franz. 1950. Psychosomatic medicine. New York, W. W. Norton.

Blumberg, E. M., P. M. West, and F. A. Ellis. 1954. A possible relationship between psychological factors and human cancer. Psychosom. Med. 16:277–86.

Cobb, B. 1952. A social psychological study of the cancer patient. University of Texas, unpublished Ph.D. dissertation.

—— 1959. Emotional problems of adult cancer patients. J. Am. Ger. Soc. 3:274–85.

—— 1955. Review of the highlights of a decade of psychological research in cancer, in R. L. Clark, Jr. and R. W. Cumley, eds., Year book of cancer. Chicago, The Year Book Publishers.

—— 1960. Some implications of psychological stress in cancer. Blackwell Memorial Lecture (unpublished), County Medical Society, Sherman, Texas.

—— 1958. Unpublished case notes. M. D. Anderson Hospital and Tumor Institute, Houston, Texas.

—— 1962. Cancer, in James F. Garrett and Edna S. Levine, eds., Psychological practices with the physically disabled. New York, Columbia University Press.

Dunbar, Helen Flanders. 1955. Mind and body: psychosomatic medicine. Rev. ed. New York, Random House.

Fisher, Seymour and Sidney Cleveland. 1956. Relationship of body image to site of cancer. Psychosom. Med. 18:304–9.

Greene, William A., Jr. 1954. Psychological factors and reticuloendothelial disease: I. Preliminary observations on a group of males with lymphomas and leukemias. Psychosom. Med. 16:220–30.

Greene, William A., Jr., Lawrence E. Young, and Scott N. Swicher. 1956. Psychological factors and reticuloendothelial disease. II. Observations on a group of women with lymphomas and leukemias. Psychosom. Med. 18:284–303.

Grinker, Roy R. 1956. Toward a unified theory of human behavior. New York, Basic Books.

—— 1956. Unpublished notes on Conference on Psychosomatic Aspects of Cancer, The University of Texas, M. D. Anderson Hospital and Tumor Institute, Houston, Texas.

Healey, John E., Jr., ed. 1970. Ecology of the cancer patient. Washington, D.C., The Interdisciplinary Communication Associates.

Huggins, C. B. and C. V. Hodges. 1941. Studies in prostatic cancer: effect of castration, of estrogen and of androgen injections on a group of women with lymphomas and leukemias. Psychosom. Med. 18:284–303.

Kowal, S. J. 1955. Emotions as a cause of cancer. Psychoanalytic Review 42:217–27.

——1956. Depression as a forerunner of cancer. Unpublished paper. M.D. Anderson Hospital and Tumor Institute, Houston, Texas.

Krasnoff, A. 1959. Psychological variables in human cancer: a cross validation study. Psychosom. Med. 21:291–95.

LeShan, L. and R. Worthington. 1955. Some psychologic correlates of neoplastic disease. J. Clin. Exp. Psychopath. 16:281–88.

—— 1956. Personality as a factor in the pathogenesis of cancer: a review of the literature. Brit. J. Med. Psychol. 29:49–56.

Luthe, Wolfgang. 1956. Unpublished notes on Conference on Psychosomatic Aspects of Cancer, The University of Texas, M. D. Anderson Hospital and Tumor Institute, Houston, Texas.

MacDonald, Ian. 1957. Psychologic reactions to radical cancer treatment, in R. L. Clark, Jr. and R. W. Cumley, eds., Year book of cancer. Chicago, The Year Book Publishers, pp. 552–56.

Renneker, R. and M. Cutler. 1952. Psychological problems of adjustment to cancer of the breast. J. Amer. Med. Assoc. 148:833–38.

Renneker, R. 1957. Psychologic impact of cancer, in R. L. Clark, Jr. and R. W. Cumley, eds., Year book of cancer. Chicago, The Year Book Publishers, pp. 547–52.

Sutherland, A. M. 1952. Psychological impact of cancer surgery. Public Health Reports 67:1139–43.

—— 1957. Psychologic care of the cancer patient, in R. L. Clark, Jr. and R. W. Cumley, eds., Year book of cancer. Chicago, The Year Book Publishers, pp. 556–57.

West, P. M. 1954. The origin and development of the psychological approach to the cancer problem, in J. Gengerelli, and F. Kirkner, eds., The psychological variables in human cancer. Berkeley and Los Angeles, University of California Press.

—— 1957. Psychologic factors and host resistance in cancer, in R. L. Clark, Jr. and R. W. Cumley, eds., Year book of cancer. Chicago, The Year Book Publishers, pp. 542–46.

West, P. M., E. M. Blumberg, and F. W. Ellis. 1952. An observed correlation between psychological factors and growth of cancer in man. Cancer Research 12:306–7.

Wheeler, J. I., Jr. and B. M. Caldwell. 1955. Psychological evaluation of women with cancer of the breast and cervix. Psychosom. Med. 17:256–68.

JOHN NAUGHTON

CORONARY HEART DISEASE *

CORONARY HEART DISEASE (CHD) describes the many varied clinical manifestations associated with atherosclerosis of the coronary arteries. The manifestations include angina pectoris, myocardial infarction, cardiac arrhythmias, congestive cardiac failure, and sudden death. A minority of investigators, this author numbered among them, prefer the term Ischemic Heart Disease (IHD) since the clinical manifestations sometimes occur in the absence of obstructive atherosclerotic lesions in the coronary arteries. Nevertheless, it is now appreciated that atherosclerosis begins in early life, at least as early as puberty, and progresses at an insidious and undefined rate over a long period of years (Enos, Holmes and Beyer, 1953; McNamara, Molot, Stremphe, and Cutting, 1971). The causal relationship of coronary atherosclerosis to disorders of myocardial function is not understood. Since it is well-established that the majority of victims of CHD have extensive obstructive disease of the coronary arteries (Baroldi, 1966), most investigators are satisfied that mechanical impedance of blood flow by plaques, thrombi, or emboli is the most likely mechanism of myocardial dysfunction.

Since World War II many investigators have attempted to unravel the mysteries of Coronary Heart Disease. Despite their apparent failure to identify etiology, they have contributed greatly to the understanding of the pathogenesis and the natural history of the disease process. Epide-

JOHN NAUGHTON, M.D., is Professor of Medicine and Director, Division of Rehabilitation Medicine, The George Washington University Medical Center, Washington, D. C.

* A glossary of medical terms is given on pp. 235–36.

miologists (Keys, Taylor, Blackburn, Brozek, Anderson, and Simonson, 1953; Kannel, Cartelli, and McNamara, 1967) contributed by identifying the "coronary prone" subject by enumerating the so-called risk factors. Included among the identifying marks are an elevated systemic blood pressure, elevation of the serum lipids (cholesterol and triglycerides), excessive obesity, diabetes mellitus, a family history of heart disease, heavy cigarette smoking, a sedentary living pattern, and certain personality traits. These factors can be identified oftentimes many years before an actual cardiac event. While the presence of any single factor increases the risk of eventually suffering from heart desease, the combination of two or more increases the possibilities several fold over the low risk enjoyed by the person devoid of these factors. Many investigators have speculated that successful modification of these factors will reduce the incidence of CHD and have developed a field of medicine identified as Preventive Cardiology. In contrast to the field of Rehabilitation Medicine, their efforts are directed toward the care of patients without identifiable impairment.

INCIDENCE

The manifestations of Coronary Heart Disease number in excess of two million new events annually in the United States. The disease process is the leading cause of death in the United States and the Western Hemisphere (American Heart Association, 1971). Its toll is highest in the middle-aged population and in men in a ratio of 9:1 over women. The acute death rate approximates 20 to 30 per cent of the total victims; the risk of death being greatest during the early minutes and hours of illness. The total annual direct and indirect cost in the United States approaches thirty billion dollars, a figure comparable to the peak annual expenditures for the Vietnam conflict. Obviously, CHD provides a great challenge and responsibility to Rehabilitation Medicine.

CARDIAC REHABILITATION

Cardiac rehabilitation is a process whereby a patient is *restored to* and *maintained at* his optimum physiologic, psychologic, vocational, and social status. Implicit in this process is the institution of those measures which will prevent progression of the underlying disease process and the development of additional impairment (Editorial, 1969).

The rehabilitative process may be instituted at any of several points in the natural history of CHD. The most obvious starting point is at the onset of myocardial infarction, but those patients with any degree of impairment manifested by angina pectoris, latent myocardial dysfunction, or arrhythmias also require rehabilitative care. The extent, form, intensity, and duration of care varies from patient to patient.

MYOCARDIAL INFARCTION

For most CHD victims, cardiac rehabilitation begins with the awareness of an acute cardiac event, usually myocardial infarction. This event is a pathological process in which myocardial muscle is destroyed by an ischemic process and the patient is impaired for a period of time ranging from as short a duration as six weeks to lifelong. The severity and duration of impairment are usually related to the extent of the muscle damage, but in many instances, it may be accentuated and aggravated by psychological rather than by physical limitations.

The rehabilitation process is divided into four stages as follows:

Stage 1   Coronary Care Unit (CCU)
Stage 2   Cardiac Rehabilitation Unit (CRU)
Stage 3   Convalescence
Stage 4   Recovery

STAGE 1

A CCU is a geographical unit equipped with specialized electronic devices for patient monitoring and staffed by specially trained physicians, nurses, and allied health personnel.

A suspected cardiac patient is usually admitted directly to this unit, and if myocardial infarction is documented, he remains there for three to seven days depending upon the seriousness of his illness and the demand for admission to the unit. While there, his cardiac rhythm is monitored continuously, and should any disturbance in rhythm occur, appropriate treatment, such as cardiac defibrillation or resuscitation, is instituted.

The Coronary Care Unit (CCU) concept has added enormously to the rehabilitation process by decreasing the mortality rate from disturbances of cardiac rhythm. A recent study reported that the mortality rate on a CCU was 17 per cent compared to a rate of 35 per cent for patients treated in open hospital wards (Hoflendahl, 1971).

While in the CCU a patient's physical activity is limited markedly. If uncomplicated and clinically stable, he is permitted to use a bedside commode for stool evacuation and by the fourth or fifth day post-infarct he is allowed to sit at the bedside to eat his meals. Socialization is usually limited to short visits by his wife and a few close friends.

STAGE 2

The Cardiac Rehabilitation Unit (CRU) is an equally specialized unit located near or in juxtaposition to the CCU. Those patients with an uncomplicated and stable course and with rehabilitation potential are transferred to the CRU. Initially, cardiac rhythm is monitored as the patient adapts to a less dependent environment, thus insuring immediate intervention if required.

A Cardiac Rehabilitation Unit (CRU) provides an environment in which each patient's ambulatory program is monitored and in which appropriate counseling of patient and spouse is rendered when warranted. The ambulatory program is increased in a gradual and progressive manner from day to day. The guidelines which dictate whether the level of activity is too severe include the onset of symptoms such as shortness of breath, chest pain and light-headedness, a heart rate in excess of 120 beats per minute, the onset of cardiac arrhythmia, or an unstable electrocardiogram (ECG). The health-care team documents these items after a patient has progressed through each new level of activity. In general, patients are actually capable of performing at higher levels of activity than are customary during this period. The average uncomplicated patient can sit erect in a comfortable chair for periods of thirty to sixty minutes, eat at his bedside, attend to his self care, and take short walks in the hospital corridor without incident by the time he is ready for discharge from the hospital.

The Cardiac Rehabilitation Unit stage begins with a patient's transfer from the Coronary Care Unit and usually terminates on the 21st or 25th day post infarct. More impaired patients require a longer hospital stay and many uncomplicated patients will be hospitalized for as short a stay as 16 to 18 days. Lown and Sidel (1969) have suggested the possibility of decreasing the hospital stay for uncomplicated patients to 12 days. This attitude contrasts sharply with that of only a decade ago, when most cardiologists insisted that the hospital phase of myocardial infarction should be minimally 42 days.

The accelerated care of myocardial infarction patients has caused some investigators to question whether detrimental effects are associated with it. Burch and DePasquale (1966) in particular have stressed the importance of considering a patient's limitations as well as his potentials, and have advised wisely that every physician should remember that it is possible to rehabilitate a patient without rehabilitating his heart. The converse is also possible, and obviously successful rehabilitation demands skillful evaluation and judgment. Despite expressed fears that accelerated programs of ambulatory care might be associated with an increased incidence of cardiac complications such as ventricular aneurysms and congestive cardiac failure, a controlled study reported that patients ambulated early were at no greater risk of developing these complications than were patients treated in a more traditional care program (Groden, 1971). The implication is that late complications of myocardial infarction are related to the amount of cardiac muscle destroyed by the ischemic process rather than to the ambulatory efforts.

While hospitalized in a CRU the patient and his spouse can receive appropriate counsel regarding dietary regulation, physical activity, sexual activity, life style, and the myriad of other questions that might come to mind. The role of the spouse is stressed in the rehabilitation process because it is she who usually buys and prepares the meals. While the role of nutrition is still undefined, each patient and spouse should have an opportunity to have their questions answered. It is generally accepted that for those patients who are overweight weight reduction should be encouraged. In this situation the nutritional counseling might be limited to that of developing a calorically balanced diet. This oftentimes will suffice to correct abnormal lipid elevations. For those patients with specific abnormalities of their lipid profiles, the dietary regimen might require curtailment of carbohydrate intake.

Good rapport and counseling is especially required for those spouses whose attitudes differ significantly from those of the health care team. It is well established that if the attitudes of the physician are diametrically opposed to those of the patient or family the efforts put forth by the health team will be thwarted when the patient returns home (New, Ruscio, Priest, Petritsi, and George, 1968).

In some institutions the CRU counseling is administered by health professionals to the patients in groups under the supervision of a physician, and in others it is still handled between physician, patient, and spouse.

STAGE 3

Convalescence begins with discharge from the hospital and lasts until a patient returns to work. Its duration usually ranges from the third-thru the eighth-week post-infarct. During this stage the patient recuperates at home, and the immediate care of the patient is transferred from the health team to the spouse and family members.

At home the patient can continue to care for himself, eat meals with the family (unless the generation gap is conflict laden), perform routine paper work, and take short walks in the house, yard and neighborhood. The spouse's role is active and reinforcing in this stage. In addition to modifying any dietary requirements, she can monitor the patient's response to varying stressful stimuli, such as physical activity, by counting the heart rate at rest and at the end of each new level of effort. She should encourage the patient to achieve a level of stress which will increase the heart rate to a level ranging from 110 to 120 beats per minute, and should advise that he decrease the magnitude of the effort if the heart rate exceeds 120 beats per munute. Should she detect an irregularity in rhythm, she should notify the physician.

STAGE 4

Recovery begins with a patient's return to work. It may be as early as six weeks in a few instances and as long as fourteen weeks for other patients, but generally begins at the eighth week. Initially, a patient returns to part-time employment, gradually increasing his working day over a period of two weeks. Again, the level to which he progresses is dictated by the presence or absence of symptoms and can be monitored physiologically by an occasional measurement of the heart rate.

Prior to entering the Recovery Stage each patient is re-evaluated by his physician. This evaluation includes: (a) an appropriate history to elicit the presence or absence of adverse symptomatology; (b) a physical examination to detect additional abnormalities; (c) a standard ECG recorded at supine rest; (d) a chest x-ray for determination of heart size; (e) and the performance of either a single-stage or progressive multistage exercise stress test. The latter is not pursued if the history and physical examination suggest a worsening of the patient's cardiovascular status.

EXERCISE TESTING

The application by clinical medicine during the past two decades of principles developed by exercise physiologists in the early part of the twentieth century has enhanced the advancement and refinement of the rehabilitation process. The development of standardized exercise tests provided a tool with which to measure the cardiovascular adaptation to varying levels of physical stress. The results are used to provide the patient with appropriate guidelines for the performance of physical activity. The introduction of exercise stress testing has had as important an impact on cardiac rehabilitation as has the introduction of the CCU to the acute care of the myocardial infarction patient.

Exercise tests (Masters and Oppenheimer, 1929) were first introduced as a diagnostic tool in clinical medicine, and over a long period of years their value in adding to the diagnostic yield of latent or overt ischemic heart disease was well substantiated. The indications for an exercise stress test now include: (a) the diagnosis of heart disease in patients with unexplained chest pain; (b) the evaluation of an individual's fitness for either work or sport; and (c) the evaluation of the effects of a specific therapeutic intervention or of a particular rehabilitative regimen (World Health Organization Technical Report, 1968).

In the clinical situation, exercise stress tests are administered preferably in a hospital facility. Bicycle ergometers, motor-driven treadmills, or steps can be used to administer a test. Each instrument offers certain advantages and disadvantages in terms of space, expense, and psychological stimulation. In the United States the treadmill is gaining popularity, whereas the bicycle ergometer is used almost exclusively in Europe. Regardless of the instrument employed, the principles used in the design and administration of an exercise stress test are similar. They include the following:

a) Every patient must have an appropriate history and physical examination prior to performance of the test.

b) A control ECG is recorded during supine rest and compared with the previous records.

c) Each patient is informed of the indications for the test, its potential hazards, and that it will be discontinued if he or she becomes symptomatic or if the physician detects evidence of adverse physiological adaptation.

d) Each test is preceded by a "warm-up" at a very low level of effort followed by a short recovery period of two to three minutes.

e) The initial workloads are relatively minimal in terms of the usual patient's peak work capacity, and the energy requirements are added gradually at periodic intervals to maintain as aerobic a performance as is possible.

f) Criteria used to terminate a test include attainment of a predetermined peak heart rate adjusted for the patient's age, the onset of arrhythmias, the development of ischemic ST-T changes, failure to increase the systolic blood pressure, and undue tachycardia.

Of the exercise stress tests developed during the past twenty years, some were of a continuous design in which each workload was added without a rest period. Others employed an intermittent design in that a rest period was interposed between each new workload. A continuous test has the advantage of conserving time, whereas the intermittent test allows the physician to make more critical observations about the patient's adaptation to each workload.

In our laboratory a motor-driven treadmill is used almost exclusively. In order to assure a testing situation which is flexible and applicable to individuals varying from the very limited to the maximally fit, the following procedure is utilized.

If the subject to be evaluated is a cardiac patient, his warm-up is accomplished while walking on the treadmill on a level grade at a speed of 1.0 mph for three minutes. During this performance, a physician observes the patient's ability to adapt to the pace of the machine as well as looking for evidences of physiologic maladjustment. This short walk is followed by a three-minute period of recovery. The patient then begins walking on a level grade at a speed of 2.0 mph. Thereafter, the workload is increased by elevating the slope of the treadmill bed 3.5 per cent every three minutes. Each workload approximates an additional increment of the resting metabolic state (MET), that is 2, 3, 4, and so on, times the energy cost of rest. He performs at each workload for three minutes to insure the development of a near physiologic steady state and to make appropriate clinical observations. This test is terminated if the patient becomes symptomatic, develops adverse signs, or negotiates a workload of 7 METS (2.0 mph on a 17.5 per cent grade; O_2 equivalent 21.5 ml/kg/min).

Patterson, Naughton, Pietras, and Gunnar (1972) reported that a performance capacity of 7 METS or greater correlated with that of Functional Class I as defined by the New York Heart Association (1964); 5 to 6 METS with Functional Class II; 3 to 4 METS with Functional Class III; and 2 METS or less with Functional Class IV. These findings are comparable to the approach to functional evaluation reported by Turrel and Hellerstein in 1958. A workload of 7 METS requires from 7.5 to 8.5 kcal per minute. A patient who performs at this level without the onset of symptoms or other adverse findings can perform most of the jobs currently available in the United States. For those patients whose job might require a higher level of sustained work the stress is increased to approximate the job situation. Admittedly, in a mechanized society there are few jobs whose demands are that strenuous. To induce a higher level of physical stress, the treadmill bed is lowered to a slope of 12.5 per cent and the speed increased to three miles an hour after the subject completes the 7 MET workload. This new level approximates 8 METS, and thereafter the speed is held constant while the slope is increased by 2.5 percent increments every three minutes. Again, each new workload increased the energy expenditure about 1 MET.

Since most healthy, sedentary middle-aged men have a peak capacity of 10 to 11 METS, and because most patients are tested at submaximal thresholds, there is little practical value for the practicing physician to employ a test design whose peak demands exceed 12 METS. The above approach to testing provides a flexibility in design which prevents the necessity of the patient running or trotting or of walking against an insurmountable grade.

PARAMETERS MEASURED DURING EXERCISE

An adequate appraisal of a patient's work capacity necessitates the recording of at least a single lead ECG and the measurement of the systemic blood pressure and heart rate during each physiologic state. In addition, we routinely record a single lead ECG, a phonocardiogram and a carotid pulse contour at supine rest immediately before and after exercise for the measurement of the pre-ejection period (PEP), and the left ventricular ejection time corrected for heart rate (LVET$_c$).

THE EXERCISE ECG

There is more information available concerning this parameter than any other usually recorded in association with an exercise stress test. In

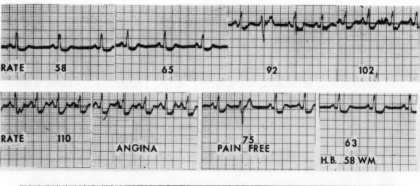

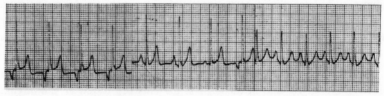

FIGURE 1. A normal exercise ECG response (lower tracing) is compared with an abnormal tracing. In the lower ECG tracing the P-wave is inverted while the patient is at rest, and becomes upright with exertion; there are no abnormal changes reflected in the QRS complex, ST-segment, or T wave. Characteristic depression of the ST-T wave indication of an ischemic response together with the appearance of premature ventricular contractions were recorded in the patient HB during exercise.

the normal situation the major changes observed on an exercise ECG are an increase in heart rate, slight elevation of the T-P baseline, and a reciprocal displacement of the ST segment at the J-junction which lasts less than 0.08 seconds. In many cardiac patients some portion of the resting ECG complex is abnormal. During exercise, each abnormal ECG complex should not change significantly from that recorded at rest. The most frequently documented abnormalities induced by exercise are depression of the ST segment in excess of 0.1 MV lasting longer than 0.08 seconds with or without inversion of the T-wave; increased conduction delay resulting in a prolongation of the QRS interval; or the onset of arrhythmias, particutarty frequent premature ventricular contractions. The onset of any of these ECG features during exercise is considered an abnormal response. Figure 1 depicts a normal and an abnormal ECG response associated with exercise testing.

SYSTEMIC BLOOD PRESSURE

Systolic and diastolic blood pressure are measured by the auscultatory technique. The systolic blood pressure normally increases in proportion to the intensity of the physical stress. We have measured a mean elevation of 7.3 mm Hg per MET in healthy subjects, and consider an elevation in excess of 15 mm Hg per MET as excessive and abnormal. In some patients with limited myocardial reserve the systolic blood pressure may fail to increase or may actually decrease. Such responses are also abnormal.

The diastolic blood pressure is not as accurately measured by the auscultatory technique as is the systolic blood pressure. Despite this handicap, there are ample data available to characterize its relative response. The usual adaptation is for the diastolic blood pressure to remain near the measurement recorded at rest (sedentary subjects and patients) or to decrease gradually as the magnitude of the physical stress is increased (athletes). If the diastolic blood pressure increased more than 10 mm Hg above that recorded in the control state, this is considered an abnormal response.

HEART RATE

The heart rate is the easiest and most accurate parameter to measure during exercise. The normal reaction is for the heart rate to increase in proportion to the magnitude of the work task. In an athlete the rate of elevation approximates four heart beats per MET; in sedentary subjects eight beats per MET; in grossly obese subjects twelve beats per MET; and in severely impaired patients as high as sixteen beats per MET. An elevation in excess of twelve beats per MET is considered abnormal. Figure 2 displays the character of physiologic responses recorded in two healthy men contrasted with two cardiac patients.

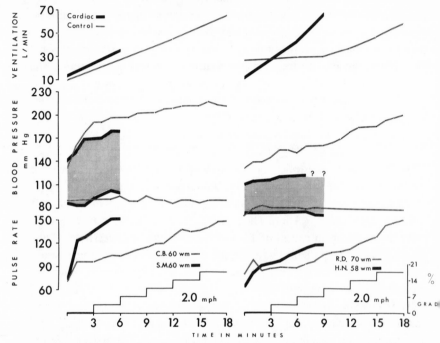

FIGURE 2. The physiologic responses of heart rate, blood pressure, and minute ventilating at rest and during exercise are compared between two healthy subjects and two cardiac patients. The work capacity of the two patients was severely limited. In addition, the character of the blood pressure response measured on patient RD was abnormal, as was the heart rate response in patient SM.

SYSTOLIC TIME TENSION INDEX (STTI)

Hellerstein (1968) reported that the STTI adequately reflected the myocardial work associated with exercise. This parameter represents the product of the systolic blood pressure and the heart rate. Its value is consistently higher in the cardiac patient than in the healthy subject while performing at comparable levels of submaximal exercise, a finding which indicates that the myocardial efficiency is reduced or impaired in cardiac patients. In addition, cardiac patients cannot achieve as high an STTI at peak workloads as can healthy subjects.

THE PHASES OF SYSTOLE

The pre-ejection period (PEP) is of longer duration and the left ventricular ejection time is corrected for heart rate (LVET$_c$) of a slightly shorter duration in cardiac patients than in healthy subjects at supine rest (Whitsett and Naughton, 1971). The PEP shortens in response to physical stress in both healthy subjects and cardiac patients, and therefore does not provide discriminatory information.

The LVET$_c$ provides discriminatory data which reflect the myocardial contractile state. This measurement is essentially unaltered in duration following physical stress in sedentary healthy subjects, while its duration shortens following exercise in healthy physically conditioned athletes (Naughton and Leach, 1971). However, the LVET$_c$ prolongs slightly following exercise in asymptomatic patients with healed myocardial infarction (Whitsett and Naughton, 1971) and markedly in patients with angina pectoris and cardiomyopathy (Pouget, Harris, Mayron, and Naughton, 1971). A shortened duration reflects acceleration of the rate of myocardial performance, whereas a prolongation indicates evidence of myocardial dysfunction. This measurement apparently provides a valuable adjunct to the appraisal of the cardiac patient whose other parameters may not be significantly abnormal during exercise.

The development and refinement of exercise stress testing provides a clinical tool for the frequent and periodic evaluation of cardiac patients by atraumatic, noninvasive techniques. As long as each patient is tested in the same manner, a determination as to whether or not his condition is stable, deteriorating, or improving can be made.

THE DEVELOPMENT OF ACTIVE
REHABILITATION PROGRAMS

The introduction of exercise stress testing confirmed the clinical observations that many patients with healed myocardial infarctions use the same physiological mechanisms to adapt to physical activity as do otherwise healthy subjects (Chapman and Fraser, 1954). These observations led to the hypothesis that cardiac patients would respond to physical conditioning in a manner similar to healthy subjects.

During the past fifteen years many reconditioning programs were conducted (Naughton, Lategola, and Shanbour, 1966; Tobis and Zohman, 1970; Rechnitzer, Yuhasz, Pickard, and Lefcoe, 1965; Varnauskas, Bergman, Houk, and Bjorntorp, 1966; Gottheiner, 1968) and the results reported. At least two of the programs were of an extended duration. The approach to reconditioning varied slightly from study to study, but in general, the programs utilized the principles of aerobic performance and did not use isometric exercises. In our programs, each patient was introduced to a regimen of walking, mild calisthenics, and throwing a basketball back and forth to his partner for the first month. As each patient's ability to tolerate more strenuous physical effort increased the walking was interspersed with fifteen to twenty seconds of jogging, the calisthenics became more arduous, and the patient was allowed to participate in ball games. The proportion of time spent walking to jogging was gradually decreased, and by the end of four months most patients were able to jog a distance of one-half mile continuously in a period of time that ranged from five to six minutes. The core attraction of the activity was the volley ball participation. The game permitted a certain degree of socialization, allowed the patients an opportunity to express a competitive spirit, and provided a form of intermittent training.

A patient's progress from one level to the next was gauged by the presence or absence of symptoms, the quality of his work-capacity evaluation, or by the quality of the responses documented while the patient was participating in the activity program. The latter is ascertained by recording an ECG and heart rate via telemetry (Figure 3).

Most patients attained a training level at which they utilized from 150 to 300 kcal per hour. The level of activity performed during ball games was regulated by matching patients with individuals of comparable skill and fitness. If the competitor excelled in fitness, he could obviously stress a patient unduly. One patient was monitored while playing "bounce ball" with five different subjects on five different days (Figure 4). The average heart rate of the patient ranged from 140 to 150 beats per minute while playing with others, while it varied from

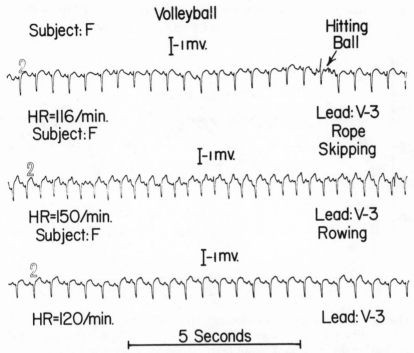

FIGURE 3. A telemetered ECG tracing recorded while a patient performed different types of exercise is depicted. The heart rate level ranged from 116 beats per minute during volley ball to a high of 150 beats per minute while skipping rope. Despite the high heart rates, the ECG response was normal.

100 to 120 beats per minute when the patient was opposing a patient of comparable clinical status. It is important for those healthy subjects who supervise the physical reconditioning of cardiac patients to remember that each patient's work capacity is limited upon entering an activity program.

Patients must be protected in an exercise program just as they are in the hospital and in the laboratory facility. Each participant is taught to perform cardiorespiratory resuscitation and how to react to an emergency situation. The gymnastic facility is equipped with emergency drugs and a DC defibrillator. The program is conducted under the supervision of a physician, and the allied health staff is trained to act as his agent in the program.

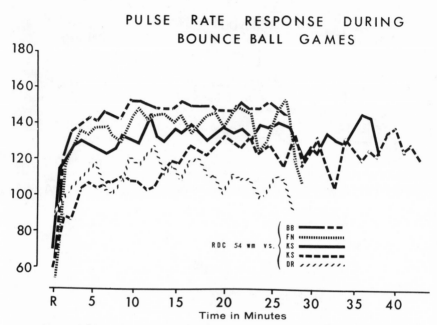

FIGURE 4. Patient RDC was monitored while playing a "bounce ball" game with healthy subjects of varying degrees of physical fitness. The figure depicts the wide variation in mean heart rates when playing with DR, a physically untrained subject compared to playing with BB, a physically fit subject.

Since many communities and medical centers lack a centralized facility in which to conduct group-exercise programs, many patients are given prescriptions and counsel for a home program by their physicians. In these instances the patient usually purchases a stationary bicycle, and is advised to increase the resistance to pedaling to that level which will produce a heart-rate response that approximates 60 to 70 per cent of that achieved during the exercise stress test. Such home programs are usually conducted for fifteen minutes a day.

Although a group program seems preferable to an individual one, this has not been substantiated. A group program always poses the problem of the ideal duration of participation. The usual approach is to recondition a patient to a predetermined level of physical fitness and to discharge him after three to four months to perform at this level independently from then on. However, since the underlying atherosclerotic process may occasion other complications in due time, some investigators have advocated an open-ended approach to physical reconditioning in which patients always perform vigorous exercise under medical supervision. It is apparent that if regular physical activity is warranted in the care of the cardiac patient, new types of facilities located in geographic proximity either to the patients' job or home must be constructed and staffed. In some cities facilities such as a YMCA or school gymnasium could be used. In addition, post-graduate training programs must include experience in exercise stress testing and in the conduct of exercise programs.

The results of physical reconditioning programs for post-myocardial infarct patients are amazingly similar from investigator to investigator. They include:

a) A decrease of the heart rate level at rest and while performing at comparable levels of energy expenditure;

b) a decrease of the systolic blood pressure at rest and while performing at comparable levels of energy expenditure;

c) a significant increase in physical working capacity;

d) a decrease in the STTI at submaximal work levels indicative of improved myocardial efficiency;

e) improvement in the ECG;

f) a shortening rather than an increase of the LVET $_c$ after exercise;

g) an improved state of well-being; and

h) significant modifications of behavioral and social patterns.

The data reported to date indicate that regular physical activity by cardiac patients significantly attenuates the morbidity. However, appropriate control studies from which to judge the effects of physical reconditioning on mortality are lacking. Gottheiner (1968) reported evidence of a decreased mortality rate in the active patients compared to sedentary patients, but a longer controlled-population study must be performed to determine the efficacy of regularly performed physical exercise.

SEXUAL ADJUSTMENT

The attitudes toward the sexual life of the post-myocardial infarct patient have changed just as dramatically during the past twenty years as has the posture toward early ambulation, exercise stress testing, and active rehabilitation programs. In the past, most physicians hesitated to concern themselves with a patient's emotional problems, especially if sex were the topic. This apparent omission in patient care was probably related to a multitude of factors, some of which included an appalling absence of scientific information dealing with the topic; an unconscious or unexpressed fear on the part of the physician that he might harm the patient psychologically, physiologically, or both; and the realization that counseling might require long and valuable time. In retrospect, this unwillingness on the part of a physician seems paradoxical, when one appreciates that most physicians are married, have fathered two or more children, and are considered "coronary prone."

More information concerning the marital adjustment of cardiac patients and the effects of a myocardial infarction on sexual performance is still needed. However, there is every reason to reassure the cardiac patient that he can expect to return to a normal sexual adjustment when he recovers. Hellerstein and Friedman (1970) reported that the return to sexual adequacy is related to the seriousness of the illness and to the presence or absence of symptoms. They reported that most cardiac patients resumed sexual relations from eight to fourteen weeks post-infarct, with the average asymptomatic patient resuming this activity at about eleven weeks and the symptomatic patients at sixteen weeks.

When monitored while engaging in sexual activity, cardiac patients were found to attain mean peak heart rate responses during orgasm of 117 ± 4.2 beats per minute, with a high in one patient of 144 beats. These levels of heart rate are maintained for ten to fifteen seconds at most and are followed by a return to 85.0 ± 3.9 beats during the second minute of the resolution phase. These data indicate that the peak oxygen cost of sexual activity requires a level of four to five METS with an average energy expenditure of three to four METS throughout the entire performance. These levels of oxygen utilization represent a modest degree of physical activity, and suggest that sexual activity can be engaged in by most patients with healed myocardial infarctions.

Some patients withdraw from sexual activity because of fear of dying. Again, there is a paucity of information with which to reassure the cardiac patient, but that which does exist is encouraging. Ueno (1963) reported that coital death occurred in only 34 of 5,559 cases of endogenous sudden death. Twenty-eight of the deaths occurred in men, and in eighteen the cause was of an apparent cardiac origin. Of the 34 deaths, 24 were related to extra-marital sexual activity, and were associated with an excess of alcohol consumption as well. It seems appropriate to state that the patient who desires to enjoy sexual activity in a compatible marital relationship runs little risk, while the patient who places himself in a potentially stressful environment increases the risk of a fatal cardiac event.

Impotence is another complication that may occur to the post-infarct patient. While Hellerstein and Friedman did not document any episodes of impotence in their series of 48 patients, instances of impotence related to the use of pharmacologic preparations such as tranquilizers (Greenberg, 1965; Pouget, *et al.*, 1971) and cardiac glycosides (Anderson, 1966) and in association with the psychological reaction to the illness are reported. While most instances of impotence are transient and can be handled adequately by the primary physician, some will require formal psychiatric counseling.

BEHAVIORAL FACTORS IN
CORONARY HEART DISEASE

Cardiac impairment of any type in an individual who was previously healthy and unlimited leads to a series of emotional reactions which in themselves might produce severe limitations and disability. However, before a physician attempts to rehabilitate a patient psychologically, it is imperative that he have an understanding of the antecedent behavioral pattern of the patient. To date this is one of the lesser explored areas in CHD.

Friedman and Rosenman (1959) contributed a valuable concept to the role of behavior in the pathogenesis of CHD when they reported that patients with CHD possess (1) a tense, sustained drive to achieve self-selected but usually poorly defined goals, (2) a profound inclination and eagerness to compete, (3) a persistent drive for recognition and advancement, (4) a continuous involvement in multiple and diverse functions constantly subject to time limitations (deadlines), (5) a habitual propensity to accelerate the rate of execution of many physical and mental functions, and (6) an extraordinary mental and physical alertness. These features characterize Personality Pattern Type A, while those patients who lack these qualities are classified as Personality Pattern Type B. The classification was further refined into categories A_1, A_2, B_3, and B_4 (Rosenman, Friedman, Straus, Wurm, and Kositchek, 1968).

Since the introduction of the Type A and Type B concepts, these same investigators have reported that in prospective studies the Type A patient not only has an incidence of CHD that approximates six times that of the Type B subject, but at autopsy the Type As have six times as severe coronary arterial atherosclerosis (Rosenman, *et al.,* 1956).

Several other investigators studied other aspects of behavior in CHD patients, and their results have supported the concepts developed by Friedman and Rosenman. Cathey *et al.* (1962) reported that cardiac patients oftentimes characterize their lives as a burden in which even success is viewed with a certain degree of dissatisfaction. They are prone to accomplish tasks "the hard way," that is, they make a task appear as work even when it is not. These investigators likened this pattern to that of Sisyphus, the Greek mythological figure who was condemned to a life of rolling a rock to the top of a hill. Every time he neared the summit, the rock rolled back down. The CHD patient was thus viewed as one "who never quite made it."

Brozek, Keys, and Blackburn (1966) administered the Minnesota Multiphasic Personality Inventory (MMPI) and the Thurstone Temperament Index (TTI) to professionals and businessmen as they began a prospective study of the influence of risk factors on the development of CHD. All subjects of the study were healthy at entry. In the ensuing years it was found that the men who succumbed to CHD had scored higher on the "hypochondriasis" scale (MMPI) and on the "Activity Drive" scale of the TTI than did the healthy subjects, who correlated with the Type A concept.

The above studies indicate that behavioral patterns must be considered a "risk factor" together with those factors previously enumerated, and they indicate that successful rehabilitative intervention must be directed at the patient's perception of his life style.

The immediate emotional impact of myocardial infarction manifests itself in depression and anxiety. These symptoms are often expressed as fear of impending death, concern over unmet obligations, and focusing on issues in the home situation which may be unrelated to the illness. The severity of the psychological impact is often blunted during the CCU Stage, when patients are constantly reassured by the presence of the staff and the continuous monitoring. However, when discharged to an open area, many patients develop overt manifestations of depression and anxiety. Klein *et al.* (1968) reported a significant elevation of cat-echolamines in CHD patients during this transition period, a finding which correlates with the patient's anxiety and insecurity. In most instances these emotional reactions are alleviated by strong reassurance on the part of the physician. However, many patients do not make their feelings known, and therefore the physician does not concern himself with them. It is well advised that the physician take a few moments each day to explore these areas so that hazardous reactions are prevented at a later date (Hackett, Cassem, and Wishnie, 1968).

The depth of the emotional reaction usually lessens as the patient's symptoms abate. However, in those patients whose precoronary personality profiles were characterized by a significant degree of depression and hypochondriasis, the cardiac event may aggravate these features to the extent of producing prolonged or permanent psychological impairment. These patients may require formal psychiatric therapy. It is very likely that many of the patients who succumb to premature and unnecessary retirement following an episode of myocardial infarction were so predisposed prior to the event. The cardiac illness simply provided the necessary catalyst to bring the reaction about.

If the patient does possess Personality Pattern A, then it is imperative that he be made aware of its features so that the characteristics might be modified. Thus far, no control studies are available concerning the effects of formal psychotherapy in modifying the personality pattern. However, Bruhn, Lategola, and this writer (1968) reported that actively rehabilitated CHD patients modified their total life style even though physical exercise was the only overt therapeutic approach employed. The sedentary patients decreased only their level of cigarette smoking. These results suggested that physical activity provided a fulcrum around which patients became more health-conscious and then modified their life style in a favorable direction. In addition, these findings demonstrated that a significant reduction in the mortality rate of exercising cardiac patients would be due to factors other than the exercise per se.

Even the selection into an active rehabilitation program is related to the precardiac behavior pattern. Patients who volunteered and adhered to the program for three months or longer invariably had a history of participation in vigorous physical activity either in the high-school or college years. Those patients who maintained or reduced their preinfarct activity levels following recovery were usually of a sedentary habitus in puberty.

The mortality statistics (Gertler, White, Simon, and Gottsch, 1964) provide ample reason for the physician to provide an optimistic psychologic picture for CHD patients. Pell and D'Alonzo (1964) reported an over-all death rate of 30 per cent in 1,331 industrial employees. Of the deaths, 25.2 per cent occurred in the first hour; 6.3 per cent during the next thirty days; and only 1.5 per cent in the second month. Of the thirty-day survivors, 90.5 per cent were alive at the end of one year. It appears that the outlook for the patients who make it to a CCU and who survive more than twenty-four hours is generally good. There is little apparent reason for a physician to reinforce a patient's dependence or levels of depression and anxiety if his clinical course is uncomplicated.

RETURN TO WORK

A primary goal of comprehensive cardiac care is the restoration of the patient to his previous occupational adjustment. The success rate is related in part to the application of the physiological and psychological techniques alluded to previously, and in part to a patient's perception of and desire to return to the job.

Most patients with uncomplicated clinical courses are able to return to those job situations which are clerical, administrative, and not physically strenuous. However, in a bureaucratic society it is often the emotional circumstances associated with the job situation rather than the physical requirements of the work which act as a deterrent to vocational rehabilitation. This is particularly true in the case of supervisor-employee conflict. When such deterrents exist (Pearson, 1963), counseling with the employer to identify a new level of responsibility and performance is warranted. If the job conflict cannot be resolved, then it is appropriate and warranted to refer the patient to a vocational counselor for prevocational evaluation and job retraining. The latter is often difficult to achieve in those CHD patients who are forty-five years of age and older because of current social attitudes toward the aging. However, there are many occupational roles in which CHD patients can perform well if an opportunity were provided. These include jobs as laboratory technicians, hospital messengers, librarians, practical nurses, and medical ombudsmen.

There are probably some job situations for which a myocardial infarction contraindicates continued performance. These include occupations in which a population group is placed at additional risk because of the unpredictability of some of the severe complications of the atherosclerotic process, namely sudden death. A myocardial infarction patient should not be re-employed as a commercial pilot or bus driver. He can, however, drive his own car and perform any occupational task which will not unduly jeopardize public safety. Since psychological reactions can affect physiological responses, those patients in whom a question of adverse adaptation needs resolution can be studied while they wear a portable monitoring device such as a Holter ECG (Hinkle, Meyer, Stevens, and Craver, 1967). While doing this each patient keeps a diary of those events which disturb him or which are associated with the precipitation of symptoms. The ECG is recorded for a period of hours and is scanned afterward. If adverse disturbances of cardiac rhythm or the onset of ischemic ST-T changes are detected which bear a relationship to job stress, the patient should be counseled to make appropriate adjustments or to do something else. If the ECG response is normal even in relation to stress, the patient is counseled as to adapting to the situation.

Pell and D'Alonzo's data concerning employability of cardiac patients (1964) indicate that although the five-year survival rate for the thirty-day survivors approximates 75 to 80 per cent, a far lower percentage of patients was employed five years after myocardial infarction. They reported that 50 per cent of the salaried and 43 per cent of the wage earners were gainfully employed.

Weaver (1961) studied the rate of absenteeism of cardiac patients and reported that it was not significantly higher in patients than nonpatients. In fact, considering the number of additional cardiac events that occurred in the patient population, it appeared that the patients worked hard at not increasing their rate of absenteeism.

SURGICAL APPROACHES TO REHABILITATION

Major advances in surgical techniques altered the course of the lives of patients whose impairments were once considered irreversible.

The most dramatic advance was the introduction of coronary bypass surgery. In this procedure a strip of saphenous vein is removed from the patient's thigh and interposed between the ascending aorta and a point distal to a major atherosclerotic obstruction in the coronary artery. This procedure is indicated for patients whose performance capacity is limited by angina pectoris. While the long-term results of this procedure are not known, there is little doubt that premature retirement for many patients has been obviated.

Extensive cardiac surgery is often warranted for CHD patients whose conditions are complicated by large ventricular aneurysms and/or large areas of nonfunctioning heart muscle, and who have thus become cardiac invalids. Such procedures include excision of the diseased areas of the heart and approximation of the viable muscle tissue. Many patients in otherwise hopeless congestive heart failure have been rehabilitated as a result of such apparently heroic interventions. A few CHD patients have required artificial valves and obliteration of a perforated area of damaged heart muscle.

Patients with pathologically slow cardiac rates and/or with complete heart block have been helped enormously by the implantation of permanent cardiac pacemakers. Their implantation has decreased the one-year mortality rate in this patient population from 50 to 15 per cent, and has made it possible for many of the patients to resume full-time employment. These patients require close surveillance and periodic monitoring to insure against battery failure. When power failure is detected, new batteries are inserted under local anesthesia. The average life time of the batteries is about twenty months.

RESEARCH NEEDS

Although cardiac rehabilitation gained momentum as a science and as an adjunct to comprehensive patient care during the past decade, there are still many questions which await answering before the critical mass of the medical community will accept it as an asset.

Still unanswered is the question of the value of an organized CRU on the patient's ultimate outcome in terms of employment, modification of life style, and psychological performance. The approach is sound and feasible. But is it needed? Does it offer a better therapeutic outcome than do the traditional approaches to postinfarct care?

More critical examination must be applied to active rehabilitation programs. It is well-documented and generally well-received that regular physical activities produce definitive physiological changes in many patients in the directions desired. But exercise can be hazardous to a patient with impairment of his "power supply," (Naughton, Lategola, and Shanbour, 1970). Is the risk of chronic exercise worth it? Enthusiasts justify active physical intervention on the grounds that the quality of life is improved, and this in itself offsets the issues of longevity and mortality. Other investigators rightfully maintain a posture that preservation and extension of life are the principal goals to be achieved. The critical answers concerning the ultimate benefit or hazards associated with exercise therapy will require a large scale, long-term study of many thousands of patients. Although obviously arduous, this research must be done if the scientific community is to be properly reassured that this approach to cardiac rehabilitation is the wisest, safest, and most effective one.

Research in the area of cardiac rehabilitation should attempt to define the basic mechanisms responsible for the physiological and psychological changes which occur as a result of the process. Just as important is the exploration of those processes which mitigate against rehabilitation, whether they be organic, emotional, or environmental.

Detailed psychosocial investigation of the patient, the family, and the job milieu are also required to answer the many unresolved questions relating to the role emotional and environmental stimuli play in aggravating or modifying the degree of cardiac impairment.

Research into the development of programs of self-education of the patient and those individuals involved in cardiac rehabilitation is needed. It is well established that failure in patient care is often related to too little time spent in communication between patient and physician. The development of programmed education concerning the approach to dietary modification, physical activity, sexual adjustment, and return to work could obviate this apparent lack of comprehensive patient education.

A pharmacopoeia of physical activity must be developed to provide the guidelines required by physicians and allied health personnel charged with the responsibility of giving the patient an activity prescription and guiding its application. As more and more patients enter activity programs, the need for specific regimens in the form of an exercise prescription will become mandatory. Such an accomplishment will be realized only through a multicenter, collaborative research effort.

Research to determine those predictors which reflect progression of the atherosclerotic process or of additional impairment seems mandatory if cardiac patients are to be placed in positions of greater responsibility. Certainly, the destiny of the United States was guided by two men chronically at risk from another cardiac event or an episode of sudden death. How can lives such as theirs and of those they are charged to serve be better protected?

SUMMARY

Cardiac rehabilitation is a process designed to achieve optimal physiologic, psychologic, vocational, and social adaptation by the patient to his environment. It is an ongoing process designed to achieve health restoration, health maintenance, and further prevention of disability and of the underlying disease process. Cardiac rehabilitation requires the interest and interaction of cardiologists, psychiatrists, psychologists, surgeons, allied health professionals, patient, and family. The advances made in all of these areas during the past twenty years have justified the identification of a discipline known as Cardiac Rehabilitation.

GLOSSARY

ANEURYSM—A sac formed by dilatation of the walls of an artery, vein, or heart chamber. In myocardial infarction, the diseased area of heart muscle may become very thin and dilated, forming an aneurysm. Such disorders may participate paradoxically in response to myocardial contraction or they may not participate at all. The dilatation of the heart muscle is labeled a ventricular aneurysm.

ANGINA PECTORIS—Chest pain typically associated with heart disease. It is usually precipitated by exercise, over-eating, emotional stress, and exposure to cold, either singly or in combination.

ARRHYTHMIA—A variation of normal heart rhythm. It may denote a "skip-beat" due to atrial or ventricular extra-systoles or a more serious disturbance such as ventricular fibrillation.

ATHEROSCLEROSIS—A condition characterized by loss of elasticity, thickening, and hardening of the arteries.

AUSCULTATORY TECHNIQUE—The art of detecting blood pressure by eliciting the Korotkoff sounds.

CATECHOLAMINES—The pressor substances norepinephrine (noradrenalin) and epinephrine (adrenalin).

CONGESTIVE CARDIAC FAILURE—A term used to describe the clinical findings associated with a loss of cardiac reserve.

DEFIBRILLATION—The process of reversing an abnormal heart rhythm.

DIABETES MELLITUS—A condition characterized by an abnormal glucose tolerance and a deficiency of insulin production.

ELECTROCARDIOGRAM—A graphic tracing of the electric current which activates contractions of the heart muscle.

EMBOLUS—A clot or other plug brought by the blood current from a distant vessel and forced into a small one so as to obstruct the circulation.

ERGOMETER—A dynamometer on which work performance is measured.

HYPOCHONDRIASIS—Morbid anxiety about health, often associated with a simulated disease and more or less pronounced melancholia.

ISCHEMIA—Local and temporary deficiency of blood. In heart disease it describes those conditions which result from an insufficient flow of blood through the coronary arteries to the heart muscle. Prolongation of the process produces conditions such as angina pectoris and myocardial infarction.

LEFT VENTRICULAR EJECTION TIME (LVET)—The duration of ejection by the left ventricle.

LEFT VENTRICULAR EJECTION TIME CORRECTED FOR HEART RATE (LVETc)—Heart rate is corrected with a regression equation and added to the LVET.

LIPID—Refers to the fats and esters with analogous properties, and usually includes cholesterol, triglycerides, free fatty acids, and phosphatides.

MET—The resting metabolic oxygen consumption expressed as ml/kg/min. At rest the measurement approximates 3.5 ml O_2/kg/min. A person with a ten MET capacity, therefore, achieves a performance level of 35 ml O_2/kg/min.

PHONOCARDIOGRAM—A tracing or record of a patient's heart sounds.

PLAQUE—A patch of atherosclerosis which produces impedance to blood flow.

PRE-EJECTION PERIOD (PEP)—The duration from the onset of ventricular depolarization until the onset of ventricular ejection. This measurement includes the electromechanical events of that period.

RESUSCITATION—The restoration to life or consciousness of one apparently dead.

SYSTOLIC TIME TENSION INDEX (STTI)—An indirect measurement of heart work. It is the product of the systolic blood pressure and heart rate.

TACHYCARDIA—Rapid heart rate. At rest a heart rate in excess of 100 beats per minute.

THROMBUS—A plug or clot in a blood vessel or in one of the cavities of the heart, formed by the coagulation of blood and remaining at the point of its formation.

REFERENCES

Anderson, T. 1966. Digitalis induced impotence. Nordic Med. 75:334.

Baroldi, G. 1966. Myocardial infarct and sudden coronary heart death in relation to coronary occlusion and collateral circulation. Amer. Heart J. 71:826.

Brozek, J., A. Keys, and H. Blackburn. 1966. Personality differences between potential coronary and noncoronary subjects. Annals of the New York Academy of Sciences 134:1057.

Burch, G. and N. DePasquale. 1966. Potentials and limitations of patients after myocardial infarction. Amer. Heart J. 72:830.

Cathey, C., H. Jones, J. Naughton, J. Hammarsten, and S. Wolf. 1962. The relation of life stress to the concentration of serum lipids in patients with coronary artery disease. Amer. J. Med. Sci. 244:421.

Chapman, C. and R. Fraser. 1954. Cardiovascular responses to exercise in patients with healed myocardial infarction. Circulation 9:347.

Editorial. December, 1969. Exercise in the prevention, in the evaluation, and the treatment of heart disease. J. S. Carolina Med. Assoc. 65:supp.

Enos, W., R. Holmes, and J. Beyer. 1953. Coronary disease among United States soldiers killed in action in Korea. J. Amer. Med. Assoc. 152:1090.

Exercise tests in relation to cardiovascular function. 1968. World Health Organization Technical Report 338:5.

Friedman, M. and R. Rosenman. 1959. Association of specific overt behavior patterns with blood and cardiovascular findings. J. Amer. Med. Assoc. 169:1286.

Gertler, M., P. White, R. Simon, and L. Gottsch. 1964. Long-term follow-up study of young coronary patients. Amer. J. of Med. Sci. 247:154.

Gottheiner, V. 1968. Long-range strenuous sports training for cardiac reconditioning and rehabilitation. Amer. J. Cardiology 22:426.

Greenberg, H. 1965. Erectile impotence during the course of tofranil. Amer. J. Psychiatry 121:1021.

Groden, B. 1971. The management of myocardial infarction: a controlled study of the effects of early mobilization. New York Heart Assembly 1:4:13.

Hackett, T., N. Cassem, and H. Wishnie. 1968. The coronary care unit: an appraisal of its psychological hazards. New Eng. J. Med. 279:1365.

Heart facts. 1971. Amer. Heart Assoc., 44 East 23d St., New York, N. Y.

Hellerstein, H. 1968. Exercise therapy in coronary disease. Bulletin of the New York Academy of Medicine 44:1028.

Hellerstein, H. and E. Friedman. 1970. Sexual activity and the postcoronary patient. Archives of Internal Medicine 125:987.

Hinkle, L., J. Meyer, M. Stevens, and S. Craver. 1967. Tape recordings of the ECG of active men: limitations and advantages of the Holter-Avionics instruments. Circulation 34:752.

Hoflendahl, S. 1971. Influence of treatment in a coronary care unit on prognosis in acute myocardial infarction. ACTA Med. Scand. 519:supp.

Kannel, W., W. Castelli, and P. McNamara. 1967. The coronary profile: twelve-year follow-up in the Framingham study. J. Occup. Med. 9:611.

Keys, A., H. Taylor, H. Blackburn, J. Brozek, J. Anderson, and E. Simonson. 1963. Coronary heart disease among Minnesota business and professional men followed fifteen years. Circulation 28:381.

Klein, R., V. Kliner, D. Zipes, W. Troyer, and H. Wallace. 1968. Transfer from a coronary care unit. Archives of Internal Medicine 122:104.

Lown, B., and V. Sidel. 1969. Duration of hospital stay following acute myocardial infarction. Amer. J. Cardiology 23:1.

McNamara, J., M. Molot, J. Stremphe, and R. Cutting. 1971. Coronary artery disease in combat casualties in Vietnam. J. Amer. Med. Assoc. 216:1185.

Masters, A. and E. Oppenheimer. 1929. A simple exercise tolerance test for circulatory efficiency with standard tables for normal individuals. Amer. J. Med. Sci. 177:223.

Money, J. and R. Yankowitz. 1967. The sympathetic-inhibiting effects of the drug ismelin in human male eroticism with a note on mellaril. J. Sex Research 3:69.

Naughton, J., J. Bruhn, and M. Lategola. 1968. Effects of physical training on physiologic and behavioral characteristics of cardiac patients. Archives of Physical Medicine 49:131.

Naughton, J., M. Lategola, and K. Shanbour. 1966. A physical rehabilitation program for cardiac patients: A progress report. Amer. J. Med. Sci. 252:545.

Naughton, J. and W. Leach. 1971. The effect of a simulated warm-up on ventricular performance. Med. and Sci. in Sports, 3:169-71.

New, P., A. Ruscio, R. Priest, D. Petritsi, and L. George. 1968. The support structure of heart and stroke patients: a study of the role of significant others in patient rehabilitation. Soc. Sci. and Med. 2:185.

New York Heart Association. 1964. Diseases of the heart and blood vessels: nomenclature and criteria for diagnosis. 6th ed. Boston, Little Brown, p. 112.

Patterson, J., J. Naughton, R. Pietras, and R. Gunnar. 1972. Treadmill exercise in the assessment of the functional capacity of cardiac patients. Amer. J. Card. 30:757-62.

Pearson, H. 1963. Stress and occlusive coronary artery disease. Amer. Heart J. 66:836.

Pell, S. and C. D'Alonzo. 1964. Immediate mortality and five-year survival of employed men with a first myocardial infarction. New Eng. J. Med. 270:915.

Pouget, J., W. Harris, B. Mayron, and J. Naughton. 1971. Abnormal responses of the systolic time intervals to exercise in patients with angina pectoris. Circulation 43:289.

Rechnitzer, P., M. Yuhasz, H. Pickard, and N. Lefcoe. 1965. The effects of a graduated exercise program on patients with previous myocardial infarction. Canadian Med. Assoc. J. 92:858.

Rosenman, R., M. Freidman, D. Jenkins, R. Straus, M. Wurm, and R. Kositchek, *et al.* 1956. The prediction of immunity to coronary heart disease. J. Amer. Med. Assoc. 198:1159.

Rosenman, R. et al. 1968. The relationship of behavior pattern A to the state of the coronary vasculature. Amer. J. Med. Sci. 44:525.

Tobis, J. and L. Zohman. 1970. Follow-up study of cardiac patients on a rehabilitation service. Arch. Phys. Med. 51:826.

Turell, D., and H. Hellerstein. 1958. Evaluation of cardiac function in relation to specific physical activities following recovery from acute myocardial infarction. Progressive Cardiovascular Diseases 1:237.

Ueno, M. 1963. The so-called coition death. Japanese J. Legal Med. 17:333.

Varnauskas, E., H. Bergman, P. Houk, and P. Bjorntorp. 1966. Haemodynamic effects of physical training in coronary patients. Lancet 2:8.

Weaver, N. 1961. Disability absenteeism of industrial workers with myocardial infarcts. Amer. Heart J. 62:457.

Whitsett, T. and J. Naughton. 1971. The effect of exercise on systolic time intervals in sedentary and active individuals and rehabilitated patients with heart disease. Amer. J. Cardiology 27:352.

CEREBRAL PALSY

ALL INDIVIDUALS with cerebral palsy have in common some disorder of posture and movement. As a consequence, cerebral palsy has frequently been considered and is sometimes appropriately categorized as primarily a physical disability. In fact, during the course of visits to public schools throughout the country in the past ten years, we note that cerebral palsy is almost invariably listed as the "major crippling disorder" found among school children in the United States.

However, due to the origin of cerebral palsy in the brain, plus the fact that the brain dysfunction occurs before the maturation of the central nervous system, cerebral palsy is uniquely different from most other physical disabilities in its impact upon the individual, his family, and the community.

DEFINITIONS

Cerebral Palsy is a general term which has been defined in several ways by many investigators, including Phelps (1947), Crothers (1951), Perlstein (1952), Courville (1954), Denhoff (1960), Ingram (1964), Bax *et al.* (1964), Keats (1965), and Cruickshank *et al.* (1966). In general, the term has been used to identify a group of disorders which have several characteristics in common:

SHERWOOD MESSNER is Director of the Professional Services Program Department, United Cerebral Palsy Association, Inc., New York, N.Y. UNA HAYNES is Associate Director of the Department.

1) A maldevelopment, injury to, or dysfunction of the developing brain may result in disorders of posture or movement.

2) Since the brain is the center not only of muscular control but also of vision, hearing, the sense of touch, intelligence, many aspects of behavior, and other functions, the neuromuscular manifestations are but one component of the disabilities which may affect the individual with cerebral palsy.

3) While there is general agreement that the initial lesion or dysfunction of the brain should not be of a progressive nature in order to be classified as cerebral palsy, the type and extent of the clinical manifestations are ever-changing as the individual grows and develops. In addition, the ultimate outcome may be favorably or unfavorably affected by environmental factors.

The definition and description used by United Cerebral Palsy Associations, Inc., are as follows:

Cerebral Palsy is the clinical picture, usually manifesting itself in childhood, with dysfunction of the brain in which one of the major components is motor disturbance.

Thus, cerebral palsy can be described as a group of conditions, usually originating in childhood, characterized by paralysis, weakness, incoordination or any other aberration of motor function caused by pathology of the motor control centers of the brain.

In addition, there may be other manifestations of cerebral dysfunction, such as learning difficulties, psychological problems, sensory defects, convulsive and behavioral disorders of organic origin.

In March 1970, at a conference held in Santa Monica, California, Denhoff (1970), described cerebral palsy as "A syndrome in which disordered central nervous system function interferes with life adjustment." This definition is helpful in prompting consideration of the broad spectrum of difficulties which may be faced during the lifetime of the individual and his family; the range of professional and ancillary personnel which may need to be mobilized on their behalf; and the variety of community facilities which may be required to provide a reasonably adequate program of services.

CLASSIFICATIONS AND TERMINOLOGY

CLINICAL

By Posture and Movement. Since the common factor of neuromuscular involvement has often been a primary consideration, classification of cerebral palsy is frequently based upon the clinical findings related to posture and movement (Perlstein, 1952, pp. 30–34) as follows:

1) Spasticity: In spasticity, the underlying component is exaggerated contraction of muscles subjected to stretch. Increased muscle tone and hyperactive deep reflexes are also noted. Sometimes, flaccidity (in which the muscles fail to respond to volitional stimulation) is classified under the broad category of spasticity, since weak stretch reflexes may be obtained as well as increased deep reflexes. Flaccidity, as such, is relatively rare. It is important to note, however, that some infants who evidence significant lack of tone during the first weeks and months of life (the "floppy baby") may later evidence athetosis.

2) Athetosis: Athetosis or dyskinesia are terms used to describe jerky, uncontrollable, irregular twisting or writhing movements of the extremities.

3) Ataxia: Ataxia is characterized by inability or awkwardness in maintaining balance or coordination.

4) Rigidity: This is a term used to describe increased resistance to passive movement. The resistance may be continuous through the entire range of movement (lead pipe rigidity) or interrupted at regular intervals by jerky movements sometimes called "cog wheel" type motion.

5) Mixed type: This classification is used when there is a combination of disorders in the same person, such as athetosis and spasticity or rigidity and ataxia.

Topographical. The clinical classifications of cerebral palsy are also delineated topographically, that is, by location of the handicap. Some of the most commonly used terms are *paraplegia* (involving legs only), *diplegia* (involving the legs primarily, but also the arms), *quadriplegia* (involving all four extremities), *hemiplegia* (in which the problem is lateralized to one half of the body, etc.). These terms are rarely used alone, but rather in conjunction with clinical classifications.

By Associated Problems. Reviewing in *Child Neurology and Cerebral Palsy* (1960) the many associated problems which are found in cerebral palsy, either singly or in combination, Ingram (1960) cites perceptual disorders causing dyslexia and dysgraphia; Paine (1960) and Tizard (1960), disturbances of sensation; Zangwill (1960), deficiencies in spacial perception; Williams (1960), disturbances of sensation, and effects of emotional factors on concept formation and perception; Skatvedt (1960), visual and auditory problems, behavior difficulties, and various levels of intellectual deficit. Cruickshank *et al.* (1966) devote a major part of their discussions to the visual, hearing, speech, language, intellectual, and behavioral disorders, any or all of which may, in effect, prove more handicapping then the neuromotor aspects. Denhoff (1967, pp. 76–77) enumerates and describes the associated problems as follows:

1) Convulsions: There are many varieties, but minor and mixed types are more common. Thirty to 50 per cent of patients have seizures or are seizure prone.

2) Sensory and Perceptual: Vision, hearing, and stereognosis may be impaired, as well as the visual and auditory perceptual-motor systems. Visual-motor perceptual dysfunction is more common than auditory-motor imperception. These systems contribute barriers to learning when they are impaired.

3) Mental Retardation: Intellectual deficit is present in about 50 per cent of cases. More or less this infers poor integration of the sensory-motor systems rather than genetic (chromosomal) causes.

4) Behavior: Early body anxiety (fear of changing position of body in space) results in fear of body movement, such as walking or falling. Later, hyperkinetic behavior (hyperactivity, short attention span, poor power of concentration, variability of mood, impulsiveness, irritability, explosiveness, and poor school work) may be present. . . . During this period, environmentally derived behavior patterns may develop, such as passivity, anxiety, attention-seeking, or aggressive attitudes.

In the proceedings of an International Study Group (1962), Ingram points out that it was the intensive and long-term study of individuals with cerebral palsy and others with major problems of epilepsy and mental retardation that first alerted clinicians to recognize finer and finer deviations from normalcy, not only in detecting aberrant neuromotor functions but also the broad spectrum of sensory-perceptual, behavioral and other barriers to learning listed above. Postulated by Goldstein (1936), and later by Strauss and Werner (1943), the concept of a syndrome of cerebral dysfunction, manifesting itself in behavioral as well as neurological dimensions, began to receive much attention. This is illustrated by reports on hyperactivity made by Anderson (1963), Eisenberg (1966), Ingram (1966), Millichap (1968); on clumsiness made by Reuben and Bakwin (1968), Walton (1963); on visuomotor disabilities made by Gordon (1968), Walker (1965); and on associated movements made by Abercrombie *et al.* (1968), Cohen *et al.* (1967), to name but a few. A great variety of new classifications is now being developed, the definitions of which are marked by considerable diversity of opinion. All in common make an effort to differentiate the sensory-perceptual or behavioral barriers to learning from the more classical facets of the syndrome. Many attempts are made to more precisely define and/or describe the population to be identified within these categories. However, there is still great controversy about the terms being used. These include: the Brain Damaged child, the Brain Injured child, Hyperkinetic Impulse Disorder, Special Learning Disability, the Aphasoid child, the Dyslexic child, the Interjacent child, the Clumsy child, the Minimally Neurologically Handicapped child, and the Perceptually Handicapped child.

Pertinent to this discussion is the fact that some children with cerebral palsy who share these particular problems are now additionally classified as "perceptually impaired," "aphasoid," "dyslexic," etc. One of the consequences of these classifications in some communities is that the child with cerebral palsy becomes eligible to attend classes more precisely designed to meet his major educational needs rather than those primarily related to his musculature. In other communities, regulations exclude any child from such classes who has a neuromotor problem except for some "clumsiness." In others, children with "mild" cerebral palsy are eligible, but those with moderate or severe neuromotor problems are rejected. Some communities are using the classifications above plus those indicating the degree of retardation, when present, or the factors of blindness, deafness, etc., rather than the physical handicap classification, to determine appropriate educational placements.

By Severity. The problems of classification relative to the severity of the various disabilities found in cerebral palsy are still under study. This makes it exceedingly important that there be a thorough description of the individual by the various professional persons involved in the diagnosis or evaluation of the child or adult with cerebral palsy and his family. For instance, a child who can walk and talk and is relatively normal in physical activities, with the exception of impairment in fine precision movement, may be classified as mild as far as the neuromuscular aspects of his cerebral palsy are concerned. However, he may concomitantly have frequent and severe seizures, or he may be totally blind and thereby severely disabled from these points of view.

As previously pointed out, to be designated as cerebral palsy the origin of the problem, that is, the dysfunction and/or known damage to the brain, should be static. However, clinical evidence of the degree, as well as the type of involvement, may change. For instance, a child whose neuromotor problem was classified as mild or moderate during early childhood might be reclassified as moderately or severely disabled later in life, if a sudden and extensive growth spurt or other unusual stress markedly impairs his ability to function. Or the reverse may be true. Solomons (1963) has called attention to the changing neurological picture observed in his series wherein a previously diagnosed abnormality such as spastic-hemiplegia was spontaneously resolved during early childhood. In other cases, orthopedic surgery, therapy, or a combination thereof may enable a child to be changed from a moderate to a mild classification. Byers (1941) states that the final classification of neuromotor aspects of disability in cerebral palsy must await developmental maturity.

In like manner, some children display an increase in attention span or a decrease in hyperactivity with developing maturity. This may occur without any apparent direct relationship to specific programs of remediation. In other instances, these changes may appear directly related to a combination of medical, educational, and home management services.

In summary, classifications as to severity, as well as other classifications are subject to change as the individual matures or as a consequence of services that have been brought to bear on his behalf.

ETIOLOGIC

Another method of classification, as outlined by Denhoff (1966, pp. 27–28), is *etiologic,* referring to the course and time of occurrence of the probable defect or injury to the brain.

Prenatal. During the prenatal period, cerebral palsy may be caused by:

1) Heredity: (a) static (familial athetosis, familial tremor, familial spastic paraplegia); (b) progressive (demyelinating diseases).

2) Acquired in utero: (a) prenatal infection (rubella, toxoplasmosis, other maternal infections); (b) prenatal anoxia (carbon monoxide or strangulation of mother, maternal anemia, hypotension, for example, following spinal anesthesia, placental infarcts, placental abruptio or kinking of the cord); (c) prenatal cerebral hemorrhage (maternal toxemia, direct trauma, maternal bleeding diathesis); (d) metabolic disturbance (diabetes, aminoaciduria); (e) irradiation (gonadal).

Perinatal. There may be obstetrical and constitutional causes:

1) Obstetrical: (a) anoxia (mechanical respiratory obstruction, atelectasis, narcotism due to drugs, placenta praevia or abruptio, maternal anoxia or hypotension, breech deliveries with delay of the after-coming head); (b) trauma and hemorrhage (dystocia, disproportions and malposition, injudicious forceps application, holding back of head, pituitary extract induction of labor, sudden pressure changes, precipitate or caesarean delivery).

2) Constitutional: (a) prematurity; (b) hyperbilirubinemia and isoimmunization (kernicterus due to Rh factor, ABO incompatability, physiologic jaundice, syphilis, and other infections); (c) hemorrhagic disease of the newborn (hypoprothrombinemia, anemia of the newborn).

Postnatal. Postnatal causes include: (a) trauma (subdural hematoma, skull fracture, cerebral contusion); (b) infection (meningitis, encephalitis, brain abscess); (c) toxic (lead, arsenic, coal tar derivatives); (d) vascular (congenital cerebral aneurism, thrombosis embolism, hypertensive encephalopathy, sudden pressure changes); (e) anoxia (carbon monoxide poisoning, strangulation, high-altitude and deep-pressure anoxia, hypoglycemia); (f) neoplastic and late developmental defects (brain tumor, cyst, hydrocephalus).

In general, it is believed that approximately 33 per cent of the cases are related to perinatal anoxia and/or trauma; about 18 per cent to prenatal infections, irradiation, drugs, etc.; about 16 per cent to postnatal infections or injury; and about 10 per cent to genetic factors. Frequently, there may be several etiologic factors involved. There are obvious values to etiologic classifications, particularly from the point of view of prevention, a matter which will be discussed later in greater detail. However, in 25 per cent to perhaps 40 per cent of the cases, the causes may never be clearly determined.

While there have been some types of brain pathology identified, such as that following oxgyen deprivation around the time of birth, a pathological report at autopsy often fails to demonstrate correlative pathology in cerebral palsy. Consequently, the term dysfunction rather than damage is usually preferred.

NOMENCLATURE

Those who are interested in studying the incidence and prevalence of cerebral palsy, the determination of relative adequacy of services, or the delineation of unmet needs, face a real problem in the great range of variability in nomenclature which obtains in this field. What one physician may describe as cerebral palsy, giving a clinical picture of the type, location, degree, cause (if known), and associated handicaps, etc., another may see in the same person and describe quite differently. The following listing of diagnostic terminology found during a study of cerebral palsy in the State of Minnesota by Wallace, *et al.* (1960, pp. 8–9), illustrates this point:

Abscess of brain
Ataxia
Birth injury
Birth stroke
Blood clot on brain
Brain injury
Brain injury from car accident
Cerebellar ataxia atypical spastic
Cerebral atrophy
Cerebral degeneration
Cerebral hemorrhage, cause of
  brain damage

Cerebral palsy spastic
  hemiplegia congenital
Cerebral palsy right hemiplegia
Cerebral palsy spastic monoplegia
Cerebral palsy spastic paraplegia
Cerebral spastic hemiplegia
Cerebral spastic infantile
  monoplegia
Cerebral spastic paraplegia
Cerebrospastic infantile hemiplegia,
  due to encephalitis
Chronic brain syndrome

Chronic brain syndrome with brain trauma
Chronic brain syndrome with epidemic encephalitis
Chronic brain syndrome with encephalitis, behavior reaction
Chronic brain syndrome following meningitis
Congenital anomalies and cerebral palsy
Congenital cerebrospastic quadriplegia
Convulsive disorder
Encephalitis
Encephalitis with brain damage
Encephalitis from scarlet fever
Epilepsy and spastic
Erythroblastosis
Hemiparesis secondary to cerebral vascular accident
Hemiplegia
Idiot with congenital cerebral spastic
Infantile quadriplegia

Jaundice at birth
Little's disease
Measles encephalitis
Mentally retarded and spastic due to brain injury
Myxedema and cerebral palsy
Paralyzed from birth
Paraplegia
Partially paralyzed and epileptic seizures
Perceptually handicapped
Post traumatic with athetoid
Post traumatic spastic
Residual hemiparesis
Retarded and spastic
Rh incompatibility
Spastic
Spastic palsy
Spastic paralysis
Spastic and deaf
Spastic diplegia
Tendencies of cerebral palsy
Tension athetoid

The educator, psychologist, speech pathologist, and other members of diagnostic and evaluation teams may use still different terms.

The authors have found, on the basis of community studies, that when an educational and/or psychologically determined (rather than a strictly medical) diagnosis is used for school placement, individuals with cerebral palsy are found not only in regular school classes, in programs for the orthopedically disabled, or in homebound class categories, but also in special educational programs for the blind or visually handicapped, deaf or hard of hearing, educable or trainable retarded, emotionally disturbed, multihandicapped, and one or another of the rapidly proliferating special programs for the "perceptually handicapped," the "brain injured," etc. Later discussion relative to the organization and delivery of services will highlight other avenues for identifying individuals with known or suspected cerebral palsy during infancy.

PREVALENCE

From the preceding discussion, it is obvious that determining the precise number of individuals with cerebral palsy is a virtual impossibility since there is so little agreement on the definition and parameters of the problem. A number of studies have been made over the past twenty-five years, both in this country and abroad, which vary greatly in the size of the cerebral palsied group in proportion to the over-all population. The most widely accepted prevalence figure is 3.5 per thousand of the general population. This would indicate that in the United States, with a population of over two hundred million, there are approximately 750,000 children and adults who have cerebral palsy. If a broader definition is utilized to include those individuals with minimal physical handicap but with varying degrees of other disabilities, the total would be significantly greater, perhaps two and a half to three times the number. Some studies of specific population groups have found a prevalence much smaller than this. On the other hand, Wishik (1956) found a much higher prevalence in a study in Georgia where, by clinical examination of a sampling of all cases reported, it was determined that there were 5.4 cerebral palsied per one thousand children under twenty-one years of age.

The United Cerebral Palsy Association has demonstrated in several communities that a conscientious job of case identification will find two individuals per thousand population under twenty-one with cerebral palsy and one individual per thousand population twenty-one and over. These figures delimit the total problem to those who have need of some kind of specialized, community-based services. Since about 40 per cent of the general population is under twenty-one years of age, and since we expect to find two individuals per thousand in this group, this would mean that in a population of 100,000 there would be eighty children under twenty-one who need local services; and in the population group over twenty-one, where we would expect to find one individual per thousand who needs local services, there would be an additional sixty individuals. This would make a total of 140 children and adults residing in any community of 100,000 who require locally based services.

EARLY IDENTIFICATION
AND PREVENTIVE IMPLICATIONS

The studies of Lilienfeld, *et al.* (1951, 1954, 1955), Anderson (1953), Rogers, *et al.* (1954), Nesbitt (1957), and others suggest that when processes responsible for infant mortality occur in lesser degrees in surviving children they may be assumed to give rise to neurological disorders in these children, including behavioral, neuromotor, and receptive dysfunctions. Contributing to disproportional perinatal loss and "at risk" status in the infants who survive are a variety of factors associated with the maternal history, including health, social and psychological status, labor, and delivery. These, plus the neonatal and postnatal syndromes which may be involved, have been compiled by Oberman (1965). A review of these factors suggests not only the potential of identifying the baby at risk but also many aspects of primary and secondary prevention worthy of attention.

PRIMARY PREVENTION

Among measures of primary prevention, Mitchell (1971) lists the importance of general health in the prospective parents; the value of good prenatal care to prevent preterm birth; prevention of Rh sensitization by the injection of anti-D gamma globulin; recognizing a contracted pelvis and carrying out a caesarian section rather than subjecting the infant to a difficult delivery; prevention of hypoxia by early detection of placenta previa; guarding against infections in the pregnant mother such as German measles, which constitutes a serious threat to the developing fetal brain by interfering with normal fetus formation during the first three months, and toxoplasmosis or listeriosis, which when acquired in the latter part of pregnancy can damage the brain. It is pointed out that there is no need to wait for new knowledge in primary prevention but rather to apply what is already known in the organization and delivery of preventive services.

Although only a small minority of cases of cerebral palsy can clearly be attributed to genetic causes, it is believed that further research in this field will have a great potential for additional preventive success.

Where obstetric standards are high, Mitchell (1971) states the major antecedent of cerebral palsy is low birth weight. The disordered brain function found in small for term babies may be of genetic or embryonic origin, or be a consequence of severe nutritional deprivation in prenatal life. However, considerably more research is needed before significant advances can be made for effective prevention.

As skill in fetal medicine increases, the fetus can be kept in a healthy state in spite of adverse environmental influences. Mitchell (1971) calls attention to intrauterine transfusion as one example of modern technology which promises rapid progress in this area. In like manner, he calls attention to the great potential inherent in the reduction of infant mortality plus the improvement in the quality of surviving infants that will become possible when the great advances which already obtain in the field of neonatology can be carried out through the advent of properly equipped hospitals, adequately staffed by qualified personnel.

SECONDARY PREVENTION

In the neonatal period, secondary prevention merges with primary prevention. The brain is still growing very rapidly in the newborn period and the infant's central nervous system is highly susceptible to damage from a variety of sources. Naturally, the small infant, born prematurely, the small for term baby, and babies known to have been stressed for one or more reasons—all require particularly careful monitoring. In addition to the factors listed in the Oberman outline of syndromes in the neonatal period, Mitchell (1971) calls attention particularly to the potential problems posed by and management required in the presence of hypoxia (oxygen-lack), hypoglycemia (low blood sugar), hyperbilirubinemia (excess serum bilirubin), and hypernatremia (high levels of plasma sodium). Although accidental injury is not so likely to occur during the first days and weeks of life, it is as important to prevent such injury and keep the baby free from infections during this period as it is in later infancy. New knowledge about the relationships of good nutrition to brain development, identified by Wigglesworth (1969), also reinforces the need for appropriate attention to these factors.

Following the neonatal period, the incidence of any serious illness, the increasing possibility of involvement in accidents, especially traffic accidents, the dangers of lead, arsenic, or other poisoning, and the tragic possibility of child neglect or of child abuse as outlined by Kempe (1962), are all factors which fall within the aegis of secondary prevention. Every effort which can be brought to bear following birth to minimize the occurrence of unwarranted secondary disabilities or the extent of a superimposed disability is included within secondary prevention by some, and identified as tertiary prevention by others.

Services which can be mobilized to help detect dysfunction and avoid or minimize the extent of secondary complications include parameters beyond the immediate medical indications and intervention outlined above. For instance, it is to be hoped that all babies, as well as those "at risk," will have a continuum of health surveillance by the pediatrician during the first years of life. The physician is in a most fortuitous position to note evidence of any previously unrecognized congenital abnormality, delays or aberrations in the normal growth and developmental patterns, a general failure to thrive, or other indications of a possible cerebral dysfunction or related developmental disability. In the United States, many of the families most at risk of having a handicapped child either do not understand the need for and value of medical surveillance of their young or cannot afford private medical care. While clinics are available to the medically indigent, they are often very crowded. In rural areas, there may literally be no clinic services available. However, in any or all of these circumstances, families usually have service available from city or county health department public health nurses or a visiting nurse service. Increasingly, these nurses are developing sophistication in the earlier detection and appropriate referral of infants who deviate from the normal (Haynes, 1967). A proliferation of day care and developmental programs is now rendering services to increasing numbers of infants and children from the high-risk population. Child developmentalists, early childhood educators, public health nurses, and certain specially trained and supervised laymen are utilizing screening tests, such as the Denver Developmental Test (1966), in conjunction with these services. These are rather broad screening tests, but their use, coupled with the adjunctive medical services, are tending to foster earlier recognition of developmental delays and/or aberrations.

SERVICES: ORGANIZATION AND DELIVERY

At the conclusion of this chapter, there is a listing of more than one hundred types of services which may be needed at one time or another by individuals with cerebral palsy and their families, or by the community in dealing with this disabling condition. These have been organized under several general headings, and have been set forth in a Chart of Program Services (pp. 287–93) which represents an effective tool for determining adequacy of services, gaps in existing services, and for long-range planning.

It can readily be noted from this chart that because of the nature of cerebral palsy a very comprehensive and far-reaching matrix of services is needed in every community. It would not be expected, nor would it be appropriate, that all of these types of services would be available in every community. Some of them are needed only at relatively infrequent intervals. These can, therefore, be utilized by a larger population or serve a larger geographical area. An example of this would be a comprehensive diagnostic and evaluation clinic that might be adequate to meet the needs of an entire state or region within a state. On the other hand, there are some types of services that, to be effective, must be located in close proximity to the individual on a periodic basis. An example would be a program of home-based services.

SERVICE SETTINGS AND PERSONNEL

In the American Edition of *Handling the Young Cerebral Palsied Child at Home,* Haynes (1970) discusses services available. She points out that since children with cerebral palsy vary both in the types and extent of their needs the family physician, the child's pediatrician or the physician at the child's health clinic may wish to supplement his own evaluation with those of other professional colleagues before developing a comprehensive plan of care for the child. In many university centers, most large cities, and some smaller towns, there are specialized diagnostic clinics for handicapped children. If these are located reasonably close to where the child lives, the referring physician may arrange for the child to obtain these evaluations as an outpatient. If the family lives in a very rural area, the doctor may suggest that the child be admitted to a medical center hospital for a few days where a diagnostic team is available to assist him with this evaluation process.

Following the initial evaluation, a program is designed to meet the child's individual needs. The referring physician usually continues to be the one to guide and supervise the manner in which this program is carried out and remains the primary resource for advice and counsel. When there is a cerebral palsy center available locally, the physician may share some of this responsibility with the medical director of such a center, but he usually continues to supervise the child's basic health needs and to care for him when he is ill.

There are a variety of professional workers to whom such physicians may delegate responsibility for aiding the family in meeting the child's daily needs. In certain stages of the child's development it may be a speech therapist, an occupational therapist, a specialist in early childhood education, or a combination of such specialists who will be working most closely with the parents on the home aspects of the child's total program. Therapy is a very important aspect of care for any child with cerebral palsy, and if there is a cerebral palsy center or other resource available locally which provides these services, therapists will frequently be the ones to help most intensively during the early childhood years.

Quite a few centers also have public health nurses who make home visits, working in close cooperation with other members of the center staff. When the family lives at a significant distance from the nearest diagnostic and treatment centers and considerable time passes between visits, the city-county health department or visiting nurse services may be utilized by the center staff to aid at home. Since the advent of Medicare in the United States, an increasing number of these agencies have added consultant therapists, nurses with special preparation in the field of rehabilitation, plus more social workers and nutritionists, enriching the services available for the home-program aspects of care.

In some rural areas, visiting clinic teams, including physicians, therapists, nurses, and social workers, are sent out by a university medical center or state crippled children's service program to counsel with local physicians, public health nurses, and the family between visits to the center. Mobile teams of therapists and nurses sponsored by the Elks

Foundation, United Cerebral Palsy, or similar agencies are available in a few states. They travel to rural homes in specially equipped station wagons to help families carry out home-management aspects of the child's program between visits to the physician or clinic.

Certain types of services, such as social case work, psychological evaluation and counseling, recreational programs, and some aspects of long-term care, may be available through generic agencies in the community. These would include family service associations, mental health and mental hygiene clinics, child guidance clinics, public welfare services, public recreation facilities, and group-work agencies. In most communities these agencies will not be serving individuals with any significant degree of disability unless the Cerebral Palsy Association has worked closely with them in developing a specific program.

MEDICAL SERVICES

A continuum of medical surveillance, with appropriate medical intervention when indicated, constitutes an important aspect of any service program for individuals with cerebral palsy.

During infancy through childhood it is the pediatrician who is usually responsible for carrying out initial evaluations, including whatever laboratory procedures he deems appropriate. Since the presenting problems may be complicated and possibly camouflaged as cerebral palsy at first, the pediatrician will not only be concerned with his initial findings but will also usually keep the child under careful surveillance at regular intervals. Some of the laboratory tests which have proved useful and may be ordered at one time or another include urine amino acids, thyroid function tests, and x-rays of the wrists for bone age. The electroencephalogram, and more rarely a pneumoencephalogram, may be indicated. From a pediatric and sometimes from a neurological point of view, certain drugs may be used, such as anticonvulsant medications. Later, muscle relaxants or behavior modifiers may be indicated, carefully prescribed and monitored, depending upon the individual needs of each child. It is also worthy of special mention that the unique medical problems presented by the individual with cerebral palsy should not obscure the basic health needs he shares with all other children and adults. These include prophylactic inoculations and other health surveillance measures of childhood and regular medical examinations to maintain health and to foster the early detection of possible illness in later life.

During the growth and developmental periods, orthopedic consultation may be indicated. In some instances orthopedic aids such as splints or braces may be utilized. In many cases, the possible value of orthopedic surgery will probably be assessed repeatedly as the child grows older. In some individuals and at certain stages of development, the orthopedist may recommend surgery, to overcome severe flexion of the knee, for example. In some cases, orthopedic surgery may eliminate the need for heavy bracing.

If there are other medical problems present such as squint, the consultation of an ophthalmologist for visual evaluation and possibly medical or even surgical management of this type of difficulty may be indicated. In like manner, a severe hearing problem may suggest the need for the services of a medical specialist in this field.

DENTAL CARE

Surveillance of dental health, plus any possible special needs which may arise due to abberrant prenatal development, abnormal muscle tension in and around the area of the mouth, etc. are part of the generic health services which are needed by all individuals with cerebral palsy. Since it proves particularly difficult for some individuals to tolerate and effectively use dentures, there is an added need for sound dental care to maintain and promote the best possible state of dental health.

SCHOOL SERVICES

For some time voluntary agencies such as the National Easter Seal Society for Crippled Children and Adults, United Cerebral Palsy Associations, Inc., and chapters of the National Association for Retarded Children have been providing nursery school services with adjunctive therapies for preschool children. Some public schools are beginning to admit handicapped children under the age of three although the great majority do not render service until the ages of five to seven years.

Children with cerebral palsy will be found in almost every type of school setting in most communities. However, those who are admitted to regular elementary or secondary classes in the public schools, or to special classes for the educable or trainable retarded, or to special classes for the blind, deaf, the visually handicapped, the hard-of-hearing, etc., tend to be almost exclusively children who have a minimal degree of physical handicap. The requirements often are that the child be ambulatory, toilet-trained, and have some method of communication. Therefore, most of the children with cerebral palsy who are attending public school classes will be found in special classes for the so-called crippled, orthopedically handicapped, or physically disabled. Furthermore, the tendency is to group together in these classes all children who have a moderate to severe degree of physical handicap, regardless of their intellectual capacities or their barriers to learning. In practice, therefore, children with cerebral palsy are taught in classes that serve individuals with a great variety of learning handicaps. If this is to result in quality education, the teacher of such classes must indeed be versatile in order to discover and cope with the many types of learning problems which these children exhibit.

Ideally, children with cerebral palsy should be placed in classes according to their abilities to learn, or their major barriers to learning. This would mean that some children, although perhaps functioning in a wheelchair but of normal or above intelligence, should be attending class with nonhandicapped children of average or above intelligence. In a few situations where this has been tried, it has been found that the disabled child may need special tutoring in order to overcome some of the deficits that have occurred in the maturation process; or the teacher may need consultation from persons specially trained for working with the physically handicapped in terms of the kind of special equipment, positioning, etc., that makes it possible for the child to function in a regular classroom.

Unfortunately, these situations are very rare because of the fact that architectural barriers make it impossible for physically handicapped children to gain access to regular classrooms, or in some instances because of administrative regulations or even legislation which prohibits children from being placed in these classes. The same principles should apply to placement of children with greater or lesser degrees of mental retardation plus a physical handicap; or those who have visual or hearing problems; but again, it is the exception rather than the rule that such children are placed in classes for the retarded, for the blind, deaf, partially sighted, or hard-of-hearing.

Many children who have the multiple handicaps indicated above are entirely excluded from public school programs because there are no special classes for them. Recently in a few states classes for the multiply handicapped are being organized, but in most instances these refer to children with a sensory disability, such as those who are deaf and blind, deaf and mentally retarded, blind and mentally retarded, etc., rather than to those who have a physical handicap in addition to one or more of the other disabilities.

As a result, many children with cerebral palsy have not had the benefit of public school services until quite recently. In a few states, legislation has been passed to make it possible for public schools to purchase educational services from voluntary agencies such as United Cerebral Palsy Associations. In New York State, for example, Assembly Bill 4407 makes it possible for the State Department of Education to contract with private schools or voluntary agencies to provide educational services for children who for any reason cannot receive these through the public school system. Some of the money for these programs comes from federal resources.

In some rural areas, children who need special class placement are serviced either in a home instruction program or are admitted to a residential school. The latter type of arrangement has also been used for children who need a great deal of special medical and therapy services or those who have unsatisfactory home or living arrangements. However, residential school placement has become less important in the total picture as communities have developed their own special daytime classes.

In some of the larger urban areas, the special classes for the crippled or orthopedically handicapped have been concentrated in one school facility, which makes it possible for ancillary therapy services to be more easily provided. One result, however, has been the almost complete isolation of these children from children who are not disabled or from children with other types of disabling conditions. Many people have felt that this segregation is undesirable for both the handicapped and the nonhandicapped. The trend, therefore, has been to locate one or more classes for the orthopedically handicapped in a regular elementary or secondary school so that much, if not all, of the child's program could be on an integrated basis. There is the further problem with special schools that concentration of all children in one place often requires many children to be transported, often over great distances. Not only does this tire the child but it also cuts seriously into the number of hours available for education.

In summary, it might be said that the ideal situation in a community would be one with a number of options available to children with special learning problems so that they might be placed in the program which could best meet their special learning needs.

SERVICES FOR OLDER TEEN-AGERS AND ADULTS

Because of the factors outlined in the previous section, there are many children with cerebral palsy who become teen-agers and adults without having had an adequate educational program. Great gaps in their information about the world in which they live make it difficult if not impossible for them to go on to higher education or to have very much hope of entering the world of work. In a few instances, programs of prevocational assessment have been made a part of the school experience; but for the most part the individual with cerebral palsy reaches chronological maturity without having had any preparation for independent living or for work. A few who have been able to complete high school and who are thought to have the capacity for college work have been encouraged by counselors to enter college. Unfortunately, many such individuals tend to develop unrealistic vocational objectives, often completely out of line with their physical, mental, and emotional capacities. A few individuals with cerebral palsy have completed college and even graduate school and find a position appropriate to their training.

The vast majority of individuals we are discussing might be characterized as "drop-outs" from the mainstream of society. Their inadequate educational experiences have been compounded by psychological and social handicaps, all of which are superimposed upon their physical handicaps.

Garrett (1963, pp. 19–20) discussed employment potential of individuals with cerebral palsy and the important variables in predicting employability.

From a theoretical viewpoint, what can one expect in regard to the employment potential of the cerebral palsied? Probably 50 per cent to 60 per cent of the cerebral palsied youngsters who present themselves for vocational rehabilitation need some type of sheltered workshop experience. About half of these will probably remain in the workshop for the rest of their lives. A very small group, perhaps about 10 per cent, is ready for placement. The rest are in need of vocational training. In other words, the role of sheltered work as a facet in the vocational rehabilitation program, particularly for the cerebral palsied, is one which cannot be overestimated.

The interesting thing is that the cerebral-palsied individual is generally less able to perform semiskilled work than either clerical or unskilled jobs, and this is largely because of the lack of the necessary dexterity required by the former. But those who are trained for clerical or unskilled jobs generally find their outlet in this field of work, whereas those who are trained at the semiskilled level usually find their outlet for work in something other than semiskilled jobs. The most important variable in predicting employability for the cerebral palsied would seem to be manual dexterity.

There are three fundamental things required for manual dexterity, and which determine whether or not a person can work. One is the ability to grasp and to hold with one hand, regardless of what position that hand might be in; second, the ability to oppose the thumb with the first and second fingers—in other words, the pinching motion with one hand; third, the factor termed two-hand coordination, which has to do primarily with speed and the ability to coordinate under pressure.

What are some of the other factors which appear to be important in ultimate work adjustment? They are what the authors would term employable skills, and these are rather simple. One is handwriting, the other is speech. If a cerebral-palsied youngster can write, the potential for vocational rehabilitation is high. Or, if a cerebral-palsied youngster can speak intelligibly, then again his vocational-rehabilitation potential is high.

Comprehensive vocational programs for disabled persons are fairly common in larger cities at present. Discussion on establishment and operation of such programs can be found in *Sheltered Workshops: A Handbook* (1966), an organizational and operational manual prepared by a committee of nationally known consultants to the National Association of Sheltered Workshops and Homebound Programs. It contains a glossary of terms and a bibliography.

Friedman (1963) describes more specifically one such program operated by United Cerebral Palsy of Philadelphia. The components are similar to other vocational service programs. They include intake and screening, counseling, testing, evaluation, personal-adjustment training, sheltered workshop, placement, and follow-up.

In a work-activities center the primary focus is on the provision of meaningful activity for enrollees. It constitutes in essence a day-care situation which may provide adequate respite for families that are attempting to care for a severely handicapped individual in the home. Thus, it also can be an alternative to institutional placement.

The emphasis in a work activities program is not on quantity of production but rather on a climate that promotes personal, social, and emotional growth. At the same time, the small amounts of money earned by the participants can be quite important both in fostering a sense of achievement and also because under certain conditions the individual can qualify for federal Social Security payments.

It would appear that much can be done to enhance functioning of severely disabled individuals in work settings. Engineers are beginning to turn their attention to the development of hardware that has the potential for increasing the productivity of such persons or that might make it possible for many individuals now excluded from work-activity centers and sheltered workshops to be served in the future. United Cerebral Palsy Associations, Inc. has initiated a pilot program along these lines under a grant from the Rehabilitation Services Administration, Department of Health, Education and Welfare.

It will be seen that programs for nonworking teen-agers and adults are an important aspect of total services. Among the major elements of such a program are social activities, recreation, independent living, adult education, hobbies, opportunities for decision-making, and for becoming acquainted with the immediate community. Independent living can be interpreted as any kind of activity which helps the individual make personal adjustments, such as cooking and homemaking, personal hygiene, skills in activities of daily living, skill in communications, the development of more adequate self concepts, peer and family relationships, and learning how to manage frustration and anxiety. Nonworking teen-agers and adults also must be helped to undertake community service in a volunteer capacity. They may need opportunities for spiritual growth. Obviously, many of the activities listed can be carried on through existing agencies and institutions in the community. Churches, neighborhood houses, settlements, counseling agencies, group-work and recreational agencies, as well as voluntary associations devoted specifically to the handicapped—all have a role to play. Unfortunately, most of the generic services in the community do not understand their role in relation to these individuals. Therefore, part of the task is one of educating community leadership, and specifically leadership of the various agencies as to the why and how of program development. It may be necessary for the specialized agency to demonstrate the feasibility of a particular kind of program and then to help one of the generic agencies carry it on. On the other hand, it probably will continue to be the responsibility of the specialized agency to support some activities, particularly for the more severely and multiply involved.

TRENDS AND ISSUES IN THE ORGANIZATION
AND DELIVERY OF SERVICES

Many of the services listed on the chart previously mentioned have been available to part of the target population for quite a few years. On the other hand, there are a number of categories which are of fairly recent development and which should be highlighted at least by listing them. Among them are a variety of patterns for residential living for adults with cerebral palsy.

RESIDENTIAL SERVICES

There are several demonstrations involving residential facilities being conducted in the United States and abroad which range from independent apartment living to residential facilities which provide total care. They include foster home placements; living in nursing homes, perhaps in a special wing for younger people; groups living in apartments with or without supportive services; hostels; wings of hospitals or convalescent homes; and, particularly in Europe, entire village complexes for the handicapped. Closely related to this is the concept of homemaker services, or home health aides. These are trained persons who come into the home of the individual or the family to perform certain duties which make it possible for the individual or the family to cope more easily with day-to-day care problems.

The residential school was one of the early service resources developed in the United States with special reference to handicapped children of normal or near normal intelligence who were previously denied service in their local public school. Residential schools are still available in many states, supported by tax monies or under the sponsorship of voluntary organizations. With the proliferation of community-based services, there is now less need for such facilities, since many children can receive the required services in their local communities. However, in some rural areas and in communities which have not yet provided the above alternatives, the residential school is still a necessary resource.

Individuals with severe and extensive disabilities, coupled with severe to profound mental retardation, have, in the past, been given minimal attention in locally based service programs, resulting in their referral to state institutions for the retarded. Through the combined interests of the personnel in these institutions, United Cerebral Palsy Associations, the National Association for Retarded Children, the American Association on Mental Deficiency, and the federal program for the developmentally disabled, a major effort is now under way to change the minimal custodial care previously offered to this population into a truly rehabilitative program.

In the local community, there is increasing evidence of shared concerns and combined programming for these individuals and their families. The National Association for Retarded Children, United Cerebral Palsy, plus tax-supported services for the retarded and physically handicapped are reducing some of the need for residential care. In a later discussion of services for infants and their families, it will be seen that these aspects of service can markedly help prevent some of the seriously handicapping and unwarranted secondary disabilities which previously required residential services away from home.

MAN-MADE ENVIRONMENT

Among the newer trends in services are such matters as architectural design to foster programming. This goes beyond the important areas of eliminating architectural barriers in access to buildings and to facilities within buildings. The newer concept is that architecture be related to the function for which the space is to be used. Also, there is increased awareness of special problems of transporting individuals with cerebral palsy, since without some type of transportation provision of services tends to be meaningless.

INFORMATION, REFERRAL, AND FOLLOW-ALONG SERVICES

Anyone, whether a professional worker, parent of a handicapped child, or others concerned, should be able to find the appropriate service at the appropriate time. However, this requires more than a superficial knowledge of the community and its resources. United Cerebral Palsy Associations has evolved the concept of an Information, Referral, and Follow-Along Service (UCPA, 1970) as a specific program component without which many other services cannot be fully utilized. It is described as follows:

Information. People come to UCP or a related agency with a wide variety of requests, problems, and needs. They must be helped to find and use effectively all of the community's relevant resources. Information related to the existence of all health and welfare services must be collected by the agency sponsoring the service and then made available. Because a wide range of resources and types of information is available, the data must be accurate, current, and carefully maintained, and readily accessible in a central information file. It should include eligibility criteria, cost, waiting time, and all other data important to clients, as well as to agencies, institutions, and organizations which are also involved in providing service.

Referral. Helping the client choose appropriate resources requires knowledge of the resources, an ability to explore the client's needs in relation to the available resources, and an evaluation of the client's ability to use the resources effectively. There must also be an opportunity for counseling, especially where resources are not available. The final choice of resources is the client's, and his full participation in the referral process must be assured.

Follow-Along. Once the referral is made, the client is entitled to a follow-through that insures his reaching the place to which he was referred and to his being accepted for service that will continue as long as necessary. The Centralized Follow-Along Service involves the maintenance of a confidential basic record for each client, with additions contributed by serving agencies.

Information in the confidential record is always available to the client, who makes the decision as to whether or not it is shared with any other appropriate resource. Follow-along will be responsible for periodic review to help if the client becomes inactive, if he is recommended for a different service, or requires additional services. When the client is recontacted, he is given another chance to use the partnership. The choice is the client's.

This type of service has many corollary values. Among them are:

1) Counseling and supportive services to clients. Many clients come hoping for the chance to clarify their problems and to be helped to a simple solution. Some persons may need a continuing relationship; others will benefit from intermittent supportive contact.

2) Coordination of services for the individual and his family. It is easy to think of family situations, for example, which require such services as a diagnostic evaluation, a school, a homemaker, a recreation group, and a dental clinic—perhaps at the same time. An Information, Referral, and Follow-Along program can undertake the meshing of services of several different agencies working with one or more family members simultaneously over a period of time. The effort is made to see the needs of the client and his family as a whole.

3) Consultive services to community agencies. The reluctance of some agencies and professionals to offer services to the cerebral-palsied person may stem from a total lack of familiarity with this group and the consequent fear about being able to meet the person's needs. For example, some registered nurses, physicians, and dentists may not have had experiences beyond their academic orientation that relate to cerebral palsy. The security of having a consultant to whom the professional person or agency can turn for advice and additional information will go a long way in overcoming the tendency to avoid serving the handicapped client at all.

4) Integration of the handicapped into the community. The ultimate objective is to assist the cerebral palsied to participate in community life to the fullest extent of their physical and mental capabilities. Community agencies can be utilized for the handicapped as well as the non-handicapped population, for example, housing, recreation, foster home

services, counseling, education, home care, homemaking service. Often the handicapped as a group are totally forgotten, and it is necessary to point out the possibility of broadening all agencies' constituencies to include the handicapped person.

5) Documentation of unmet needs. This program offers the most efficient way to help develop the data by providing firsthand evidence concerning the unmet needs of the handicapped individual and his family.

6) Coordinated life span program and protective services. United Cerebral Palsy affiliates have a special obligation to see that the individual with cerebral palsy gets the service he needs as he moves either from one age level of competency to another or from one social and emotional situation to another. The physically disabled adult has the ultimate human right to manage for himself when he can, as well as the right to have protective services when he cannot. Protective services can be described as a constellation of services designed to help individuals retain or achieve competence to manage their own affairs or to act on behalf of those incapable of managing for themselves. Many requests for long-term planning stem from a request for immediate service, which will reveal the multiplicity of the problem. It is therefore an aspect of service that must be offered to all, including those who may not be aware of its availability. Parents should be informed that long-range planning as well as protective service planning is possible at any time. Central to the program is the affiliate's reaching out for a periodic evaluation, even after a child goes away to school or an adult enters a residential facility.

SERVICES FOR INFANTS AND THEIR FAMILIES

The importance of early educational intervention for infants and young children has been strengthened by the evidence that infants demonstrate learning during the first few days and weeks of life (Crowell, 1971; Haith, 1971; Kessen and Salapatek, 1971; Caviness and Gibson, 1964). This learning has been measured by their differential behavioral and physiological responses to the presentation of visual and auditory stimuli.

Starr (1970), Hunt (1961), Hebb (1947, 1955), and others have theorized regarding the importance of infancy and early childhood as the critical period during which the child develops basic schemes for handling information. The sensory-motor stage (birth to eighteen months) provides the basic framework by which the child begins to respond and adapt to his environment. The ability of an infant to develop appropriate voluntary movement in early infancy as discussed by Luria (1957) points up the need for specific attention and services adequate to meet the special problems of babies identified as having neuromuscular aberrations and/or delays.

New knowledge about the relationships of good nutrition to brain development (Wigglesworth 1969) also presents a challenge in achieving adequate programming for infants with cerebral dysfunction. The early amelioration or resolution of problems in sucking and swallowing, which occur with frequency in this population, may be a critical component in helping the baby attain adequate nourishment in relation to brain development, as well as the more immediately recognized basic health goals of such intervention.

The studies of Gesell (1941) and his colleagues (Gesell and Amatruda 1947; Gesell, *et al.*, 1960), plus many additional contributions to the literature in the past decade, have called attention to the deleterious effect of environmental deprivation and stress on the normal infant. It is axiomatic that these factors can significantly interfere with the disabled infant's achievement of his potential. Less frequently recognized and duly considered is the potentially harmful effect of an aberrant baby upon his parents and other family members. Brazelton (1961) has described the interaction of a "difficult" infant—the strong influence he wields in determining the nature of the mother-child relationship—and how the resulting problems in this relationship tend to reinforce the difficulties of the child in psychosocial as well as physical adaptation to the environment. Gallagher (1956) and other investigators have clearly defined the impact of parental rejection or oversolicitude upon the handicapped child. These detrimental attitudes may well originate long before the diagnosis of exceptionality in the child is made. If persistent and unresolved, they may complicate or even negate all succeeding efforts toward habilitation.

It is factors of this type which prompted the Early Care Task Force of United Cerebral Palsy Associations to study the nature and extent of services currently available for such infants and their families. The authors have personally visited a broad range of programs in a variety of university and community settings sponsored by voluntary and official agencies throughout the United States. It was found that there are still comparatively few providing more than the basic diagnostic and evaluation services, with some therapy consultation and/or direct therapy utilizing an approach which will be discussed in a later section of this chapter. In general, very little if any attention is directed to the cognitive development of the infant or other parameters of service which extend beyond the more strictly medical aspects. However, there are a few highly innovative new approaches which are worthy of careful review.

From 1962 to 1969 Jones *et al.* (1962, 1969) called attention to the comprehensive approaches to services for children (eighteen months to three years of age) being developed at the University of California in Los Angeles. These have now been adapted for babies under two years and their families. Denhoff and Robinault (1960), Denhoff and Langdon (1966), and Denhoff (1967) traced the evolution of the program at Meeting Street School in Providence, Rhode Island, which had previously concentrated on the preschool and older group but later added an active and comprehensive service for infants under two years of age. In both of these programs the critical component of the cognitive development of the child is stressed. They have found ways to meet broad spectrum needs without excessive or inconsistent handling; and they stress the importance of service to the family.

In 1970 United Cerebral Palsy Associations, Inc., and the Western Interstate Commission on Higher Education jointly sponsored an interdisciplinary conference to develop appropriate guidelines in the evolution of a "curriculum" for infants under two years of age who have known or suspected cerebral dysfunction (Hensley and Patterson, 1970). Identifying as a central theme the cognitive development of infants, Robinson (1970) reviewed research in cognition and the implications for early care, suggesting that carefully planned experiences must be initiated as early as possible and that high priority must be assigned to symbolic and communication skills and to the basic concepts and skills which enhance their emergence. Strothers (1970) emphasized the role of the psychologist as a psychometrist and clinician, developmental theorist and experimentalist, and most importantly as a humanist. Connor (1970) presented a curriculum concept which reviews the kaleidoscope of instructional behavior with the teacher-competency roles based upon the Taxonomic approach of Tannenbaum (1969). In a review of current practices in infant programs, Rembolt (1970) pointed out that a program based on planned activity can achieve desired objectives and is preferable to an unplanned, random response program. In addition, he highlighted the importance of careful evaluation of the infant's developmental stage, determining what systems are intact and functioning at any given point in time, defining goals and the sequence of steps to their attainment, and helping the child overcome barriers, rather than directing attention primarily to the categorical disease as such.

Just as there are many educational approaches which can be utilized in the development of a curriculum for the infant, there are also many systems of therapy as reviewed by Gillett (1969). Jones (1970) has called special attention to the so-called neuro-developmental or neuro-physiological approach of Bobath (1967) and Finnie (1970), which has appeared useful in a number of settings. While stressing the discrete body of knowledge and skill which can be brought to bear by the individual members of the interdisciplinary team, Jones also calls special attention to the way physical and occupational therapists can be taught by medical specialists and speech therapists how to improve defects in the oral pharyngeal area and thus integrate this as part of their other interaction with a baby. This example of sharing of knowledge and skills to reduce the number of people actually handling an infant will be discussed later. Referring to the work of Kagan (1966) that states that the first eighteen months of life in the normal infant is one of tremendous development in both perceptual and motor development as well as personality development, Jones emphasizes the importance of providing as normal an experience as possible for the handicapped child. She also stresses that adaptation of the child to the mother and the mother to the child may be more difficult if the child has a physical handicap, and feels it may well be more crucial in such cases than when the child is normal. The mother or other immediate caretakers are considered key persons in the infant service program.

Working in concert with the parents as well as with the child, six of the basic areas of infant service in these programs include: talking to the baby; providing opportunities to exercise emerging sensory-motor functions; encouraging the baby's efforts; paying attention to all factors related to adequate nutrition; dealing with a baby in distress; and providing continuity in a few basic and warm relationships.

Denhoff (1970), in reviewing the services for infants at Meeting Street School, highlights the concentration which is placed upon body awareness and control, visual-perceptual motor skills and language. The Home Development Guidance Program of this agency is a comprehensive plan of developmental guidance to encourage maturation, especially at critical periods, and it incorporates family guidance within the framework of child care. The program emphasis is directed to the family role in the nurturance of the baby, using the strengths within the family's own life style—supporting, teaching, counseling, guiding, and in general re-emphasizing the Center's concept that management programs must be moved out of the hospital and clinic to the kitchen and the living room.

FACILITIES

There is considerable divergence of opinion among agencies and professional workers as to the need for building specialized facilities to serve individuals with cerebral palsy and related disorders. On one hand, there is a great temptation for agencies which raise their own money to build centers dedicated to their particular type of clientele. On the other hand, many agencies have found that it is possible to utilize existing facilities such as neighborhood houses, churches, schools, etc., to program effectively for the special needs of the cerebral palsied.

The widespread concept that all services in a particular community for the disabled should be under one roof contains a number of fallacies. First, it tends to result in less flexibility in programming because a service developed within a particular facility is not as easily "spun off" to another agency when this might be appropriate. Second, it inevitably involves the identification of the handicapped as "special," whereas there needs to be real effort to normalize the lives of and services for these individuals. Third is the belief that centralization is more efficient. This has not proven to be valid. Although it may have been proposed as an expedient to foster the more efficient use of professional personnel, this does not necessarily follow. Studies of so-called comprehensive facilities serving all handicapped have indicated that even this may be a mirage. Mere size or "comprehensiveness" does not in itself ensure the efficiency of operation nor the nonduplication of services. We have noted even within one facility that various departments are not really aware of what other departments are doing, nor are they communicating with one another.

It must be recognized that most agencies dealing with people, such as schools, churches, settlement houses, scout troops, and others, have long adapted to the need for neighborhood orientation. Therefore, the move toward centralization of services for the handicapped is contrary to the general patterns of our society. Also at issue is the matter of attitudes in the community toward the disabled. If the handicapped person is ever to be accepted as a contributing member of society, the mechanisms now making for isolation and segregation must be altered.

One of the major hurdles that prevents decentralization of facilities is the reluctance of highly trained professional staff to become adjusted to traveling to several different locations. That it can be done has been demonstrated by a number of agencies. A UCP affiliate, such as the one in Los Angeles, has operated as many as eight different centers in different geographical locations within the county. One interesting by-product of such a system is that it has motivated highly trained therapists and teachers to develop their skills as consultants to other staff and to families. Since under this system staff members do not have the opportunity of working with children on a five-day-week basis, but rather may see them only once or twice a week, it becomes necessary for them to impart a greater measure of their knowledge and skills to the other people who are in contact with the children or adults on a more consistent basis. In the face of increasing shortages of professional personnel, this type of activity has special advantages.

PLANNING OF SERVICES

It will be noted that an entire section of the Chart of Community Services is concerned with community organization and planning for services. These might be considered as indirect services, as contrasted with the direct "laying on of hands."

In recent years a mystique has grown up in nearly every field around the concept of planning for services. To some extent, planning has become an end in itself rather than a means for delivery of quality services. Nevertheless, some amount of planning is necessary if we are to avoid complete fragmentation of programs and utter confusion on the part of the client and his family.

The specialized agency concerned with services for the cerebral palsied must be a part of whatever community planning bodies are in existence. Otherwise, the unique needs of the cerebral palsied will not usually receive adequate attention. On the other hand, planning for more specific aspects of services must begin with and, to a large extent, be confined within the cerebral palsy agency itself. If such planning is based on up-to-date knowledge about the over-all pattern of services and facilities in the community, and if planning is done on an interprofessional basis within the agency, it will ensure to a large degree that the planning will be in harmony with both the needs of the target population and the over-all pattern of services in the community.

As an example of the process of planning and its relation to a program for the cerebral palsied, one might consider the recent developments within the field of mental health and mental retardation planning. As a result of the emphasis by the federal government in the early sixties on the importance of mental retardation, there evolved a process whereby each state was encouraged to develop a plan for services to individuals with mental retardation. Although possibly everyone recognized that at least half of the individuals with cerebral palsy are also mentally retarded, there was almost no effort on the part of those taking the initiative in planning to include representatives of the agencies serving the cerebral palsied. In a few states, United Cerebral Palsy Associations were able to have representation and a voice in the process of mental retardation planning; but for the most part these plans were drawn up by those who had little or no primary concerns about the significant numbers in the mentally retarded population who also have physical handicaps. As a result, most of the state plans did not make provision for these individuals.

In the late 1960s it became apparent that there were many needs in common among individuals with cerebral palsy, individuals with epilepsy or other types of central nervous system disorders, and individuals with mental retardation. The concept of developmental disabilities evolved slowly, and in 1970, through a cooperative effort of the various agencies, a federal law was passed, Public Law 91–517, called the Developmental Disabilities Community Facilities and Construction Amendments of 1970. This legislation now provides a broad base for services to the mentally retarded, the cerebral palsied, those with epilepsy, and those having other neurological handicaps related to mental retardation. Again, this legislation will be implemented through a planning process at the state level, and there is an opportunity for those concerned with cerebral palsy to get in on the "ground floor," since it is mandated that this group shall be included. There is, of course, much concern on the part of those primarily working with the mentally retarded that the services and thrust will be weakened because of the broadening of this program. This concern is not well founded. Cooperative planning and, in many cases, cooperative programming by the various agencies, should result in a much more effective delivery system for all concerned.

APPROACHES TO SERVICE

Since many of the various types of service discussed previously are to be found in rehabilitation centers, it may be of interest to review briefly, the way services may be provided in such settings.

MULTIDISCIPLINARY

One method previously used in rehabilitation centers was the multidisciplinary approach. This was a type of assembly-line activity wherein the individual was diagnosed and evaluated by a variety of consultants in the fields of medicine, therapy, social work, and/or vocational rehabilitation. Unfortunately, this type of approach often resulted in a rather inflexible arrangement wherein each professional worker operated more or less on his own and usually lacked adequate communication with his colleagues. This reduced the opportunities for sharing each other's interests and concerns or working together in a coordinated fashion toward immediate and long-range goals. The individual and his family were often confused by the apparently conflicting statements and recommendations made by the various multidisciplinary consultants.

INTERDISCIPLINARY

The "interdisciplinary" approach has now largely supplanted the multidisciplinary concept of service in most rehabilitation centers. Here, representatives from the multiple-specialty areas meet together to exchange information, discuss various approaches to rehabilitation, and work cooperatively in the design and implementation of the program. It is significant to note, however, that each member of these professional teams still "does his own thing" on behalf of the individual, whom he chiefly treats on a one-to-one basis.

While the following illustration offers relatively narrow interpretations of the role of individual staff members, it is not unusual to find one patient who is individually treated with considerable intensity and for long periods of time by a staggering number of people in this interdisciplinary approach. For example, problems with ambulation are referred to the special attention and intervention of the physical therapist; hand and arm function to the occupational therapist; the speech needs to the speech therapist; continuing education to the teachers; diversional requirements to the recreation, music, and other workers; social and family concerns to the social and group workers; psychological and related needs to the psychologist and/or psychiatrist. Thus, one individual with multiple disabilities may be handled, manipulated, talked to, and moved about for hours, every day or many times a week, by no less than three and often as many as six or more professional persons.

It is difficult to deny any individual the broad spectrum of knowledge and skill now available in the scientific community to aid him in attaining the highest possible degree of rehabilitation. When all of the specialists involved make a real effort to meet, effectively communicate, and coordinate activities on his behalf, many of the service recipients have attained a high degree of rehabilitation through this type of interdisciplinary approach.

However, there is increasing concern on the part of thoughtful members of interdisciplinary teams, and particularly on the part of specialists in child growth and development, regarding the impact upon a child multiply disabled by cerebral palsy or a related disorder early in life when he is constantly subjected to so much individualized intervention by so many authoritarian adults for such a significant part of his total childhood. Since the child with cerebral palsy or related disability is not sick in the usual sense of the word, some questions are asked. Is it really necessary to segregate him from normal peers for so large a part of his day or week? Is it necessary to provide him with the habilitation services he needs? What does it do to his developing self-image to spend so much of his childhood in a tile-walled, hospital-like milieu, surrounded by uniformed personnel? This is the situation which obtains in most rehabilitation centers, whether they are located in a hospital or in a separate building. Is it necessary for therapists to work in the hospital or a rehabilitation setting to provide quality service to such children? If the child is seen by his family and the community as one who needs to be in a hospital or rehabilitation-center setting most of the time, what does this do to their attitudes toward and feelings about him, if and when he is eventually referred out of the rehabilitation unit and tries to join the mainstream of normal community living?

"CROSS-DISCIPLINARY"

One adaptation of the interdisciplinary model has recently been developed in an attempt to solve the problems outlined above. This adaptation is termed "cross-disciplinary." The expanding body of scientific knowledge continues to increase the potential contributions of physicians, of physical, speech, and occupational therapists, of nurses, social workers, and psychologists, as well as early childhood educators. They can provide comprehensive diagnostic, evaluative, and broad habilitative services for handicapped infants and their families, preventing many unwarranted secondary disabilities and fostering the optimum potential for development. However, infants cannot tolerate excessive, frequent, or inconsistent handling by a variety of specialists.

In the cross-disciplinary approach, representatives of all concerned professional disciplines contribute to the differential aspects of diagnosis and evaluation, the selection and testing of the intervention which each deems appropriate to the age and stage of the baby's development, in much the same manner described in the "Interdisciplinary Approach." However, instead of each professional person rendering direct service, they teach and help the parent and one of the team members, or both, to carry out the appropriate regimen, and to do so in a functionally integrated manner. The multihandicapped baby is then handled by only one, two, or possibly three people. These "primary programmers" are sensitive to the baby and/or family needs and may obtain specialized consultations between regularly scheduled evaluations at appropriate intervals.

The cross-disciplinary concept of service also provides a more normative environment for disabled children who may spend a large segment of their childhood in a predominantly medical-type milieu. Great care is being exercised to maintain the beneficial aspects of the interdisciplinary approach while simultaneously reducing segregate handling of each aspect of the disability. Normal peer relationships are fostered throughout the child's day and due attention is focused upon the family role. In Claremont, California, the Danbury School is a public elementary school which was designed to serve normal children as well as those with varying degrees of physical and other handicaps. Physically handicapped infants are accepted with their parents for medical and therapy services as soon as they are referred by the California Crippled Children's Services. When deemed ready to participate, the children attend the educational classes at three years of age. While they may need specific medical intervention in a hospital or other medical setting from time to time, a major part of their childhood and programming takes place at school, supplemented by homebased services.

The staff of the school consists of a principal, teachers, occupational, physical, and speech therapists, a part-time orthopedist and pediatrician, a school nurse, several children's aides, and the usual secretarial and custodial staff complement. The program is a joint and cooperative function of the Department of Public Instruction, with added special education services provided by the state. The California Crippled Children's Services is responsible for the adjunctive medical and therapy components of the services rendered.

One distinctive feature of this school is the fact that the architectural design encourages and enhances new approaches in the way professional personnel work together on behalf of handicapped children. It looks like and is accepted by the community as a school, not a medical center. Therapy equipment occupies part of the classroom space. Therapists and teachers work together in a team-teaching concept to provide an integrated therapeutic approach, with the children in the classroom setting. Office space is shared, thus not only helping to facilitate formal sessions of joint planning for the child's total daily experiences but also encouraging continuing interaction between staff members on an informal basis throughout the day. The fact that their office windows view the teaching areas also means that therapists who are not already involved in a team-teaching situation may observe and quietly step in during a class period to adjust a child's prosthesis, help place his hands and arms in a more functional position, or have a quiet word with the teacher about the therapeutic goals to be included in that period (that is, the need for the child to lock braces, to stand up in the standing table a few minutes, be more encouraged to speak). The open design of the building also encourages both formal and informal integration of children, including those with and without handicaps, into small joint-interest or activity groupings several times a week, or daily in some instances. While it is possible for a therapist to draw a curtain and be alone with the child in a therapy area for special evaluation, trying out a new modality, or conducting some other special function, it is very interesting to note the continuous integration of therapy by teachers and aides as well as therapists. The therapist selects, tries out, and then teaches her colleagues the proper procedures, after which much therapy takes place during daily experiences without withdrawal of the child from the classroom milieu.

Naturally, there are times when the skill of a therapist must be used on a one-to-one basis with a child. For example, a speech therapist may withdraw to a private room to provide a special stimulation of the oral-pharyngeal area to facilitate tongue and throat action just before lunch. However, a continuation of the cross-disciplinary concept may also be seen when the therapist talks with the child about a new word the teacher introduced that morning.

It is patent that a variety of interdisciplinary team members have been developing new ways to share the implementation of joint goals through the cross-disciplinary approach and without continuous, intensive, and segregated "laying on of hands." Admittedly, the staff of this school is made up of professional persons with sufficient ego strengths and security in their professional competence to facilitate role sharing.

This program is not being presented as the ultimate or indeed the only answer to a variety of new child and family-centered approaches which are now evolving in the United States. However, it does serve to illustrate ways in which some private and some tax-supported agencies are demonstrating that a broad habilitative approach can be effected without undue handling by adults and that many children with disabilities need not develop a self image colored by living a large part of their childhood surrounded by uniformed adults in a hospital-like environment. Interaction with normal peers can also be effected within the same environment where the required habilitation program takes place when both normal and handicapped children are served in the same school. All of these factors have special relevance in considering the future organization and delivery of services in the United States.

RESEARCH

NATIONAL INSTITUTE OF NEUROLOGICAL DISEASES AND STROKE

This agency, which is part of the National Institutes of Health, U.S. Department of Health, Education and Welfare, supports a great deal of basic research related to the nature and functioning of the central nervous system. Specifically, in relation to cerebral palsy, is the collaborative study being conducted by this Institute on the Etiology of Cerebral Palsy and other Neurological and Sensory Disorders in Infancy and Childhood. This has been in operation since 1959 and involves intensive monitoring of 60,000 pregnancies, including follow-up of the children for as long as seven years. Some of the findings have been previously discussed in the section on Early Identification and Preventative Implications.

UNITED CEREBRAL PALSY RESEARCH AND EDUCATIONAL FOUNDATION

After several years of profitable investment in promoting basic research in the area of cerebral palsy, the Foundation has recently elected to establish new priorities for support. The overriding and principle direction will be toward the support of any worthwhile, well-constructed research which bears directly and immediately on the problem of the prevention or treatment of cerebral palsy.

Highlighted among these priorities are the following:

Prematurity. Prematurity is unquestionably the number-one enemy among the causes for cerebral palsy. This, coupled with the rising incidence of prematurity, particularly among the deprived segment of the community, requires increased emphasis directed toward the prevention of prematurity and improving the methods of managing the premature, high-risk infant after birth.

One research grant has supported the work of Dr. Kenneth Ryan, Chairman of the Department of Obstetrics and Gynecology of the University of California at San Diego, who has been exploring the hormonal control of the length of pregnancy. His investigations are indicating that the fetus itself may be exerting some control of its own destiny as it relates to the time it decides that it should be born. The fetus supplies certain precursors of the hormone estrogen manufactured by the placenta. As the fetus grows it supplies more of these substances. The time comes when the level of estrogen reaches a critical point (in relation to other parameters) that inititiates the onset of labor. These investigations of Dr. Ryan hopefully will lead to further understanding of factors which initiate labor and finally to means of delaying the onset of labor when it occurs prematurely.

Dr. Joseph Dieniarz, Director of the Laboratory of Uterine Physiology of the Michael Reese Medical Center in Chicago, is approaching this problem directly. He is assessing different treatment techniques that will inhibit contraction of the uterus. Each treatment is evaluated by the incidence of successfully maintained pregnancies and the degree of delay obtained in imminent premature labors, as compared with a group of premature labors without any treatment.

Infections Affecting the Brain. While we have come close to being able to prevent German measles with the use of a vaccine, there are undoubtedly a host of other viral agents which are capable of producing cerebral palsy. Some of these are very poorly understood, and may well turn out to be more frequent causes for cerebral palsy than German measles itself. In addition, there are other infections, particularly in very young children, which may produce brain damage and cerebral palsy. Oftentimes, these infections may be mild or inapparent, yet resulting in severe residual brain damage.

Dr. Heinz Eichenwald, Professor and Chairman of the Department of Pediatrics of the University of Texas Medical School at Dallas, has observed an increased incidence of neurologic impairment in children who gave histories of relatively minor diarrheal infections during their infancies, even though the infection did not involve the brain. A similar phenomenon has been described in mice who after a barely symptomatic intestinal virus infection have developed irreversible damage to their brains.

Dr. Richard Johnson, the Dwight D. Eisenhower United Cerebral

Palsy Professor of Neurology at the Johns Hopkins School of Medicine, is studying viral infections in the mother which cause the brain and spinal cord to develop in a malformed fashion. Understanding the mechanisms by which infections of the immature nervous system lead to malformations may in turn lead to more specific preventative measures.

Obstetrical and Newborn Factors. In the area of prevention, the Foundation is also providing research support into investigations of obstetrical factors around delivery which might place the infant at risk of developing brain damage and of factors affecting the status of the newborn which might predispose him to cerebral damage.

Some examples of research strategies covering this early period of life include the following:

Dr. Mary Ellen Avery, Chairman of the Department of Pediatrics at McGill University, is exploring the use of a specific hormone which appears to accelerate the maturation of the lung. This may prove to be useful in the prevention of respiratory difficulties in prematures who cannot absorb enough oxygen because of the immaturity of their lung cells. The persistence of the latter difficulty causes damage to brain cells when they do not receive enough oxygen.

Dr. Sidney Carter, United Cerebral Palsy Professor of Neurology at Columbia University, along with Dr. Stanley James, Professor of Anesthesiology, are measuring many chemical factors monitoring brain waves, electrocardiographs, and the speed of conduction of nerves. Many of these tests are being done while the fetus is in utero, while being delivered, and on the newborn infant while he is in the nursery. These studies are conducted to enable recognition at the earliest time when a baby is experiencing distress so that appropriate corrective measures can be taken prior to the onset of irreversible brain damage.

Jaundice in the Newborn. While we have come close to solving problems due to Rh blood group incompatibilities, there are other blood-grouping incompatibilities and other causes of jaundice which may be more insidious, more difficult to detect, and capable of producing equally serious brain damage. New methods of treating these conditions, if detected early, make it increasingly imperative that we move ahead with significant research in this area.

The UCP Foundation is supporting three research teams who are investigating a new approach to preventing the brain damage that ensues when a baby becomes excessively jaundiced. In 1958 Cremer in Great Britain suggested that intense light could reduce the blood level of bilirubin, the pigment responsible for damage to the brain as well as the yellow color of the skin. Although phototherapy is now a standard treatment for jaundice in many centers, there previously had been very little critical evaluation of the potential dosages and dangers of this seemingly simple treatment.

ORGANIZATIONS RELATED TO PROBLEM
OF CEREBRAL PALSY

THE AMERICAN ACADEMY FOR CEREBRAL PALSY

A professional membership organization that concerns itself primarily with the medical and therapeutic aspects of services. Recently the Academy has been extending its areas of interest to educational, psychological, and vocational aspects of services, as well as to family problems, and to a limited extent the problems of nonworking adults with cerebral palsy. Address inquiries to the Administrative Office, 1255 New Hampshire Ave., N.W., Washington, D.C.

UNITED CEREBRAL PALSY ASSOCIATIONS, INC.

A national voluntary agency devoting its total concern to individuals with cerebral palsy and to their families. There are about 300 local and state affiliates of the national organization which support or provide a variety of service programs—all of the more than 100 services listed in the UCPA chart (pp. 287–93) are being provided somewhere in the United States by one or more of the affiliates. Address inquiries to United Cerebral Palsy Associations, Inc., 66 East 34th St., New York, N.Y.

THE NATIONAL EASTER SEAL SOCIETY
FOR CRIPPLED CHILDREN AND ADULTS

Supports a large number of therapy or rehabilitation centers providing a variety of services to individuals with cerebral palsy, as well as to people with other disabling conditions. Address inquiries to the National Easter Seal Society for Crippled Children and Adults, 2026 Ogden Ave., Chicago, Ill.

THE NATIONAL CEREBRAL PALSY SECTION OF THE
CANADIAN REHABILITATION COUNCIL FOR THE DISABLED

Coordinates services for the cerebral palsied in Canada. Address inquiries to the Council at 165 Bloor St. East, Toronto 5.

THE INTERNATIONAL CEREBRAL PALSY SOCIETY

Recently formed as a successor to the World Commission on Cerebral Palsy that had functioned as a branch of Rehabilitation International. Sponsors conferences and other educational opportunities for people working with cerebral palsied individuals around the world. Address inquiries to the Society at 12 Park Crescent, London, W.1.

REFERENCES

Abercrombie, M. L. J. 1968. Some notes on spatial disability: movement, intelligence quotient and attentiveness. Develop. Med. Child Neurol. 10:206.

Anderson, G. W. 1953. Current needs for research on the obstetrical factors in cerebral palsy. Cerebral Palsy Review 14:3–8.

Anderson, W. 1963. The hyperkinetic child: a neurological appraisal. Neurology 13:968.

Bax, Martin C. O. 1964. Terminology and classification of cerebral palsy. Develop. Med. Child Neurol. 6:295–97.

Bax, Martin C. O. and R. C. MacKeith, eds. 1960. Child neurology and cerebral palsy. Little Club Clinic, Devel. Med. no. 2, National Spastics Society, London.

Bobath, B. 1967. The very early treatment of cerebral palsy. Develop. Med. Child Neurol. 9:373–90.

Brazelton, T. B. 1961. Psychophysiologic reactions in the neonate: the value of the observation of the neonate. J. of Pediatrics 38:508.

Byers, R. K. 1941. Evolution of hemiplegias in infancy. Amer. J. Disc. Children. 61:915.

Caviness, J. A. and E. J. Gibson. 1964. Visual and tactual perception of solid shape. Ithaca, N.Y., Cornell University, unpublished doctoral.

Cohen, H. J., L. T. Taft, M. S. Mahadeviah, and H. G. Birch. 1967. Developmental changes in overflow in normal and aberrantly functioning children. J. Pediatrics 71:39.

Connor, F. P. 1970. Education for the very young handicapped child: A curriculum concept, pp. 71–85, in Hensley and Patterson, eds.

Courville, C. B. 1954. Cerebral palsy. Los Angeles, San Lucas Press.

Crothers, B. 1951. Clinical aspects of cerebral palsy: life history of disease. Quarterly Review of Pediatrics 6:142–48.

Crowell, D. April 1971. Project to study infant's responses to stimuli. Personal communication.

Cruickshank, W., ed. 1966. Cerebral palsy: its individual and community problems. Syracuse, Syracuse University Press.

Denhoff, E. 1970. Meeting Street School Home Developmental Guideline Program, in Hensley and Patterson, eds.

—— 1967. Cerebral palsy, the preschool years. Springfield, Ill., Thomas.

Denhoff, E. and M. Langdon, eds. 1966. Cerebral dysfunction: a treatment program for young children. Clinical Pediatrics 6:332.

Denhoff, E. and I. P. Robinault. 1960. Cerebral palsy and related disorders. New York, McGraw-Hill.

Eisenberg, L. 1966. The management of the hyperkinetic child. Develop. Med. Child Neurol. 8:593.

Finnie, N. R. 1970. Handling the young cerebral palsied child at home, in U. Haynes, ed.

Frankenburg, W. K. and J. B. Dodds. 1966. Denver developmental screening test manual. Denver, University of Colorado Medical Center.

Friedman, Dale. 1963. Work evaluation technique leading to organization of a workshop, in O'Brien, ed.

Gallagher, J. H. 1956. Rjecting parents. Exceptional Children 22:273.

Garrett, J. 1963. The cerebral palsied adult, pp. 19–20, in O'Brien, ed.

Gesell, A. 1941. Developmental diagnosis. New York, Harper, p. 277.

Gesell, A. and C. S. Amatruda. 1947. Developmental diagnosis. New York, Paul Hoeber.

Gesell, A., H. M. Halverson, H. Thompson, F. L. Ilg, B. M. Castner, and L. B. Ames. 1960. The first five years of life. New York, Harper.

Gillett, H. E. 1969. Systems of therapy. Springfield, Ill., Charles C. Thomas.

Goldstein, K. 1936. Modifications of behavior consequent to cerebral lesions. Psychiatric Quarterly 10:586.

Gordon, N. 1968. Visual agnosia in childhood. Develop. Med. Child Neurol. 10:377–79.

Guide for an information, referral and follow-along service in a United Cerebral Palsy affiliate. 1970. New York, United Cerebral Palsy Associations, Inc.

Haith, M. 1971. Visual perception in newborn infants. Personal communication.

Haynes, U. 1967. A developmental approach to casefinding, PHS document 2017. Washington, D. C., Superintendent of Documents, U. S. Government Printing Office.

Haynes, U., ed. 1970. Handling the young cerebral palsied child at home. New York, Dutton.

Hebb, D. O. 1947. The effects of early experience in problem-solving at maturity. The Amer. Psychologist 2:306–307.

—— 1955. Drives and the C.N.S. (conceptual nervous system). Psychological Review 62:243–54.

Hensley, G. and V. Patterson, eds. 1970. Interdisciplinary programing for infants with known or suspect cerebral dysfunction. Boulder, Colo., Western Interstate Commission for Higher Education.

Hunt, J. M. 1961. Intelligence and experience. New York, Ronald Press.

Ingram, T. T. S. 1966. The neurology of cerebral palsy. Archives of Diseases of Childhood 41:337.

—— 1964. Pediatric aspects of cerebral palsy. Edinburgh, Livingstone, p. 1.

—— 1962. In minimal cerebral dysfunction. Clinics In Developmental Medicine 10:10–17. London, Spastics Society with Heinemann.

—— 1960. Perceptual disorders causing dyslexia and dysgraphia, pp. 97–104, in Bax and MacKeith, eds.

Jones, M. H. 1969. Early identification of children with potential learning problems. B. K. Keogh, ed. Los Angeles, University of California, Department of Education.

—— 1970. A program profile for infants and young children with physical handicaps, pp. 31–50, in Hensley and Patterson, eds.

Jones, M. H., W. H. Wenner, A. Toozek, M. Ariadne, and M. L. Barrett. 1962. Pre-nursery program for children with cerebral palsy. J. Amer. Women's Med. Assoc. 17:713–19.

Jones, M. H., M. L. Barrett, M. Delsasso, and E. Minter. December, 1969. The young handicapped child and the triumverate: parent-child-professional staff. Presented at Special Conference on Early Childhood Education, New Orleans, La.

Jones, M. H., C. Olonoff, and E. Anderson. 1969. Two experiments in training handicapped children at nursery school, in Planning for better living. Clinics in Developmental Medicine 33:108–22. London, Spastics International Medical Publications.

Kagan, J. 1966. Psychological development of the child; I. Personality, behavior, and temperament, pp. 326–67, in Falkner Frank, ed., Human development. Philadelphia, Saunders.

Keats, S. 1965. Cerebral palsy. Springfield, Ill., Charles C. Thomas.

Kempe, C. H., F. Silverman, F. Steele, W. Droegemueller, and H. K. Silver. 1962. The battered child syndrome. J. Amer. Med. Assoc. 181:17.

Kessen, W. and P. Salapatek. 1971. Response of newborns to horizontal and vertical edges. J. Experimental Child Psychology.

Lilienfeld, A. M. and E. Parkhurst. 1951. Study of association of factors of pregnancy and parturition with the development of cerebral palsy. Amer. J. Hygiene 53:262.

Lilienfeld, A. M. and B. Pasamanick. 1954. The association of maternal and fetal factors with the development of epilepsy. I. Abnormalities in the prenatal and perinatal periods. J. Amer. Med. Assoc. 155:719.

Lilienfeld, A. M., B. Pasamanick, and M. Rogers. 1955. Relationship between pregnancy experience and development of certain neuropsychiatric disorders in childhood. Amer. J. Pub. Health 45:637.

Luria, A. R. 1957. Experimental analysis of the development of voluntary action in children. Paper read to the 15th International Congress of Psychology, Montreal.

Millichap, J. G. 1968. Drugs in management of hyperkinetic and perceptually handicapped children. J. Amer. Med. Assoc. 206:1527.

Mitchell, R. G. 1971. The prevention of cerebral palsy. Devel. Med. Child Neurol. 18:137–46.

Nesbitt, R. E. 1957. Prenatal loss in modern obstetrics. Philadelphia, Davis.

Oberman, W. 1965. Personal communication, U. S. Department of Health, Education and Welfare, Welfare Administration, Children's Bureau.

O'Brien, S. B., ed. 1963. Total life planning for the cerebral palsied. New York, United Cerebral Palsy Associations, Inc.

Paine, R. S. 1960. Disturbances of sensation in cerebral palsy, pp. 105–9, in Bax and MacKeith, eds.

Perlstein, M. A. 1952. Infantile cerebral palsy, classification and clinical correlations. J. Amer. Med. Assoc. 149:30–34.

Phelps, W. M. 1947. Cerebral palsy, in A. O. Whipple, ed. Nelson new loose-leaf surgery. New York, Nelson, pp. 180–O–180–S.

Rembolt, R. R. 1970. Programing for infants with cerebral dysfunction: an overview, pp. 1–20, in Hensley and Patterson, eds.

Reuben, R. N. and H. Bakwin. 1968. Developmental clumsiness. Pediat. Clin. N. Amer. 15:601.

Robinson, H. B. 1970. Research in cognition, pp. 51–55, in Hensley and Patterson, eds.

Rogers, M. E., A. M. Lilienfeld, and B. Pasamanick. 1954. Prenatal and paranatal factors in the development of childhood behavior disorders. Baltimore, Johns Hopkins University School of Hygiene and Public Health.

Sheltered workshops: a handbook. 1966. Washington, D. C., National Association of Sheltered Workshops and Homebound Programs.

Skatvedt, M. 1960. Non-motor defects in cerebral palsy, pp. 115–19 in Bax and MacKeith, eds.

Solomons, G., R. H. Holden, and E. Denhoff. 1963. The changing picture of cerebral dysfunction in early childhood. J. Pediat. 63:113–20.

Starr, R. H. Feb. 12–14, 1970. Cognitive development in infancy: Assessment, acceleration, and actualization. Paper presented at the Merrill-Palmer Institute Conference on Research and Teaching of Infant Development.

Strauss, A. A. and H. Werner. 1943. Comparative psychopathology of brain-injured child and traumatic brain-injured adult. Amer. J. Psychiat. 99:835.

Strothers, G. R. 1970. Role of psychologist in programing for infants with known or suspected cerebral dysfunction, pp. 61–71, in Hensley and Patterson, eds.

Tannenbaum, A. J. 1969. The taxonomic instruction project: A manual of principles and practices pertaining to the content of instruction. Report to U. S. Office of Education.

Tizard, J. P. N. 1960. Some aspects of disorders of sensation, pp. 120–22 in Bax and MacKeith, eds.

Walker, M. 1965. Perceptual, coding, visuo-motor and spatial difficulties and their neurological correlates. Develop. Med. Child Neurol. 7:543–48.

Wallace, H. 1960. A study of cerebral palsy. Minnesota School of Public Health. Minneapolis, University of Minnesota, pp. 8–9.

Walton, J. M. 1960. Clumsy children, p. 24, in Bax and MacKeith, eds.

Wigglesworth, J. S. 1969. Malnutrition and brain development. Develop. Med. Child Neurol. 11:792–803.

Williams, J. 1960. The effect of emotional factors on perception and concept formation in cerebral palsied children, pp. 115–19 in Bax and MacKeith, eds.

Wishik, S. M. Feb. 1956. Handicapped children in Georgia: a study of prevalence, disability, needs, and resources. Amer. J. Pub. Health, 46:195–203.

Zangwill, O. L. 1960. Deficiency of spatial perception, pp. 133–136 in Bax and MacKeith, eds.

UCPA CHART OF PROGRAM SERVICES: MIDDLETOWN *

Service Categories	0–18 mos.	19 mos.–3 yrs.	3.1 yrs.–5 yrs.	5.1 yrs.–10 yrs.	10.1 yrs.–16 yrs.	16.1 yrs.–21 yrs.	21 and over
COMMUNITY ORGANIZATION AND PLANNING FOR SERVICES							
Community Councils	G	G	G	G	G	G	G
Inter-Agency Cooperation	G	G	G	G	G	G	G
Directory of Resources	G	G	G	G	G	G	G
Statistics	I	I	I	I	I	I	I
MR and MH Planning	N	N	N	N	N	N	N
Regional Medical Planning	?	?	?	?	?	?	?
Funding	N	N	N	A	A	N	N
Professional Services Program Committee	N	N	N	N	N	N	N
Licensing: *Certification; Accreditation*	?	?	?	?	?	?	?
Periodic Evaluation	W	W	W	W	W	W	W
Legislative Action	W	W	W	W	W	W	W
Insurance: *Health; Accident; Liability*	N	N	N	N	N	N	N
Equipment: *Special; Loan*	I	I	I	A	A	I	I
Architecture: *Program; Home Adaptations; Barriers*	W	W	W	W	W	W	W
Transportation: *Mass; Special; Volunteer*	I	I	I	I	I	I	I
MEDIA							
News Sheets	G	G	G	G	G	G	G
Instructional Materials	I	I	A	A	A	I	I
Audio-Visual Aids	I	I	A	A	A	I	I
PROFESSIONAL EDUCATION-PERSONNEL TRAINING							
Public Education	W	W	I	A	A	A	A
Schools and Colleges: *Information;*						A	I

(UCPA CHART, continued)

Service Categories	0–18 mos.	19 mos.–3 yrs.	3.1 yrs.–5 yrs.	5.1 yrs.–10 yrs.	10.1 yrs.–16 yrs.	16.1 yrs.–21 yrs.	21 and over
Affiliation							
Inter-Agency	N	N	N	N	N	N	N
Intra-Agency	W	W	W	W	W	W	W
Staff: *Orientation and Inservice*	G	G	G	G	G	G	G
Staff: *Program Skills*	G	G	G	G	G	G	G
Staff: *Administrative Skills*	I	I	A	A	A	A	N
Professional Education	N	N	A	A	A	I	N
Volunteer: *Training*	G	G	G	G	G	G	G
Contact Care Personnel: *Training*	W	W	W	W	W	W	W
Religious Counselors: *Orientation*	I	I	A	A	A	I	I
HOUSING							
Long Term: *Public; Private*	I	I	I	I	I	I	I
Short Term: *Emergency; Vacation*	N	N	N	I	I	I	I
Residence for Working Adult	X	X	X	X	X	N	N
LONG TERM CARE							
Planning for the Future	W	W	W	W	W	W	W
Program: *Life Enrichment*	X	X	X	X	I	I	I
Medical Management	X	X	X	I	I	I	I
Personal Interest: *Big-Brother Program etc.*	X	X	X	W	W	W	W
Home Service	N	N	I	I	I	I	I
Visiting Nurse Service	?	?	?	?	?	?	?
Residence: *Adapted; Foster/Nursing Home;*	?	?	?	?	?	?	?
Public	X	X	I	I	I	I	I
Legislation	W	W	W	W	W	W	W

	C1	C2	C3	C4	C5	C6	C7	C8
Guardianship: *Person; Property*	W	W	W	W	W	W	W	W
Financing	W	W	W	W	W	W	W	W
SOCIAL SERVICES								
Information and Referral	I	I	I	I	I	I	I	I
Follow-Along Service	N	N	N	N	N	N	N	N
Case Finding	W	I	I	A	A	I	I	I
Case Register	N	N	N	N	N	N	N	N
Case Work Services	G	G	G	G	G	G	G	G
Parent Counseling	G	G	G	G	G	G	G	G
Individual Counseling	X	X	X	X	I	I	I	I
Group Counseling	X	X	X	X	N	N	N	N
Home Maker Services	?	?	?	?	?	?	?	?
PREVENTION								
Immunization: *Staff and Public Education and Implementation*	I	I	I	A	A	I	I	I
Secondary Disabilities: *Priorities*	?	?	?	?	?	?	?	?
Mothers-at-Risk: *Follow-up*	X	X	X	X	X	W	W	W
Infants-at-Risk: *Follow-up*	W	W	X	X	X	X	X	X
Professional Education: *Interdisciplinary*	G	G	G	G	G	G	G	G
MEDICAL SERVICES								
Detection and Case Finding	I	I	A	A	A	I	I	I
Developmental Examination: *Motor; Vision; Hearing*	W	I	I	I	X	X	X	X
Diagnosis and Short-Term Goals: *Parent Guidance*	W	I	A	A	A	I	I	I
Specialty Consultation	I	I	A	A	A	I	I	I

	0–18 mos.	19 mos.–3 yrs.	3.1 yrs.–5 yrs.	5.1 yrs.–10 yrs.	10.1 yrs.–16 yrs.	16.1 yrs.–21 yrs.	21 and over
MEDICAL SERVICES							
Drug Rx	I	I	A	A	A	I	I
Dental Examination and Care	W	W	I	I	I	I	W
Physical Therapy } EVALUATION	W	W	A	A	A	W	W
Occupation Therapy } EVALUATION	W	W	A	A	A	W	W
Speech and Hearing } AND THERAPY	W	W	A	A	A	I	I
Nursing Care	I	I	I	I	I	N	N
Surgery: *Orthopedic; Neurologic*	G	G	G	G	G	G	G
Rx Aids: *Hearing; Glasses; Braces*	W	W	A	A	A	I	I
Rx Equipment	W	W	I	I	I	W	W
Periodic Medical Re-Evaluation	I	I	A	A	A	I	I
Hearing and Vision Re-Checks: *Preschool; Prevocational*							
Seizure Control Re-Checks	I	I	A	A	A	I	I
Physical Capacity: *Prevocational Checkup*	X	X	A	A	I	I	I
Periodic Health Re-Checks: *Teens; Adults*	X	X	X	X	I	I	I
Public Health Case Register: *Official*	W	W	W	W	W	W	W
Research—Related to Care	?	?	?	?	?	?	?
Psychiatric Consultation	N	N	I	I	I	N	N
PSYCHOLOGICAL SERVICES							
Development Assessment and Goals	I	I	A	A	A	I	I
Tests: *Intelligence; Personality*	I	I	A	A	A	I	I
Retest and Re-Evaluation: *Preschool; Preteen; Prevocation etc.*	I	I	A	A	A	I	I
Consultation: *Staff: Inter Agency*	N	N	N	N	N	N	N

EDUCATIONAL SERVICES, etc. table (rotated on page):

Counseling: Individual and Group	W	W	W	W	W	W	W
Psychotherapy	X	X	X	X	I	I	I
Perception: Tests and Remedial Recommendations	W	W	I	I	I	N	N
EDUCATIONAL SERVICES							
Evaluation: Communication and Academic Achievement	X	I	I	A	A	A	I
Learning Problems and Goals: Review and Remediation							
Prenursery and Nursery Groups	X	I	I	A	A	I	I
Baby Programs	X	N	A	X	X	X	X
Preschool Readiness Programs: Kindergarten; Ungraded	N	X	X	X	X	X	X
Day Care and Developmental Programs	X	X	A	A	X	X	X
Regular Schooling: Public; Private	X	I	I	A	A	N	N
Special Class: Public School; Private Agency	X	X	I	A	A	I	X
Special School	X	X	I	I	I	N	X
Residential School	X	X	I	I	I	N	X
Home Instruction	X	X	N	N	Z	N	X
Prevocational Goals and Experiences: Preteen; Teenage; Late Teen	X	X	I	A	A	I	X
Continuing Education Adult	X	X	X	X	I	X	I
RECREATIONAL SERVICES							
Friendly Visitation	W	W	W	W	W	W	W
Adapted Sports: Swimming; Bowling;	W	W	W	W	W	W	W

	0–18 mos.	19 mos.–3 yrs.	3.1 yrs.–5 yrs.	5.1 yrs.–10 yrs.	10.1 yrs.–16 yrs.	16.1 yrs.–21 yrs.	21 and over
RECREATIONAL SERVICES							
Physical Education	X	X	I	A	A	I	I
Group Activities: *Scouts; Adapted Games; Trips; etc.*	X	X	X	I	I	I	N
Hobbies and Creative Activities	X	X	X	A	A	A	I
Spectator Sports	X	X	X	I	I	I	I
Day Camping	X	X	X	A	A	I	N
Resident Camp	X	X	X	I	I	I	N
Family Activities	X	X	N	N	N	N	N
VOCATIONAL SERVICES							
Prevocational Assessment: *Preteen; Teen*	X	X	X	X	I	I	X
Vocational Evaluation	X	X	X	X	X	A	I
Goals, Guidance, Counseling	X	X	X	X	I	A	I
Personal Adjustment Training	X	X	X	X	X	I	I
Training for Skills	X	X	X	X	X	W	W
Work Activity Program: *Part-time; Full-time*	X	X	X	X	X	A	A
Work Experience: *Volunteer; Paid*	X	X	X	X	X	I	I

Sheltered Employment: *Workshop; Small Business*   X   X   X   X   N   N   N

Special Placement Employment   X   X   X   X   N   N   N

Home Employment   X   X   X   X   N   N   N

Source: Professional Services Program Dept., United Cerebral Palsy Associations, Inc., 66 East 34th Street, New York, New York 10016

* Population: 150,000
Estimated Number of CPs: 210
Number of CP Children (Identified): 75
Number of CP Adults (Identified): 25

Legend: A = Adequate   G = Available Generally
        I = Inadequate   (Not Related to age groups)
          (Something being done)   X = Not Applicable
       N = Not Available   ? = Do Not Know
       W = Nothing Being Done

LEONARD DILLER

HEMIPLEGIA

HEMIPLEGIA IS KNOWN to be the largest residual problem following a cerebrovascular accident. Although commonly thought of as a disease, it is not. It is rather a disability that is caused by a disease or accident involving the brain, commonly termed "stroke," "shock," or apoplexy. The disability that results from the brain injury—hemiplegia—takes the form of paralysis of greater or lesser degree on the side of the body opposite the site of the brain damage. If the paralysis is not total, it is termed paresis. Although hemiplegia is commonly associated with old age, it strikes at all ages and most often at birth and in middle and old age. When hemiplegia occurs in childhood, it is usually categorized as one of the cerebral palsies. Since the cerebral palsies are comprehensively discussed in the chapter on the subject by Messner and Haynes, the focus of the present chapter is on hemiplegia in adulthood.

INCIDENCE

Kurtzke and Kurland (1970) note that stroke occurs in about 1,500,000 Americans annually. In the 70 per cent of stroke victims who survive, it is estimated that their diagnosis, treatment, and rehabilitation costs at least $440,000,000 a year. It is further estimated that secondary losses due to premature death and disability are equivalent to more than 179,000,000 man-hours, or $700,000,000 annually.

LEONARD DILLER, Ph.D., serves as Chief of Behavioral Sciences, Institute of Rehabilitation Medicine, New York University.

The incidence of hemiplegia following stroke is difficult to assess. In Adler's (1969) survey of 5,000 survivors of stroke in Israel during a four-year period, 46 per cent had a permanent hemiplegia and 43 per cent had a transient paresis. Estimates of the number of hemiplegics in this country range from 1,000,000 (Harris and Towler, 1955) to 4,000,000 (Howard, 1960). Extrapolating from a different set of data, Waylonis, Becker, and Krueger (1970), in a study of 106 stroke victims admitted to hospitals in a midwest county with a population of 100,000, suggest an annual incidence of 200,000 to 300,000 survivors of stroke in this country, with the majority of these patients having residual hemiplegia.

It is hard to estimate how many hemiplegics are of working age. However, Gulliksen (1970) states that there are 250,000 between the ages of eighteen and sixty-five in this country. Kurtzke and Kurland (1970) have reviewed the incidence of cerebrovascular disease in different countries and point out enormous variations between cultures. For example, in Japan there is reported to be a much higher incidence of stroke than in other countries. This may be due in part to the fact that death due to cerebral hemorrhage is considered a mark of honor.

As previously mentioned, hemiplegia strikes at all ages, the incidence following a bimodal distribution. By far the greatest incidence occurs in people over fifty years of age. As Harris and Towler (1955) note, increasing the life expectancy in our society has unfortunately been shadowed by an increasing incidence of cerebrovascular disease.

DEFINITION, CLASSIFICATION, DESCRIPTION

A paralytic stroke may be defined as a neurologic disorder of abrupt development due to a pathologic process in blood vessels (American Heart Association, 1956 and 1958). In addition to its focal etiology, the notable feature of a stroke is its chronological profile. This is characterized by abrupt onset and rapid progress, the symptoms reaching a peak in seconds, minutes, or hours. If not at once fatal, a partial or complete recovery occurs in a period of hours, days, weeks, or months. A careful history will reveal that in some cases the disease advanced with slow progression by a series of small strokes. The stroke itself may vary in pattern and severity from a violent assault in which the person falls in his tracks, deprived of sense and motion with one arm and leg paralyzed—apoplexy means "to be struck down"—to a very slight deficit or derangement in speech, thought, voluntary motion, sensation, or vision.

To distinguish reversability due to the characteristics of the disease as opposed to reversability due to intervention, the following categorization has been adopted in the field: (1) *Transient ischemic attack* (TIA): a sudden cerebral episode with distinct neurologic deficit which disappears in minutes or hours. (2) *Steadily progressive from onset* (SPO): a serious neurologic deficit which progresses steadily in a "stuttering" fashion over a number of days. (3) *Single catastrophic episode* (SCE): a definitive neurologic deficit of severe degree which appears to have become stationary.

While the chronological pattern can be discerned from the history, evidence for the focal character of the brain damage is manifested by the nature of the motor paralysis. Hemiplegia is thought to be a consequence of damage to a specific area of the brain, the motor cortex, and adjacent subcortical structures that play important roles in the regulation of voluntary movement. As previously stated, if the paralysis is not total, it is then known as paresis; hence the term hemiparesis is used to refer to weakness or partial paralysis of one side of the body.

Hemiplegia affects voluntary movement of both the affected arm and leg. Contractures are a frequent problem (Rusk, 1971, 3rd ed.), for in the human body the muscles pulling the limbs toward the body are generally stronger than those pushing the limbs away from it. The hemiplegic will therefore show a characteristic stance, with the paralyzed arm flexed at the elbow, wrist, and fingers, the shoulder rotated inward to the middle of the body, the lower extremity and hips rotated inward, and the knee and ankle flexed. In walking, the hemiplegic will tend to swing the affected leg outward in a semicircle.

Although the hemiplegia is the primary disability, paralysis is seldom the only symptom. Spasm and contractures may interfere further with voluntary motion. There is often residual weakness of the lower two-thirds of the face so that the nasolabial fold appears flattened; and, when the patient talks, the mouth turns down on the involved side and pulls to the uninvolved side. Vasomotor changes on the affected side occur so that the skin of the affected side eventually becomes dry and cold. Very often changes in response to sensation are present. The hemiplegic may show dulled response to touch, temperature, and pain on the affected side. Vision and hearing may be impaired in both gross and subtle ways. Food no longer tastes the same. The patient may chew food properly only on one side of his mouth. Despite diminished sensation, complaint of intractible pain may be present. This may be accompanied by uncontrollable weeping. Minor personality changes (Harris and Towler, 1955), irritability, lethargic states, psychotic manifestations, and lapses in memory and judgment may appear. In 50 per cent of the hemiplegics—usually those associated with a right-sided paralysis —aphasia will occur. Whereas hemiplegia is basically a motor disability, more often than not it involves a whole psychomotor symptom complex.

SPECIAL CONSIDERATIONS IN THE
REHABILITATION PICTURE

THE QUESTION OF BRAIN DAMAGE

In hemiplegia, while it is clear that brain damage occurs in all cases, mental and behavioral functioning are not always adversely affected. Indeed, the varieties of responses are very great. It may help us understand these responses by considering some of the distinguishing traits of hemiplegics with and without mental and/or behavioral dysfunction. The former are commonly referred to in the literature as "organic brain-damaged"; the latter as the "nonorganic." Although these terms shall be used here for convenience sake, it must be stressed that they refer to mental and behavioral function rather than to actual brain damage. "Organic" refers to alterations in behavior and thought characteristically associated with brain damage. "Nonorganic" refers to the fact that mental and behavioral functioning appear to remain intact following brain damage.

We may then ask three pertinent questions: How often is organic behavior manifested in hemiplegia? Why is it present in some cases and not in others? What are the phenomena and problems associated with organic behavior? In answer to the first question, three independent studies (Birch and Diller, 1959; Weinblatt, 1959; Diller, Buxbaum, and Chiotelis, 1972) report that about half the hemiplegic subjects exhibited organic behavior. To answer the question of why organicity occurs in some people and not in others involves the whole concept of brain function. As previously indicated, not all brain-damaged people behave the same way. Let us, therefore, ask: Are there any basic attributes of brain function that, when impaired, result in uniform behavioral disturbances? Among the factors that warrant considerations are: size of lesion, site of lesion; nature of damage; age at which damage occurred; duration; and premorbid personality, intellect, and education.

Size of Lesion. For well over a century debate has raged over whether the amount of brain tissue that is destroyed, damaged, or diseased is or is not related to the amount of behavioral disturbance. The evidence thus far indicates that the size of the lesion per se is not the relevant factor in disturbances involving the "simple behavioral functions," that is, sensation, locomotion, etc. However, whether the size of the damage is related to disturbances of the "higher level functions" such as planning ability, motivation, etc. is still under dispute. While there are some who present evidence that a direct relationship exists (Chapman, Thetford, Beden, Guthrie, and Wolff, 1958), there is also evidence that an individual may be hemiplegic as a result of a hemispherectomy (removal of one side of the brain) yet show no basic impairment in higher-level functions (Bruell, Albee, and others, 1958; Goldstein, Goodman, and King, 1956).

Location of Lesion. Location of lesion can present a highly important factor. As already noted in the case of hemiplegia, damage to the left side of the brain is associated with right-sided paralysis and aphasia, while damage to the right side of the brain is associated with left hemiplegia and spatial disturbances (Reitan and Fitzhugh, 1971). Typically, the individual right hemiplegic profits more from nonverbal instructions. The individual with left hemiplegia profits from verbal directions (Fordyce and Jones, 1966). Hemispheric differences also suggest other correlates of interest. (1) Some observers have suggested that in left hemiplegia the primary defect is in the registration of visual stimuli. The patient fails to scan his visual environment. However, registration of auditory stimuli and retention of both visual and auditory stimuli once the information is in the system may be quite intact. The right hemiplegics are able to register visual stimuli but have difficulty in registering auditory stimuli and retaining stimuli in both modalities (Diller and Weinberg, 1970). Different patients may therefore fail the same task for different reasons and should therefore be taught in different ways. (2) Left and right hemiplegics have more accidents in rehabilitation programs than other disabled people (Diller and Weinberg, 1970). The frequency and pattern of accidents are related to impairments in information processing. (3) Left hemiplegics differ from right hemiplegics in affective styles. Left hemiplegics typically respond with patterns of denial. Right hemiplegics respond with anxiety.

Nature of Damage. It has been suggested that if we view brain damage not in terms of the locus or size of the lesion but in terms of the nature of the lesion, meaningful insights into the behavioral consequences of brain damage can be educed (Birch and Diller, 1959). For example, brain damage that is due to a specific, focalized, clean-cut lesion, such as that generally induced by surgery or an embolus, may cause a subtractive loss wherein only specific functions (not "high-level ones") are impaired. On the other hand, brain damage due to additive or disruptive lesions, which tend to occur when neurochemical or electrical forces of the brain are impaired, affects the brain in areas far removed from the size of the damage and tends to interfere with the functioning of the personality as a whole (Rosenzweig, Krech, and Bennett, 1960). This proposal has been advanced to explain the observation that an epileptic who suffers from increased seizures owing to scar tissue following surgery will perform better when the scar tissue is removed (Penfield and Jasper, 1953). The anomaly here is that more intact functioning occurs following seemingly increased brain-tissue destruction (of the subtractive type) than existed before when an additive lesion interfered with functioning. In other words, absent tissue is better than sick tissue. In general, hemiplegias occurring in arteriosclerotic populations would tend to show additive-type losses because arteriosclerosis can produce widespread changes all over the brain (Birch and Diller, 1959).

Age of Onset. The author has found no studies comparing hemiplegics in terms of age of onset. However, a number of interesting observations have been made: (1) the incidence of spastic hemiplegic in infantile cerebral palsy is relatively large, representing nearly one half of the spastic cerebral palsied in one large study (Perlstein and Hood, 1957); (2) while only 10 per cent of cerebral palsy is postnatally acquired, nearly one third of the spastic condition is postnatally acquired (Perlstein and Hood, 1957); (3) spastic hemiplegics show a delay of about nine months in walking and in speaking first words when compared with normal children, with the delay seemingly more closely related to intelligence and emotional factors than to the physical handicaps (Perlstein and Hood, 1957). One study comparing adult hemiplegics with brain-injured children on a series of perceptual tasks found many similarities (Belmont, 1957).

Duration. In the recovery of skills following brain damage, the rate of recovery is greater the closest to the time of onset. The maximum rate of recovery occurs during the first three months. However, this must be qualified in two important ways. First, recovery may differ for different systems of disturbance, for example, language, visual, motor. Second, while the rate of recovery slows down, specific skills continue to be learned as the patient adapts to his residual disability.

ORGANIC AND NONORGANIC REACTIONS

Whereas we have discussed organic and nonorganic reactions as if they were mutually exclusive, we should repeat that this is an oversimplification. In point of fact, there is probably a continuum, with organic and nonorganic at opposite ends, rather than a pure dichotomy. What are the reactions of the typical organic and nonorganic hemiplegic? These may be summarized under the following major categories: (1) life rhythms; (2) psychological functions; and (3) contacts with environment.

Life rhythms. Many hemiplegics complain of difficulties in sleeping and eating. These complaints occur with equal frequency among the organic and the nonorganic and may be related to problems of aging. The organic, however, tends to report disruption of toilet habits. In addition, he complains of somatic pains, disturbances, odd sensations, and is irritable with people and events in his environment. As a matter of fact, these varied complaints are as characteristic of the organic as is their absence in the nonorganic (Weinblatt, 1959). Organic patients require sameness of environment and regress in skills if a physical therapist is changed. The nonorganic patient is not perturbed by change. Nonorganics do not regress when therapists are changed (Diller, Buxbaum, and Chiotelis, 1972).

Psychological functions. The organic may be compared with the non-organic on a number of important psychological dimensions, including (1) perception, (2) thinking, (3) learning, (4) the emotions.

1) *Perception.* In contrast with the nonorganic, whose perceptions are basically unimpaired, the perception of the organic is marked by insecurity, fragmentation, and impotence. When presented with a task requiring the organization of a pattern of stimuli, the organic will complain about his inability to perform rather than proceed to try to solve the problem. These complaints are similar to the ones encountered when he faces complex tasks in his environment. Whereas perception refers to the pattern or meaning of sensation, it is quite clear that not only physical stimuli but also psychological stimuli can be "perceived." For example, one can perceive a feeling tone or a subtle communication between people. Psychologists have used the Rorschach inkblot test for many years as an index for organicity, because it is a complex perceptual task (Evans and Marmorstein, 1964). Although we lack a viable taxonomy of perception and its pathology, the past decade has seen a number of attempts to arrive at a more analytic view of perceptual breakdown in brain-damaged people. A perceptual problem may be related to specific defects in sensation (De Renzi and Faglioni, 1965) or a defect in integrating information from two sensory modalities (Birch and Belmont, 1962). It is also important to see if the breakdown is in the organization of the sensory inputs (afferent organization) or in integrating the information for action (Bortner and Birch, 1960). While psychologists used to equate perceptual problems with disturbances of figure ground relationships (Allen, 1962), this view appears to be giving way to more sophisticated and analytic information-processing concepts which may be more relevant for rehabilitation. For example, how does a hemiplegic search his environment? In any event, perceptual difficulties are one of the signal characteristics of organic hemiplegics (Birch and Diller, 1959).

2) *Thinking.* Thinking disturbances also distinguish organic and nonorganic hemiplegics. Organics have difficulty in assuming the "abstract attitude." This is reflected in difficulties in assuming a definite mental set; accounting to themselves for their actions and thoughts; shifting

from one aspect of a situation to another; keeping in mind various aspects of the task; grasping the essentials of a problem or a Gestalt; voluntarily evoking previous images; assuming an attitude toward the possible future other than the immediate concrete present; detaching themselves from the outer world; grasping conceptual symbols; and identifying common properties in diverse settings (Goldstein, 1959). Thus, the organic hemiplegic is preoccupied with his pain because it is immediately present in his environment. He finds it hard to talk about his future plans because he cannot consider anything beyond his immediate sensations and environment. Other examples of such concrete thinking are readily apparent in rehabilitation. The physiotherapist who asks the hemiplegic to walk to the end of the parallel bars while she tends to another patient may find that the hemiplegic has continued to walk back and forth on the parallel bars until told to stop (Belmont, Ambrose, Benjamin, and Restuccia, 1969). Various sensory paresthesias are accepted as real because of their immediacy. The patient performs well in one setting but not in another so that, when a program is changed, he becomes irritable and upset.

3) *Learning.* Some psychologists have pointed out the consequences of concrete thinking for learning (Mednick and Freedman, 1960). People who think concretely cannot generalize or transfer the meaning of stimuli and experiences from one learning situation to another. The hemiplegic who can solve a space problem with one occupational therapist may be unable to solve the same problem with another. The context and the conditions of learning are much more influential in organic than nonorganic hemiplegics. Hemiplegics both older and younger condition to positive verbal reinforcers, but not to negative (Halberstam and Zaretsky, 1969). This is probably a reflection of the patient's low self-esteem. However, if a patient can move his paralyzed hand, he can be conditioned to withdraw his hand from shock (Halberstam, Zaretsky, Brucker, and Guttman, 1971).

4) *Emotional reactions.* The most common reaction to hemiplegia is depression. Depression occurs equally often in organic and nonorganic patients. The difference between the two lies in the fact that depression may appear to be all-pervasive in organic cases because of the inability of such patients to shift their thinking and take their minds off their disability. Common sources of depression are the disability itself and the

loss of mastery associated with the disability. This sense of loss often revives all other losses experienced in life so that the patient feels overwhelmed by loss. For example, a female hemiplegic was able to say that she felt depressed because her paralysis reminded her of the time she spent in a concentration camp and of her husband's death following her arrival in America. In some hemiplegics weeping frequently occurs. The weeping may be related to mood or emotional state but may also be on an organic basis. In the latter instance, it is thought to be part of a syndrome resulting from damage or irritation to the thalamus, or due to a release of control of higher (cortical) centers. The syndrome is accompanied by spontaneous pain and overreaction to stimuli where there is normally a diminution of stimulus sensitivity. Some believe that this weeping syndrome represents a type of social adaptation in dependent, worrisome people, serving to call attention to the disability, and is not a direct consequence of organic damage (Weinstein, 1955).

Anxiety is also a common reaction in hemiplegia. It is significantly more marked in organic than in non-organic patients and appears to be one of the organic's distinguishing characteristics. The anxiety may be free-floating, fixed on somatic preoccupation, or experienced as a general uneasiness about the environment, and it is often total and profound as if the person were experiencing a series of catastrophes. At times it is founded on fear of a second stroke.

Denial of the disability may be viewed in two ways. In overt denial the patient literally denies the presence of a disability. Patients with paralysis have been known to deny their disability even though it is public and visible. Overt denial is rare, in rehabilitation settings. It generally occurs soon after the stroke and reflects the presence of diffuse brain damage. It is rare in rehabilitation settings when it is displaced by covert denial. An interesting example of overt denial which does take place in a rehabilitation setting is the fact that when asked "Do you read a newspaper?" most patients with visual field defects will claim that they do. When tested, they are unable to read and offer feeble excuses which turn out to be invalid. For example, "I can read but I don't want to because I forgot my glasses." When the glasses are brought, it turns out that the patient can't read. The patient admits the presence of the disability but then refuses to think about it or plan ahead. Covert denial of disability is generally fostered by the fact that improvement continues at a slow pace, so that the patient interprets slight changes as continued hope for his full recovery. Covert denial of disability occurs in nearly half of left hemiplegics when seen one month after admission to a rehabilitation program. When seen a year and a half after discharge it is still present in one quarter of the patients. Among right hemiplegics it is difficult to assess the evidence of denial since many are aphasic and don't speak.

5) *Dependency*. Many patients are dependent following a stroke for realistic reasons. However, a good number develop unrealistic dependencies which may interfere with rehabilitation. Sometimes this may reflect an exaggeration of premorbid dependency needs which may have existed or may have been suppressed prior to the cerebral vascular accident. Because a stroke may cause regression in emotions as well as skills, psychological dependency is common.

PREMORBID PERSONALITY, INTELLIGENCE, AND EDUCATIONAL LEVEL

The question arises whether premorbid personality, intelligence, and education affect reaction to brain damage. In the field of physical disabilities, it is often suggested that individuals with premorbid life patterns of high achievement and drive possess the greatest rehabilitation potential. Empirical evidence as well as common sense testify to this. Churchill, Pasteur, and Mach led productive lives following hemiplegias. Working with animals, Harlow found that those which received more training before experimentally induced brain damage were able to learn more effectively. "The educated man can face arteriosclerosis with confidence—if results from animals can be extended to man" (Weinstein and Teuber, 1957a and 1957b). However, this glibly applied generalization should be seriously questioned in dealing with hemiplegics. Observers have noted that people with consistent histories of successful vocational attainment may fail to adapt to hemiplegia and do poorly in rehabilitation. This is thought to occur in people who attain success at the price of denying their needs in other areas, for example, those who have limited cultural interests, lack close interpersonal relationships, or are unable to admit illness or personal weakness (Weinstein and Kahn, 1955). In such cases, adaptation occurs not by accepting the disability but through denial. Denial, in fact, may be a characteristic defense in this type of personality structure. While premorbid personality, therefore, is an important consideration in evaluating response to a disability, its relationship to current functioning in hemiplegia must be very carefully evaluated. In general, it can be said that premorbid personality and intelligence are important—but they may be vitiated by a diffusion of large lesions in the brain, by lesions strategically placed, or by the nature of the lesion. All of these may interfere with the person's ability to act or to think. In cases where the damage is small, of a subtractive nature, and of a stable character, the effects of brain damage appear to be less potent. Under the latter circumstances, the total individual becomes a more important determinant than the specific characteristics of the damage. One very difficult problem to assess is the actual extent of intellectual decline where no tests were conducted prior to the stroke. Some have suggested that education and vocational level reflect valid measures of premorbid intelligence.

Motivation. Whereas depression and anxiety often interfere with motivation, they sometimes serve to increase it. The rehabilitation process itself affects motivation. In about one third of hemiplegic patients it serves to increase motivation. However, sometimes it has the opposite effect when the patient realizes he will not make the recovery he hoped for. Increased motivation in the course of rehabilitation tends to occur in nonorganic patients (Weinblatt, 1959). Since organic patients tend to be highly anxious, they also tend to be highly aware of failure. Consequently, attempts to motivate such patients by arousing anxiety only lead to more failure. On the other hand, some studies show that "urging" instructions on simple tasks rather than relaxing or supportive ones are more effective (Benton, 1960; Blackburn, 1958; Blackburn and Benton, 1955). At the present time, therefore, it is difficult to generalize about what kind of incentives best influence performance for what kind of patient. One of the major problems of motivation with hemiplegics is the narrowing of interests and goals following paralysis. Both depression and organicity serve to narrow the individual's values, goals, and preoccupations, while concrete thinking serves to influence a patient to fixate on a goal long after it is clear that it is not feasible. Despite this, it can be shown that hemiplegics respond to incentives, including token reinforcement, if they understand the nature of the incentive.

Intelligence and Verbal Skills. Is hemiplegia associated with changes in intelligence? The answer depends on which groups of hemiplegics are being considered (for example, right vs. left, young people vs. old people) and which type of test is being used to measure intelligence.

Since most young hemiplegics who have been studied generally have been bracketed with the cerebral palsied, it is difficult to isolate a specific group. Some generalizations appear warranted concerning hemiplegics up to the age of sixteen years: (1) They appear to be slightly higher in intelligence than the other types of cerebral palsied. (2) Approximately 35 to 40 per cent of congenital hemiplegics test in a defective range (Rusk, 1971), whereas 20 per cent test in the normal or higher range (Perlstein and Hood, 1957). (3) There appear to be no differences in intelligence between right and left hemiplegics (Wood, 1959).

In adults the matter is a little more complicated. Most observers agree that right hemiplegia is associated with deficits in verbal skills. This deficit may be associated with aphasia. However, it sometimes occurs even when aphasia is not manifested clinically. In regard to left hemiplegia, verbal skills appear to be intact, while performance skills are more impaired in patients with visual field defects than in those without such defects. One must be careful about generalizing from these studies, however, as many right hemiplegics with aphasia who might show impairment in performance tasks were excluded from the studies because they were unsuitable. This differential patterning has given rise to a considerable body of speculation that suggests that different sides of the brain are involved in verbal skills as opposed to performance or spatial skills (Heilbrun, 1956; Hirschenfang, 1960a and 1960b; Masland, 1958; Reitan, 1955). From a practical standpoint the differential in skills is important because: (1) some areas of rehabilitation require verbal as opposed to performance skills (for example, speech therapy vs. occupational therapy) and (2) the manner of teaching motor skills should be examined for its dependence on verbal instructions as opposed to motor instructions.

BODY IMAGE

The term "body image" has become very popular in current psychology in referring to the concepts a person may have about himself and his body. It is less commonly known that the term had its origin in studies of brain-damaged people who literally acted as if they had lost familiarity with their bodily parts. To account for this phenomenon a British neurologist, Henry Head, postulated that in growing up we form a body schema that may be impaired when the brain is injured (Weinstein and Kahn, 1955).

Hemiplegics commonly suffer from disturbances in body image or body schema. These disturbances are more common in organics than they are in nonorganics and may involve the physical body, the spatial surroundings, and the ego. In regard to the physical body, we find in hemiplegics: (1) inability to follow instructions pertaining to parts of the body (Rusk, 1971), (2) inability to localize body parts or distances on the body correctly (MacDonald, 1960; Birch, Proctor, and Bortner, 1961), (3) denying or misrepresenting the presence of a paralyzed limb (Bender, 1952), and so forth. In regard to location in space, we find that hemiplegics may easily become lost in new surroundings or ignore or distort objects that confront them on their paralyzed side. Some hemiplegics report difficulty in driving a car following their disability because they do not trust their spatial judgment. In a survey of 525 physically handicapped people who had undergone a special driver-training program, left hemiplegics had more difficulty than any other handicapped group (Bardach, 1971). A simple test which elicits the problem is to ask the patient to drive a figure eight in a large space such as a supermarket parking lot. Finally, disturbances in ego functioning generally accompany body-image problems. These are manifested by feelings of low self-esteem and inadequacy. Frequently, they are related to sexual problems.

Disturbances in body image may pose major problems in rehabilitation. The hemiplegic who is not aware when his foot hits the ground may be afraid of falling. The patient may forget to lock his brace because he is unaware of his left side. It is our impression that body image disturbances are manifested differently in right and left hemiplegics. Right hemiplegics have difficulty in carrying out verbal directions involving their bodies, whereas left hemiplegics have difficulty in localizing themselves in space (Masland, 1958).

THE REHABILITATION PROCESS

The first stage in the rehabilitation of the hemiplegic is to maintain life and restore physiologic balance. When this is accomplished the immediate goals of a rehabilitation program are as follows: (1) to prevent and to correct any deformities that have developed; (2) to retrain the patient in walking; (3) to retrain the affected upper extremity to its maximum degree of usefulness; and (4) to teach the patient to perform the eventual activities of daily living. In about half the patients retraining of speech skills is necessary. The long-term vocational rehabilitation results may be divided into the following categories: (1) patients able to return to full-time work either in the previous job or in another job; (2) those able to return to part-time work in ordinary employment, sheltered work, or home work; (3) those capable of independent self-care; and (4) those who will require care (American Heart Association, 1956 and 1958).

MEDICAL-PHYSICAL STAGE

From the medical standpoint, once the physician has decided that the symptoms are due to cerebrovascular accident two questions of particular importance arise in diagnosis and prognosis, namely: (1) which part of the vascular system was damaged; and (2) why did the stroke occur. The answer to the former can be inferred from a careful evaluation of the neurological symptoms, for these occur in relation to the specific parts of the brain that have died and ceased to function because their particular vascular supply system has been choked. In regard to the origin of the stroke, the physician tries to deduce whether the damage is due to the blocking of a blood vessel by a thrombus (clot) or an embolus (floating clot) or whether it is due to the rupture of a blood vessel (hemorrhage). Whereas it was formerly believed that most strokes were due to hemorrhage, it is now generally recognized that cerebral thrombosis ranks first in cause, cerebral hemorrhage second, and cerebral embolism third (Merritt, 1951).

The differential diagnosis of the causes of the hemiplegia is important, particularly in the early stages, for a number of reasons (Harris and Towler, 1955). First, rates of survival and recovery differ according to cause. Those due to hemorrhage have a grave prognosis, with a 60 per cent mortality rate in the first week. Strokes due to thrombus or embolus have a better prognosis, with a much lower mortality rate—thrombosis having a mortality rate of 30 per cent during the first week and embolism even less. Second, the varieties of treatment and medication vary with etiology. Ingenious neurosurgical techniques are currently applied to remove clots or replace diseased segments of an artery by arterial grafts. In addition, powerful drugs are now at hand which alter the coagulability of the blood, dilate blood vessels, suppress infections, reduce cerebral blood pressures from dangerously high levels, or elevate them after circulatory collapse. These procedures are sometimes hazardous, and partially effective for selected patients (Millikan, 1970). Once administered, some of these drugs have to be continued over a lifetime. Hence, the hemiplegic may require medical care for the rest of his life.

Rehabilitation procedures are also influenced by etiology. Such procedures for hemiplegia due to thrombosis or embolism can be instituted within the first week of the disability, whereas patients with hemiplegia due to hemorrhage may have to wait up to six weeks. It is difficult to forecast how much spontaneous recovery will occur. Some recovery may be due to the gradual clearing of cerebral edema and circulatory disturbance, altered intracranial pressure, and return of function of cellular elements that have suffered reversible damage.

The most intensive efforts in the treatment of cerebrovascular diseases have been made in the past decade through the establishment of stroke centers and regional medical programs for heart disease, stroke, and cancer. Information concerning the location of such centers can be obtained from the Social and Rehabilitation Service, Department of Health, Education and Welfare, Washington, D.C.

The medical examination is also concerned with several dimensions in addition to etiology. These include: (1) inquiry into associated medical conditions, for example, diabetes, high blood pressure, heart disease, hypercholesterolemia, etc. because there is a high incidence of associated medical disturbances (Bauer, 1970). (These conditions may be of intrinsic importance for the patient's health and also relevant in terms of preventing future stroke and the pace of physical activity in a rehabilitation program.); (2) assessment of different motor and language systems. (This must often be explored in greater depth by rehabilitation specialists, for example, physical, occupational, and speech therapists in planning a rehabilitation program.); (3) neurologic examination to survey the patient's sensory, motor, language, and thought processes. (Detailed evaluation of all of these behaviors and conditions may involve several medical specialties, including neurology, internal medicine, and physiatry. Other health specialists who may be involved are physical, occupational, and speech therapists and nurses.)

The medical specialist who guides the patients' programs in a medical rehabilitation setting is the physiatrist. He is trained to evaluate the hemiplegic patient and work with the members of the rehabilitation team to help the patient in his recovery. (Since physiatry is a young specialty not so well known as some of the other medical specialties, it may be noted that if there is no physiatrist in the local community one can write to the American Academy of Physical Medicine and Rehabilitation of the American Congress of Rehabilitation Medicine, 30 North Michigan Avenue, Chicago, Illinois 60602 for information.)

Medical planning is important not only in terms of long-term prognosis but it also applies to short-term management with regard to a number of issues. Should treatment be conducted on an inpatient or outpatient basis? How much? How long? When should the patient be involved in discussing job or business-related matters? Should the patient walk with or without a cane? These are only a sample of the many types of questions which arise in the management of the hemiplegic patient.

In regard to *physical treatment,* the extent of disability resulting from the cerebral lesion is first measured by a series of tests, which include muscle examination to determine the power of both the affected and the unaffected muscles, the range of motion in the joints, and the patient's proficiency in activities of daily living (Rusk and Marx, 1953; Rusk, 1971). The importance of preventing and treating deformities cannot be overstressed (Peszczynski, 1954). The principal deformities are a frozen shoulder and a shortened heel cord. Heat, massage, and stretching are generally useful in treating the deformity.

In ambulation a careful analysis of the hemiplegic's gait, including the swinging and stance phase, is a necessary prerequisite for a training program. A knowledge of body mechanics as well as of corrective procedures for pathological movement is used by the physician to prescribe a series of exercises and mechanical appliances, including braces, wheelchairs, or special lifts for the shoe. The retraining activities are carried on for the most part by a physiotherapist. The gait of a hemiplegic, its pathology and its treatment, has been the subject of a number of detailed studies (Peszczynski, 1954).

In treatment it is important to begin training the unaffected arm as rapidly as possible, for very often the unaffected arm must be used to take over the functions of the affected arm in caring for daily needs. Furthermore, the unaffected arm is often used in ambulation training, the patient holding a cane in his unaffected hand to control his walking. Training of the affected arm is started while the patient is developing one-handed skills with the unaffected arm. If the affected arm is flaccid, a re-education program similar to that used in poliomyelitis is started. If the arm is spastic, treatment starts at the shoulder and proceeds distally to the fingers. Occupational therapy is of particular value in arm retraining as it combines exercise and retraining with interesting activity (Ayres, 1960; Reynolds, 1959). The fingers of the spastic hemiplegic are most difficult to re-educate for any useful purpose. If useful function is ever attained, it represents a great expenditure of time and much concentrated effort by the patient (Rusk, 1971). It is of interest to note that many of the tasks used by occupational therapists to elicit purposeful movement involve psychomotor skills (Carroll, 1958; Rusk, 1971). Proficiency in their execution resembles proficiency on performance tests of intelligence. A number of occupational therapists have pointed out that perceptomotor rather than manual skills seem to be crucial for success in retraining hemiplegics (Williams, 1967). They have noted a very curious fact: left hemiplegics who still retain use of their dominant hand tend to do poorer than right hemiplegics who have not only lost use of the dominant hand but often demonstrate aphasia.

Speech therapy for those hemiplegics suffering from language disorders is integrated into the rehabilitation program.

MANAGEMENT OF PERSONAL REACTIONS

Of key importance in the rehabilitation of hemiplegics is the reaction of the patient himself. Because a cerebrovascular accident strikes with frightening suddenness, a person may find his whole way of life changed in a moment. What is the impact on him? How does he perceive the cause, the deficits? What does he expect that the goals of rehabilitation are?

Perceived Cause. A key question patients ask themselves is: Why did this happen to me? The answers they give are highly varied and serve as useful cues to the way patients define the disability. Whereas this same question is posed by many disabled people, the answers are more striking in hemiplegia by reason of a number of distinctive circumstances. A stroke happens mysteriously and suddenly, giving the person no time to adapt. The "stroke" itself is usually thought of as caused by "high blood pressure and repressed rage"—a view that is common in both folklore and medicine although the evidence for it is far from conclusive (Seidenberg and Ecker, 1954; Horenstein, 1970). Many hemiplegic patients with brain damage respond in regressed, primitive ways that are reflected in their beliefs, for example, the female patient who thought her hemiplegia was due to childbirth many years before, or the male who believed it was due to his visits to a prostitute. In general, the perceived cause may reflect not only the direction of an individual's anger, whether toward himself or others, but also the level of rational control over his beliefs, whether on a level of perceptual maturity or perceptual primitiveness. Individuals who state that their stroke was an act of nature or who are able to cite medical reasons for its happening tend to have more mature beliefs than those who personalize and tend to have more primitive beliefs and defense systems.

Perceived Deficits. How does the hemiplegic experience his paralyzed limb? Many hemiplegics report different sensations and awareness on the involved side of the body. A common tendency is to push the affected side out of awareness (Nathanson, Bergman, and Gordon, 1952; Weinstein and Kahn, 1955), for example, "I felt like I didn't have a right side at all." "At first it felt as if it wasn't my arm, as if it was out in the air." "I didn't feel like I had an arm." "It seemed like something attached that wasn't mine." "I didn't even know I had it; I would go to sleep at night and I couldn't find it." Another reaction, although less common, is to invest the disabled member with personal meanings, for example the woman whose husband had died in bed next to her commented: "My arm felt funny. Like somebody else's arm. I thought it was my husband's arm. I kept feeling it and started to get up to look at it." In general, this type of overt denial occurs more often during the acute stage of the illness. As rehabilitation progresses, the denial becomes less overt and is manifested in indirect ways, such as refusing to think about the future (Ullman, Asnenhurst, Hurwitz, and Gruen, 1960; Ullman, 1962).

Both the perceived cause and the perceived disability are related to what the hemiplegic expects of the rehabilitation program. Many patients who cannot accept their disabilities invest them with private meanings and look for irrational solutions to their problems. They look for complete cure rather than for an opportunity to help themselves. Such people tend to alternate between denial and depression because they cannot accept the goals of the rehabilitation program since these goals often fall below their expected criterion of complete recovery.

The patient's perception of progress. Since rehabilitation is a complex affair involving the coordination of different systems of treatment for several aspects of a disorder ranging from motor to vocational, the question may be raised as to how does one judge progress. Tamerin (1964) has shown that there are gradients of estimates of progress depending on behavior. For example, patients judge that they have made more progress than do physicians, and physical therapists in turn judge a greater degree of progress than do occupational therapists. Of even greater interest are the reasons offered for progress. Patients often attribute their progress to God. Their therapists involve mundane factors such as motivation and muscle strength. But what does the patient mean by God? Probing suggests that the reply does not appear more in one religious denomination than another, nor among those known to the chaplain as opposed to those not known.

SPECIAL CONSIDERATION IN MANAGEMENT

Although it is difficult to generalize about principles of management or cite specific techniques that may be unique to hemiplegia, a number of considerations might prove helpful in framing a course of treatment. Those hemiplegics who respond in a nonorganic way can be treated the same as any other group of disabled. Those who respond in an organic way may require special management, with their rehabilitation program and goals generally more limited, and with fewer activities prescribed.

Special attempts are made to keep the environment constant for the organics so that therapists and classes remain stable. A great effort is made at drill and repetition in teaching. Many trials are necessary for the organic hemiplegics to attain mastery in a skill, and these trials should be spaced rather than massed together. Training materials should be life-like and meaningful, and it is important that the patient be made aware of his progress as well as of immediate goals. Staff members are encouraged to build warm, personal relationships with the patients. They are told about the patients' psychological problems so that they will not personalize aggressive or abusive behavior that may be directed against them. They are also informed that firmness is as important as gentleness in patient management. A firm physiotherapist presents a fixed predictable stimulus figure in a world that has become otherwise distorted.

In regard to counseling and psychotherapy, hemiplegics generally require environmental information and supportive help. Although depression is common, support rather than insight therapy is warranted, for the depression is often on a realistic basis. Because many hemiplegics struggle with problems of dependency at the same time that they require supportive therapy, special care must be taken so that the patient does not become unnecessarily dependent on the therapist or counselor.

THE FAMILY ROLE

Families play a vital role in rehabilitation of hemiplegia. While the professional worker may be concerned with such aspects of the patient as his motor status or his employment, in the mind of the patient the family ranks first or second. Family involvements may be looked at in several ways. When the patient is admitted to a rehabilitation program the family goes through a crisis just as the patient does. Part of the crisis involves changes in role relationships imposed by the disability and part involves surrendering traditional functions to rehabilitation caretakers. Patients from close-knit families have more support and more clearcut situations to return to. Hirshenfang, Shulman, and Benton (1968) in a survey of 140 families drawn from a heterogeneous urban area found that 80 per cent had concrete problems such as need for help in obtaining appliances or referrals to community agencies or they required casework help in social and marital problems. Patients who did not return home after their discharge suggest a problem of major magnitude in this area. Adler has noted the frequency of behavioral disruption when the patients return home. Some families have difficulty in mobilizing themselves to adapt to the new role. For example, the hemiplegic patient who no longer can go to work imposes a physical and psychological drain on the wife. She is often burdened with the problem not only of finding substitute financial support but also how to keep the patient occupied all day. The most common complaint of hemiplegics who have left rehabilitation programs is the void in their leisure-time activities and the wish for more treatment in the hopes of ultimate complete recovery (Powell, et al., 1971).

In considering family adaptation we must note that hemiplegia usually strikes middle-aged and old people. The hemiplegic may not recover sufficiently to be completely independent in activities of daily living, so he requires help. Families become frightened because there may be some mental changes or because the patient's depression may transmit a sense of hopelessness. Since the deficits may be multiple—ranging from gross to subtle—they are hard to assess so that some are over-estimated while others are overlooked. The family may also be afraid of another stroke. Finally, the family may have to adjust to the effects of visual field problems, for example, in a left-sided field defect (left hemiplegia) the patient may ignore objects, including even a plate of food, on his left side.

The responses of families are quite varied. In general where family relations have been strained hemiplegia causes a further strain. Sexual impotency, associated with feelings of low self-esteem and depression, is not uncommon. Some patients with premorbid sexual difficulties are now relieved to use their disability as an excuse to avoid sex. Where marital problems have existed before, they now become magnified. In one case, marital infidelity on the part of the male who was hemiplegic had occurred some thirty years before the cerebrovascular accident; it now becomes the source of bitter conflict. Where marital relations had been good, they can be fully resumed after a period of adjustment. In general, the resolution of the multiple marital problems posed by hemiplegia will depend on the dynamics of the marital relationship. When the family cannot take the person back, he becomes a custodial problem. This looms as an ever-increasing choice because of the advanced age of many hemiplegics.

While the importance of predisability family relationships are apparent, they appear in subtle as well as gross ways. For example, nurturant and dependent wives minimize the severity of their husbands' aphasia (Buxbaum, 1967). It is of course unclear whether the wives are distorting or whether in fact dependent wives do elicit more communication from their aphasic spouses. Diller, Ben-Yishay, Weinberg, Goodkin, *et al.* (1971) have developed a method of using wives as speech therapists for their aphasic husbands. The method has several virtues. First, it is closer to the naturalistic situation than the rehabilitation setting. Second, it involves the wives in a constructive way. Goodkin notes that in a number of cases where predisability relationships were severely strained the treatment broke down. It is also of interest to note that when wives offer feedback of errors in speech, one can distinguish two kinds of critical comments. The first type is objective. For example, when the patient substitutes the wrong word or perseverates, the wife says, "let's try it again," or helps supply the correct word. Another type is subjective, where the wife may tell the patient making the same error, "you're no good," or "what's the matter with you today?" Nurturant wives bring about more change in functional communication than non-nurturant wives do. Adler's work (1970) with a large sample also notes that where predisability in family tensions existed, the prognosis was worse than if good relationships were present.

SOCIAL CLASS

Social class interacts with family life in a profound way. Powell *et al.* (1971) and Lee (1958) have shown that low socioeconomic families place a higher percentage of patients in chronic disease settings and nursing homes following rehabilitation than do middle-class families. Interviews with low socioeconomic patients indicate that the greatest worry of the patient during rehabilitation is where he will go when rehabilitation is finished. Family ties in low socioeconomic patients appear to be weaker. There is a much higher percentage of single and widowed people. In addition, physical facilities in the home are much more limited. While middle-class hemiplegics may continue in supportive rehabilitation following formal discharge, lower-class patients do not.

Social class appears to play a role in rehabilitation not so much in terms of motor recovery of activities of daily living but in other dimensions. First, in aphasia education level may be related to extent of recovery. Second, patients from middle-class backgrounds tend to assume more initiative than do patients from lower-class backgrounds. It is of interest to note that while brain damage may alter motor function and aspects of cognitive functions, attitudes toward authority and dependency and value systems remain consistent with premorbid personality rather than disability. For example, with regard to attitudes toward authoritarianism, hemiplegics in a private hospital setting differ from those in a city hospital setting. The difference is maintained even when the patients are seen a year after discharge. Similar patterns are found with regard to the patients' attitudes toward medical responsibility. Lower-class patients place the physician in the role of an unquestioning authority, believing that none of his recommendations are to be questioned. Middle-class people see the physician much more as a sharer of responsibility (Powell, 1971).

VOCATIONAL PROBLEMS

Vocational planning must take into account the limitations imposed by the disability. Work history, vocational goals, motivation, and environmental alternatives that enter into vocational planning are aiso involved. Planning should begin as early as possible. Moreover, one of the major tasks is to induce patients who are still preoccupied with physical cure to think about the future.

Careful individual evaluation, using standard vocational tests, is often not as fruitful in assessment as are prevocational work-sample tasks. While stress is placed on training the individual for one-handed activities, the most important use of these tasks is to assess and encourage motivation.

Vocational placement is influenced by the fact that, in certain sections of industry with deeply ingrained and systematized personnel practices, employment of hemiplegics can be achieved only with the greatest of difficulty. A set of specific objections, not only from management but also from line supervision, exists, centering primarily around increasing the liability ratio and the manufacturing costs for the industry. In general, the barriers affecting the use of hemiplegics in industry are: (1) the medical policy of the company; (2) the size of the company;

(3) the additional demands of job-related tasks; and (4) the attitudes of personnel. An active placement program is often necessary to break down these barriers (Howard, 1960).

While the social context of employment is of critical importance, certain factors specific to hemiplegia may be noted. These pertain to cognitive intactness. For example, in a survey of hemiplegics at the Institute of Rehabilitation Medicine who were referred for vocational counseling and placement, it was found that of those left hemiplegics who did not return to work fifteen out of sixteen had perceptual problems. Of the nineteen who returned to work, fifteen did not have perceptual problems while four did. This distinction did not hold with regard to right hemiplegics. However, severe aphasia appeared to be associated with failure to return to work (Weisbroth, Esibill, and Zuger, 1971).

Vocational counseling and placement should be individualized in a number of ways. First, there should be no time limits set in terms of fixed number of counseling sessions. Patients must often be seen over prolonged periods of time; while medical rehabilitation may be completed in three months, vocational may take a year. Second, placement often requires accompanying the patient to the job and establishing an atmosphere which is uncritical and supportive. This is necessary because the hemiplegic is often slow in performing mental tasks and may make errors. Even relatively intact patients experience feelings of failure because they cannot perform at their former levels of competence. The accountant who adds slowly, the clerk who makes spelling errors because of perceptual difficulties, and the salesman who does not trust himself in driving a car are all actively sensitive to feelings of failure. They all need a great deal of support in the early stages. Often they require trial placements or simulated work experiences.

RESEARCH

A number of substantive areas of research have emerged in the past several years.

PREDICTING THE OUTCOME OF REHABILITATION

The length of time for medical rehabilitation varies from several weeks to several months. Prediction of outcome and duration of medical rehabilitation treatment have received increasing attention in the past fifteen years. Early students of the problem noted a number of prognostic cues which augured well for the rehabilitant: younger rather than older; absence of sensory deficit; milder degree of paralysis; no incontinence; and absence of mental confusion. Prognosis is possible because recovery proceeds in a gradual, stepwise fashion rather than by leaps and bounds. Bard and Hirschberg (1965) showed that all subjects who recover use of the arm have some movement during the first week. Some have implicated single cognitive and/or perceptual factors, such as performance on a block design test (Lorenze and Cancro, 1962) or performance on the rod and frame test (DeCencio, Leshner, and Voron, 1970). Others have attempted to interrelate features of behavior in terms of neurological patterns, such as temporal lobe involvement (Van Buskirk and Webster, 1955), or have attempted to use multivariate techniques to take all of the known factors reported in the literature. One research group used more than 600 variables which have been alleged to be useful in clinical predictions (Anderson, 1970). These variables include medical, social, psychological, and speech factors. Ben-Yishay, et al. (1970) were able to predict duration of medical rehabilitation and proficiency in self-care activities for left hemiplegics with some success by using a variety of psychometric tests which were combined into a regression equation. For example, it was found possible to predict duration of rehabilitation within one month with an accuracy of 80 per cent. It should be noted that this prediction has been demonstrated for left hemiplegics. For right hemiplegics the matter is more complicated, first because the criteria for discharge are related to improvement in language skills which may proceed at a different pace from motor skills, and second because the organization of abilities differs for right and left hemiplegics. For example, it has been shown that learning a seemingly simple skill, such as transferring from a wheelchair to a regular chair, occurs at the same rate in left and right hemiplegia. However, it is correlated with different abilities for the two groups. They learn to transfer equally well, but for different reasons (Diller, Buxbaum, and Chiotelis, 1972).

EXPERIMENTS IN COGNITIVE REMEDIATION

Active intervention attempts have been demonstrated in the past decade. Some report successful outcomes in remediation of cognitive impairments by training in scanning behavior (Diller, *et al.*, 1971), saturated cuing on block designs (Ben-Yishay, 1971), and operant conditioning (Goodkin, 1966). While special education in this country has concentrated its efforts on children with impairments, and while neurologists and clinical psychologists have been preoccupied with diagnoses, there is increasing pressure to alleviate and remedy problems in perception and thinking, which are so important in this condition. This field will grow in the next decade.

There should be a word of caution concerning this concerted interest in attacking some of the core problems in neuropsychology from a therapeutic standpoint. In a complex field there is a tendency to apply a treatment approach derived from one body of experience to another without realization until after the fact. For example, hemiplegics have been shown to improve their performance while breathing enriched oxygen (Ben-Yishay, *et al.*, 1967) but not when it is under great pressure (Sarno, *et al.*, in press).

SOCIAL INTERVENTION

There is increased interest in the patient as a consumer. This is seen in the use of education groups for wives of aphasics, the publication of a book about stroke for use of the family (Sarno and Sarno, 1969), and experiences with therapeutic communities in rehabilitation settings which include sizeable numbers of hemiplegics (Kutner, *et al.*, 1970). These efforts suggest a groping for alternative styles of rehabilitation.

One of the greatest needs of older hemiplegics is the development of ways of developing roles and activities for those who are unable to return to work. Complaints of boredom, listlessness, and fatigue are common among those who do not return to work. Even those who do return find a void in their lives. Facilities for post-rehabilitation programs for hemiplegics might be one answer to the problem. Many medical rehabilitation settings offer extended care programs. These programs fill a semitherapeutic need. However, there is additional need for community facilities which need not be related to medical institutions, but may be integrated into other settings, such as social clubs, churches, and community centers. Along these lines, architectural and social barriers present formidable problems to overcome.

OTHER NEEDED RESEARCH

There is need for methods of assessing cognitive changes in mild strokes. This may be particularly pertinent in high-level individuals whose impairments may be slight and go undetected by standard tests.

There is greater need to educate physicians, health-care workers, and social workers to become more actively involved with stroke patients. Such patients are often shunted aside because of the slow, undramatic changes in their condition. Part of the problem may well be related to the larger attitudes of a society which tends to avoid involvement with the aging.

SUMMARY

In summary, hemiplegics constitute the second largest disability group in medical rehabilitation settings. When we consider that many require the assistance of one to four persons until they become independent, the impact of the disability can be more fully appreciated.

There is a large gap between existing needs and requests made for rehabilitation services for stroke patients. A stroke patient in need of rehabilitation often fails to obtain the type of services from which he could benefit optimally, although he may be receiving the best services available in a given community. The type of rehabilitation service available to the stroke victim may depend on a variety of factors, among them (1) financial resources supporting such rehabilitation services as research, vocational rehabilitation, geriatrics (Medicare), welfare (Medicaid), crippled children's services, and the like; (2) breadth of experience and attitudes of the key personnel of the rehabilitation services; (3) attitudes of the community toward priorities in the area of health delivery; and (4) availability of trained personnel.

Practice has shown that one of the greatest deficiencies in the area of stroke rehabilitation concerns judgment as to which patient will profit from available rehabilitation services and the decision as to when rehabilitation therapy should be modified or discontinued.

There is both undertreatment and overtreatment in the rehabilitation of stroke patients. Most overtreatment is the result of a lack of knowledge; anxiety about pleasing the patient, his family, or his physician; or overtly conscious economic abuse (comparatively rare). Undertreatment is most often due to lack of knowledge, lack of interest, lack of facilities, or lack of financial resources. Undertreatment is much more prevalent than overtreatment.

The Joint Committee on Stroke has recommended that medical rehabilitation be incorporated into the care of all stroke victims when needed. The pattern of incorporation is to depend on the size of the hospital in accordance with the following scheme: (1) large hospitals (500 beds or more) and teaching centers; (2) medium-sized hospitals (200 to 500 beds); (3) small community hospitals (50 to 200 beds); (4) community hospitals (fewer than 50 beds); and (5) very small hospitals (fewer than 20 beds). A minimum team in hospitals of smaller size would include physicians, nurses, social workers, and physical therapists. In larger institutions psychologists, rehabilitation counselors, and occupational and speech therapists would be included. Smaller settings might function more effectively by having access to more disciplines on a consultant basis. Where large rehabilitation teams are impractical, the organization of a rehabilitation advisory committee is strongly recommended. The committee would aim to facilitate case finding, early referral, adequate contacts with the family, vocational and social resources, and follow up. The Association of Rehabilitation Centers has developed standards for professional staffing and space requirements for accreditation of rehabilitation facilities.

Along with the interest in the upgrading of rehabilitation services and in the development of more adequate and regular delivery systems of care, there have been various attempts to develop alternative models or to apply rehabilitation approaches in different types of settings. A number of programs report success with rehabilitation activities in nursing homes (Kelman and Muller, 1962; Kelman and Wellner, 1962; Gordon and Kohn, 1966); geriatric wards of hospitals (Rae, Smith, and Lenzce, 1962); and in general medical wards (Adams and McComb, 1953; Carroll, 1962; Feldman, et al., 1962). Rehabilitation has been tried by delivering teams to home visits in both urban (Ragoff, Cooney, and Kutner, 1964) and rural settings (DeLagi, et al., 1962).

In addition to medically oriented rehabilitation programs there is need for the use of vocationally oriented rehabilitation programs, resident-care facilities, and the full array of social agencies.

REFERENCES

Adams, G. F., and S. B. McComb. 1953. Assessment and prognosis in hemiplegia. Lancet 256:266–69.

Adler, E. 1969. Stroke in Israel 1957–1961. Jerusalem, Polypress Ltd.

Allen, R. 1962. Cerebral palsy, in J. F. Garrett and E. S. Levine, eds., Psychological practices with the physically handicapped. New York, Columbia University Press.

American Heart Association. 1956. Cerebral vascular disease, 1st conference transactions. New York, Grune and Stratton.

—— 1958. Cerebral vascular disease, 2nd conference transactions. New York, Grune and Stratton.

Anderson, Elisabeth K. 1971. Sensory impairments in hemiplegia. Arch. Phys. Med. 52:293–97.

Anderson, T. P., N. Bourestom, and F. R. Greenberg. 1970. Rehabilitation predictors in completed stroke. Final report SRS-RD-1757-m-68-C3.

Ayres, A. J. 1960. Occupational therapy for motor disorders resulting from impairment of the central nervous system. Rehab. Lit. 21:302–11.

Bard, G., and G. G. Hirschber. 1965. Recovery of voluntary motion in upper extremity following hemiplegia. Arch. Phys. Med. 46:567–72.

Bardach, Joan L. 1971. Psychological factors in the handicapped driver. Arch. Phys. Med. 52:328–32.

Bauer, R. B. 1970. Relative influence of anatomical and nonanatomical factors in behavioral change, in A. L. Benton, ed., Behavioral change in cerebrovascular disease. New York, Harper and Row, pp. 195–201.

Belmont, I., J. Ambrose, H. Benjamin, and R. D. Restuccia. 1969. Effect of cerebral damage on motivation in rehabilitation. Arch. Phys. Med. 50:507–511.

Belmont, L. 1957. A comparison of the psychological effects of early and late brain damage. New York University, unpublished Ph.D. dissertation.

Bender, M. B. 1952. Disorders in perception. Springfield, Ill., Charles C. Thomas.

Benton, A. L. 1960. Motivational influences on performance in brain damaged patients. Amer. J. Orthopsychiat. 30:315–22.

Ben-Yishay, Y., L. Diller, I. Mandleberg, W. Gordon, and L. J. Gerstman. 1971. Similarities and differences in block design performance between older normal and brain-injured persons: a task analysis. J. Abnorm. Psychol. 78:17–25.

Ben-Yishay, Y., A. Haas, and L. Diller. 1967. The effects of oxygen inhalation on motor impersistence in brain-damaged individuals: a double-blind study. Neurology 17:1003.

Ben-Yishay, Y., L. Gerstman, L. Diller, and A. Haas. 1970. Prediction of rehabilitation outcomes from psychometric parameters in left hemiplegics. J. Consult. Clin. Psychol. 34:436–41.

Birch, H. G. and L. Belmont. 1964. Auditory-visual integration in normal and retarded readers. Amer. J. Ortho. Psychiat. 34:852–61.

Birch, H. G. and L. Diller. 1959. Rorschach signs of organicity: A physiological basis for perceptual disturbance. J. Project. Techn. 23:184–97.

Birch, H. G., F. Proctor, and M. Bortner. 1961. Perception in hemiplegia: IV. Body surface localization in hemiplegic patients. J. of Nervous and Mental Disease 133:192–202.

Blackburn, H. L. 1958. Effects of motivating instructions on reaction time in cerebral disease. J. Abnorm. Soc. Psychol. 56:359–66.

Blackburn, H. L. and A. L. Benton. 1955. Simple and choice reaction time in cerebral disease. Confinia Neurologica 15:327–38.

Bortner, M. and H. G. Birch. 1960. Perceptual and perceptual-motor dissociation in brain damaged patients. J. of Nervous and Mental Disease, 132:49–53.

Bruell, J. H., G. W. Albee, et al. 1958. Intellectual functions in a patient with hemispherectomy. Paper read at American Psychological Association meeting.

Buxbaum, Joan. 1967. Nurturance as a factor in wives' judgment of severity of spouses' aphasia. J. Consult. Psychol. 31:240–43.

Carroll, D. 1962. The disability in hemiplegia caused by cerebrovascular disease: Serial studies of 98 cases. J. Chron. Dis. 15:179–88.

Carroll, V. B. 1958. Implications of measured visuospatial impairment in a group of left hemiplegic patients. Arch. Phys. Med. 39:11–14.

Chapman, L. F., W. N. Thetford, L. Beden, T. C. Guthrie, and H. G. Wolff. 1958. Highest integrative functions in man during stress, in Association for Research in Nervous and Mental Disease. Brain and human behavior: Proceedings of the Association, December 7–8, 1956. Research Publications 36. Baltimore, Williams and Wilkins, pp. 491–534.

DeCencio, D. V., M. Leshner, and D. Voron. 1970. Perception and ambulation in hemiplegia. Arch. Phys. Med. 51:105–10.

DeLagi, E. F., R. H. Manheimer, J. Metz, S. B. Bellos, and F. D. Greene. 1962. Rehabilitation of the homebound in a semi-rural area. J. Chron. Dis. 12:568.

DeRenzi, E. and P. Faglioni. 1965. The comparative efficiency of intelligence and vigilance tests in testing hemispheric cerebral damage. Cortex 1:410–33.

Diller, L., Y. Ben-Yishay, J. Weinberg, R. Goodkin, L. J. Gerstman, W. A. Gordon, I. Mandleberg, P. Schulman, and N. Shah. 1971. Final report: studies in cognition and rehabilitation in hemiplegia. SRS-RD-2666-P.

Diller, L., J. Buxbaum, and S. Chiotelis. 1972. Learning and functional motor skills in hemiplegia. J. Genet. Psychol. Monog. 85, 249–86.

Diller, L., and J. Weinberg. 1970. Accidents in hemiplegia. Arch. Phys. Med. 51:358–63.

Evans, R. B. Y. and J. Marmorstein. 1964. Rorschach signs of brain damage in cerebral thrombosis. Perceptual and motor skills 18:977–88.

Feldman, D. J., P. R. Lee, J. Unterecker, K. Lloyd, H. A. Rusk, and A. Toole, 1952. A comparison of functionally oriented medical care and formal rehabilitation in the management of patients with hemiplegia due to cerebrovascular disease. J. Chron. Dis. 15:297.

Fordyce, W. E. and R. H. Jones. 1966. The efficacy of oral and pantomime instructions for hemiplegic patients. Arch. Phys. Med. 47:676–80.

Goldstein, K. 1959. Brain damage, in S. Arieti, ed., American handbook of psychiatry. New York, Basic Books.

Goldstein, R. L., A. C. Goodman, and R. B. King. 1956. Hearing and speech in infantile hemiplegia before and after left hemispherectomy. Neurology 6:869–75.

Goodkin, R. 1966. Case studies in behavior research in rehabilitation. Pcpt. Mot. Skills 23:171–82.

Gordon, E. E., and K. H. Kohn. 1966. Evaluation of rehabilitation methods in the hemiplegic patient. J. Chron. Dis. 19:3–16.

Gulliksen, G., Jr. 1970. Behavioral change in cerebrovascular disease, in A. L. Benton, ed., Psychosomatic and vocational rehabilitation. New York, Harper and Row, pp. 106–10.

Halberstam, J. L., and H. H. Zaretsky. 1969. Learning capacities of elderly and brain damaged. Arch. Phys. Med. 50:133–39.

Halberstam, J. L., H. Zaretsky, B. Brucker, and H. Guttman. 1971. Avoidance conditioning of motor responses in elderly brain-damaged patients. Arch. Phys. Med. 52:318–28.

Harris, J. H., and M. D. Towler. 1955. Intracerebral vascular disease, in A. B. Baker, ed., Clinical neurology. New York, Harper.

Heilbrun, A. B. 1956. Psychological test performance as a function of lateral localization of cerebral lesion. J. Comp. Physiol. Psychol. 49:10–15.

Hirschenfang, M. S. 1960a. A comparison of WAIS scores of hemiplegic patients with and without aphasia. J. Clin. Psychol. 16:351–52.

——— 1960b. A comparison of Bender Gestalt reproduction of right and left hemiplegic patients. J. Clin. Psychol. 16:439.

Hirschenfang, M. S., L. Shulman, and J. G. Benton. 1968. Psychosocial factors influencing the rehabilitation of the hemiplegic patient. Diseases of the nervous system 29:373–79.

Horenstein, S. 1970. Effects of cerebrovascular disease on personality and emotionality. In A. L. Benton, ed., *Behavioral change in cerebrovascular disease*. New York, Harper and Row, Hoeber Med. Div.

Howard, J. A. 1960. A demonstration and research study of the rehabilitation of the physically rehabilitated hemiplegic in a workshop setting. Unpublished report to U.S. Office of Vocational Rehabilitation, Washington, D.C.

Kelman, H. R. and J. N. Muller. 1962. Rehabilitation of nursing home residents. Geriatrics 17:402–11.

Kelman, H. R. and A. Wellner. 1962. Problems in measurement and evaluation of rehabilitation. Arch. Phys. Med. 43:172–80.

Kurtzke, J. F. and L. T. Kurland. 1970. Epidemiology of cerebrovascular disease, in R. G. Siekert, ed., *Cerebrovascular survey report*. Rochester, Whitney Printers and Stationers, pp. 163–75.

Kutner, B., P. Rosenberg, R. Berger, and A. S. Abramson. 1970. A therapeutic community in rehabilitation medicine. New York. Albert Einstein College of Medicine of Yeshiva University.

Lee, P. R. et al. 1958. An evaluation of rehabilitation of patients with hemiparesis or hemiplegia due to cerebral vascular disease. Rehabilitation Monograph No. 15. New York, Institute of Physical Medicine and Rehabilitation.

Lorenze, E. and R. Cancro. 1962. Dysfunction in visual perception with hemiplegia: its relation to activities of daily living. Arch. Phys. Med. Rehab. 43:512–18.

MacDonald, J. C. 1960. An investigation of body scheme in adults with cerebral vascular accidents. Amer. J. Occup. Ther. 14:75–79.

Masland, R. 1958. Central nervous system, higher functions. Ann. Rev. Physiol. 20:533–57.

Mednick, S. A. and J. L. Freedman. 1960. Stimulus generalization. Psychol. Bull. 57:169–201.

Merritt, H. H. 1951. Cerebral vascular accidents, in R. L. Cecil and R. F. Loeb, eds., Textbook of medicine. Philadelphia, Saunders, pp. 1458–69.

Millikan, C. H., 1970. Anticoagulant therapy in cerebrovascular disease, in R. G. Siekert, ed., Cerebrovascular survey report. Rochester, Whitney Printers and Stationers, pp. 218–27.

Nathanson, M., P. S. Bergman, and G. G. Gordon. 1952. Denial of illness: its occurrence in 100 consecutive cases of hemiplegia. Arch. Neurol. Psychiat. 68:380–87.

Penfield, W. and H. H. Jasper. 1953. Epilepsy and the functional anatomy of the human brain. Boston, Little, Brown.

Perlstein, M. A. and P. Hood. 1957. Infantile spastic hemiplegia. Amer. J. Ment. Defic. 61:534–68.

Peszczynski, M. 1954. Ambulation of the severely handicapped hemiplegic adult: (1) Early management, (2) Gait training. Paper read at American Congress of Physical Medicine and Rehabilitation, 32d, Washington, D.C.

Powell, Ruth B., L. Diller, R. Grynbaum, and H. Rusk. 1971. Rehabilitation performance and adjustment in stroke patients: a study of social class factors. (In press).

Rae, J. W., E. M. Smith, and A. Lenzce. 1962. Results of a rehabilitation program for geriatric patients in county hospitals. J. Amer. Med. Assoc. 180:563–66.

Ragoff, J. B., D. V. Cooney, and B. Kutner. 1964. Hemiplegia: a study of home rehabilitation. J. Chron. Dis. 17:539–50.

Reitan, R. M. 1955. Certain differential effects of left and right cerebral lesions in human adults. J. Comp. Physiol. Psychol. 48:474–76.

Reitan, R. M., and K. B. Fitzhugh. 1971. Behavioral deficits in groups with cerebral vascular lesions. J. of Consulting and Clinical Psychology 37:215–23.

Reynolds, G. M. 1959. Problems of sensorimotor learning in the evaluation and treatment of the hemiplegic patient. Rehab. Lit. 20:163–72.

Rosenzweig, M., D. Krech, and E. L. Bennett. 1960. A search for relations between brain chemistry and behavior. Psychol. Bull. 57:476–93.

Rusk, H. A. 1971. Rehabilitation medicine: A textbook on physical medicine and rehabilitation. 3d ed. St. Louis, Mo., C. V. Mosby.

Rusk, H. A. and M. Marx. 1953. Rehabilitation following cerebrovascular accident. Southern Med. J. 46:1943–57.

Sarno, J. E. and M. T. Sarno. 1969. Stroke. New York, McGraw-Hill.

Sarno, J., H. Rusk, L. Diller, and M. Sarno. In press. The effects of hyperbaric oxygenation on the mental and verbal ability of stroke patients.

Seidenberg, R. and A. Ecker. 1954. Psychodynamic and arteriographic studies of acute cerebral vascular disorders. Psychosom. Med. 16:374–92.

Tamerin, J. S. 1964. Perception of progress in rehabilition. Arch. Phys. Med. 45:17–22.

Ullman, M. 1962. Behavioral changes in patients following strokes. Springfield, Ill., Charles C. Thomas.

Ullman, M., E. M. Asnenhurst, L. J. Hurwitz, and A. Gruen. 1960. Motivational and structural factors in denial in hemiplegia. Arch. Neurol. 3:306–18.

Van Buskirk, C. and D. Webster. 1955. Prognostic value of memory defect in rehabilitation of hemiplegics. Neurology 5:407–11.

Waylonis, G. W., A. E. Becker, and K. C. Krueger. 1970. Stroke in a midwestern county. Arch. Phys. Med. 51:651–55.

Weinblatt, B. A. 1959. The role of the organization of intellectual and emotional processes as it relates to performance on a physical rehabilitation program. New York University, unpublished Ph.D. dissertation.

Weinstein, E. A. 1955. Symbolic aspects of thalmic pain. Yale J. Biology and Medicine 28:465–70.

Weinstein, E. and R. Kahn. 1955. The denial of illness. Springfield, Charles C. Thomas.

Weinstein, S. and H. L. Teuber. 1957a. Effects of penetrating brain injury on intelligence test scores. Science 125:1036–37.

——— 1957b. The role of preinjury education and intelligence level in intellectual loss after brain injury. J. Comp. Physiological Psychology 50:535–39.

Weisbroth, S., N. Esibill, and R. R. Zuger. 1971. Factors in the vocational success of hemiplegic patients. Arch. Phys. Med. 52:441–46.

Williams, N. 1967. Correlation between copying ability and dressing activities in hemiplegia. Amer. J. Phys. Med. 46:1332–38.

Wood, N. E. 1959. Comparison of right hemiplegics with left hemiplegics on motor skills and intelligence. Perceptual and Motor Skills 9:103–6.

JOSEPH M. WEPMAN

REHABILITATION AND THE
LANGUAGE DISORDERS

WHEN AN ADULT suffers brain impairment from a stroke, a head injury, or neurosurgical intervention, in addition to a variety of physical and psychological aftereffects, he is likely to show some type of language disorder. Because of the vital role that language comprehension and use plays in man's day-by-day interpersonal relations these language disorders may well become the primary dysfunction needing resolution in the patient's over-all rehabilitation effort. Much of what is expected of him by the professional team engaged in his rehabilitation therapy, as well as the expectancy of others in his social milieu, is dependent on the patient's ability to understand instructions, relate his feelings and attitudes to his listeners, describe his pains and limitations. The language-disordered patient is less likely to be able to assist in his own recovery and respond to self-care programs. He is more likely to feel frustrated and even negativistic toward efforts to help him when he perceives a mismatch between what he wants and the instructional and social goals of his therapist, his family, and his friends.

As will be seen, the language disorders demonstrate a wide variety of verbal insufficiencies. It is therefore most important in rehabilitation practice to include a careful study of the residual language ability of the patient. Each member of the rehabilitation team must not only be

JOSEPH M. WEPMAN, PH.D., is Professor of Psychology, Surgery, and Education and Director of the Speech and Language Clinic, University of Chicago, Chicago, Illinois.

alerted to the fact of a language disability but also to the form and degree the handicap takes in each instance. While it is possible to characterize the language disorders in any number of ways, such classifications are only minimally useful since each category describes such a wide spectrum of behavior. More important than classification is an adequate description of the patient's residual communication ability. Here are the guidelines for understanding the patient's rehabilitation needs as related to his ability to express himself and to comprehend others.

INCIDENCE

Some ten years ago it was estimated that over a million adults suffered from aphasia or associated language disorders in the United States alone. This is now probably an underestimate since, as time goes on, medical and surgical procedures improve and more and more people live to the age when "strokes" are more common. While it is estimated that some twenty million people in this country are sixty-years old or older, in twenty-five years the figure in that age range is more likely to be thirty million. With the age increase there is expected to be a correlated increase in the number of strokes. As our society becomes more technological and urbanized, the pressures under which we live also increase. One of the major predictors of stroke is said to relate to just this factor—living under conditions of stress. Since at least 50 per cent of stroke patients are likely to show some language disorder, the incidence in the population is bound to increase. Rather than the million aphasic patients postulated a decade ago, a better guess (no vital statistics are available to make the figure more exact) is that with each decade the total increases by no less than 20 per cent. In the ten-year span since the previous estimate it is probable that the figure is now closer to one and a quarter million and is constantly on the rise.

The foregoing estimates of incidence are based on the "stroke" population. The figures increase if one adds to the number those who have suffered brain impairment from head injury accidents, especially from the ever-increasing frequency of automobile accidents and from gunshot wounds related to national tendencies for combat. It is probably fair to guess that the total number of aphasic adults of all ages lies somewhere between one and one half and two million.

Again, large-scale vital statistics are lacking, but clinical experience indicates that about 75 per cent of all aphasic adults are male. This would be in keeping with the fact that three of every four stroke patients are male.

While the tendency for strokes to occur increases with age, a not inconsiderable number of patients seen are in the thirty- and forty-year-old group—again, increasing in number with each passing decade.

Most language-disordered adults show concomitant physical and psychological problems. However, about two out of ten show no other evident problem. For these latter few the rehabilitation process can be limited to the recovery of language and treated solely from that viewpoint. But for the greater number by far—eight out of ten—the language disorder must be treated as an integral part—perhaps the single most important part—of the total recovery and rehabilitation process. Without belaboring the point it should, nevertheless, be kept in mind that it is of little value to succeed in overcoming a language problem if the patient remains physically and/or psychologically debilitated. The reverse, of course, is equally true. It is of little value to overcome a physical disability or a psychological aftereffect of brain injury if the patient is unable to communicate. Considering the number of patients with multiple problems, physical, psychological, and linguistic, it is most important that each rehabilitation worker be alerted to and ready to assist in the totality of rehabilitation. The goals of self-care are really only satisfactorily achieved when the "whole" person is rehabilitated.

CLASSIFICATION AND DESCRIPTION

This section is devoted to discussion and categorization of language disorders. By understanding the definitions, the not inconsiderable professional literature on the subject should become more helpful. Most importantly, however, studying the illustrations and descriptions of the verbal behavior of the patients permits a finer understanding of the patient and his potential for self-care.

Certain rather limited generalities about brain injuries and their effect on language are of interest. For all but a few patients the symbolic verbal disorders—the aphasias—occur only when the neural disturbance is in the left hemisphere. Some research indicates that right hemispheric impairments also produce language handicaps, but these are likely to be less pervasive and less specifically damaging to the over-all communication effort. Close study of these patients shows that they may lose some of the abstract quality of their speech without losing the ability to speak.

The following description and definitions are based solely upon a consideration of the linguistic nature of the language disorders. In a later section, the relation of these disorders to some of the daily living and rehabilitation problems of the patients will be discussed.

APHASIA

Aphasia designates any disorder of the abilities necessary to formulate verbal symbols due to organic impairment of the central nervous system. The defect in symbol formulation should be differentiated from language and speech disorders ascribable to faulty innervation and ordering of the musculature of speech, dysfunction of the peripheral sense organs, or general mental deficiency.

This definition agrees with Head's (1926) classical concept that ". . . by symbolic formulation . . . I understand a mode of behavior in which some verbal or other symbol plays a part between initiation and execution (p. 527)." Language is conceived as consisting of three processes, each of which is believed to be acquired separately by the child developing language and is potentially sufficiently independent of the other two so that it may be uniquely impaired. In the order of their function, these three processes are:

1) Recognizing and comprehending an incoming signal by associating it with a previously acquired concept.
2) Attaching a previously acquired verbal symbol having an accepted phonemic or orthographic form to such a concept.
3) Imbedding such a symbol into a previously acquired and relatively automatized grammatical matrix.

These three processes can be identified by the concept of language expressed by Charles Morris (1938), who saw the act as being divisible into three relationships, which he labeled the pragmatical, semantical, and syntactical dimensions of semiosis (the science of signs). He defined these briefly as (1) *pragmatics,* the relation of signs to interpreters, (2) *semantics,* the relations of signs to the objects to which the signs are applicable, and (3) *syntactics,* the relations of signs to other signs.

Research has shown that one way to differentiate the symbolic disorders associated with impairment of the central nervous system is to classify them on the basis of the loss or dysfunction of one or more of the three processes. When more than one is distorted, the process most severely affected should be considered basic, but other impairments should also be noted.

Pragmatic Aphasia. Pragmatic aphasia designates disruption of the first process: a disorder of symbol formulation in which the patient cannot organize and regulate his expression in relation to a given stimulus.

Patients in this category exhibit the following abnormalities: (1) they convey little meaning in their speech; (2) they are constricted in their vocabularies, using fewer low-frequency words than would be expected in the light of their premorbid education and vocations; (3) they show an excessive use of neologisms (meaningless verbal efforts apparently substituted for specific substantive words); (4) they have inadequate feedback along all modalities, rarely recognizing their own inability to communicate satisfactorily or their errors, either neologistic or otherwise, in word usage; and (5) not infrequently they substitute or insert inappropriate substantive words.

However, (1) they are able to maintain a flow of language; (2) they retain the melody and pitch changes of normal speech; and (3) statistically, they have a normal distribution of the various parts of speech.

It is important to note that as these patients recover the ability to comprehend and react to incoming stimuli they tend to use fewer neologisms but continue to substitute and insert inappropriate words in their speech.

Samples of the speech of a pragmatic aphasic subject illustrate a typical response to a visual stimulus (Card 1—TAT):

"Well, here's the, the, uh. I sayed is the one thing that bothers me sustained. The only thing that I ever have and. I camp I was a boy whom. I were when I was a little boy many years ago. I never keep a curb of anything, aside. Till a I never have as a boy, I never had as a young boy. I never years ago I remembered anything, from any breathe of a thing. If I be a good sleed, I can't camp the inglund. Yes, I can patliteray what it is num, but I cannot I'll might take the word mishlaush he wrote."

To an auditory stimulus ("Repeat the word 'fish'."):

"I can't find a word of it. I can't word a murd in to go into things. I might have caught a word here, by accident, but I do not accidentally find what is a samplimay. What is a light marchavee and I never had this as a little boy."

Semantic Aphasia. Semantic aphasia designates a disruption of the second process; a disorder of symbol formulation in which the patient has difficulty in attaching a meaningful verbal sign to a previously acquired concept; impairment of the ability to recall and use previously acquired verbal forms applicable to such a concept.

Patients in this category exhibit the following abnormalities: (1) they have great difficulty remembering and using once-familiar proper names or substantive words (that is, nouns, verbs, adjectives) except, possibly, the most frequent and general, such as *man, thing, nice, good, do, is,* and *like;* (2) when trying to recall words of this type they frequently employ pauses, hesitation forms ("uh, well"), repetition ("the . . . the . . ."), or phrases indicating their inability to recall ("I know what it's for but I can't tell you"); (3) in place of a word which they cannot recall they sometimes employ circumlocutions ("you write with it" for *pencil*), or vocal and body gestures (buzzing and stretching out arms to indicate *airplane*).

However, they often retain the use of the highly frequent function words (articles, demonstratives, pronouns, prepositions, etc.,) and highly frequent substantive words as indicated above; and to a large extent they retain the flow, the melody and pitch changes, and the grammatical structure of normal speech except when interrupted or deflected by their inability to recall and use a desired word.

This type of disorder has traditionally been labeled "anomia" or absence of nouns, but in actuality it affects all substantive words of low frequency. Since, in general, the semantic aphasic fails to communicate much specific information to the listener, his verbal attempts achieve little or no reward, and consequently, unless he improves, he is likely to use less and less speech.

The following are samples of the speech of a semantic aphasic patient:

"Yes! We . . . when I know. If I know what they're good, they're wonderful. I can, we have everything. Why don't I say what we have, because we have all the, that goes with . . . but, good, they're good. They're good to me.

She's a good one; I like her. And then I had another one and she comes different on her time. Each one, and they're very good. Oh, we've had them a long time anyway. They're wonderful; I love them. And they're always anxious to face what they're doing, if they have something to do or anything. And . . . I'd like to tell what they say. Why don't want to say that one? I know what she feels. Like she wants to, she wants me to know. I want to say 'em like say, but it must be, did she, no I know I know. All very funny, I almost would say it would come."

Syntactic aphasia. Syntatic aphasia designates disruption of the third process: a disorder of symbol formulation in which the patient is unable to use his previously acquired grammatical structure.

Patients in this category exhibit the following abnormalities. (1) They tend to misuse, and, more often, omit altogether, the function words (articles, demonstratives, pronouns, prepositions, auxiliary verbs, etc.,) and grammatical inflections (markers of tense, plurality, etc.), and consequently, (2) they cannot form sentences or smaller syntactic constructions such as prepositional phrases and noun or verb phrases, but they speak telegraphically, using single substantive words; (3) they retain little of the melody of speech, although rising and falling pitch are often used accompanying single words.

However, they may retain many substantive words (nouns, verbs, adjectives), and they often retain certain automatic phrases, such as "I don't know" and a few very minimal sentence types like "It's a man" or "It's old."

Here are samples of the speech of a syntactic aphasic patient:

QUESTION	RESPONSE
Where is your daughter?	"New Orleans . . . home . . . Monday"
Will she stay home?	"No . . . No . . . No . . . bridesmaid . . . working . . . married . . . no . . . no . . ."

To the first free-response item on the Language Modalities Test for Aphasia (Wepman and Jones, 1961), a picture of a poker game, one such patient responded: "Poker . . . man . . . fun . . . all night."

Jargon aphasia. Jargon aphasia is a disorder of symbol formulation and expression in which previously acquired sequences of phonemes making up intelligible units of speech are no longer available, and unintelligible ones (that is, jargon) are used in their stead.

Patients in this category use almost exclusively sequences of phonemes which are unlike any specific words of their previously acquired language, but which generally follow the over-all phonemic patterns of that language (its consonants, vowels, and their permitted combinations), as well as its accentual and pitch patterns, indicating that their attempts at language probably are meaningful to them.

Individual jargon aphasic patients, as they improve, are found to be most like one or the other of the types previously described, as recall for recognizable words becomes available. However, clinical experience indicates that the most frequent words of the language and the syntax are most often recovered. Jargon expressions often are retained as neologisms after comparatively complete recovery from this stage or type of aphasia.

In this connection, there is a seeming relation between jargon and apraxic speech, but this appears to be more apparent than real. The two are not difficult to differentiate. The jargon aphasic patient retains verbal facility, melody, and often pitch changes, while the apraxic patient, seeking motor patterns, usually retains none of these. The important distinction, from clinical experience, is that jargon aphasia appears to be a symbolic-process disability stemming from the inability to recall phonemic patterns, while the apraxias are motor defects of a person who retains the symbolic formulation capacities but cannot organize and utilize the musculature of expression.

Global aphasia. Global aphasia is a disorder of language in which the patient is unable to respond verbally to stimuli except, perhaps, with an automatized word, phrase, or phoneme sequence.

Patients in this category evidence little or no understanding along any modality and little or no ability to communicate. Comprehension, where it exists, is generally limited to the specific, immediate concerns of the patient, and an examiner or therapist is likely to be able to communicate with the patient only if he happens to touch upon a patient's immediate concern.

Often such patients rely on primitive gesture and facial expressions to indicate their needs. In some there is evident retention of a meaningful automatic phrase or word. Sometimes these are used appropriately and sometimes they are so automatized that they are used indiscriminately. They often consist of such negative words or phrases as "no" or "I don't know," frequently spoken even when the patient intends an affirmative answer. Most global aphasic adults, in their attempts to speak, will reiterate at least a single phoneme sequence which may contain pitch changes as though some basic feeling were being expressed. These may vary from such combinations of sounds as "che-che" or "puta-puta" to longer vocalizations. These are distinguishable from the previously described jargon by the constant repetition of the same phrase and the comparatively limited length of utterance.

An interesting but as yet only partially validated hypothesis about the symbolic verbal disorders has been given considerable attention in clinical and research efforts. If one compares the five types of aphasia presented above in the order of severity the following sequence is observed: (1) global, (2) jargon, (3) pragmatic, (4) semantic, and (5) syntactic. The severity is considered in terms of communicatability. Thus, the global aphasic has the greatest difficulty, the jargon aphasic next, and, continuing through the list, the syntactic patient least.

It has been suggested that a regressive phenomenon may be operative here, that is, the amount of loss of communicatability may be increased as one goes down the five-part chain. Some patients show this sequence of events very clearly by the manner of their recovery. Thus, a global patient at one point in time, as he improves, often goes through a jargon phase, a pragmatic phase, a semantic phase, and finally a syntactic phase, in that order. The observation of such changes with time and therapy makes the initial localization of trauma less important, providing only a starting point for therapy.

The regression hypothesis gains additional credence where one compares the five types in the ascending order of severity with the development of language in children. The table shows this most clearly.

TYPES OF APHASIA AND THE
DEVELOPMENT OF LANGUAGE

Aphasia Types	Developmental Stages
Global	Speechless
Jargon	Preverbal speech
Pragmatic	Fortuitous word formations
Semantic	Nominal language
Syntactic	Grammatical expression

(Adapted from Wepman and Jones, 1964)

The theory would hold that an adult tends to lose most readily that part of his language he had acquired last. The effect of this possibility on therapy is dramatic. It removes the effort from any attempt to teach words—to teach a lexicon of communication. Rather, it points to the need to establish in therapy the process or language level at which the patient can function and assists him in developing that process to some degree of fluency until he is ready to undertake the next process.

NONSYMBOLIC LANGUAGE IMPAIRMENTS

Before discussing specific language therapy for aphasia, the rehabilitation worker as well as the family and friends of the patient should recognize that nonsymbolic language impairments may also be present. In some patients these will be the sole disturbance; in others they may occur concomitantly with the symbolic aphasias and complicate an already complex condition.

Agnosia. Agnosia is the inability to transmit incoming stimuli along a specific modality sufficient to arouse a meaningful state or associations to the presenting signal; the inability to imitate, copy, or recognize stimuli, or to match them with identical stimuli.

In the present schema the term agnosia is reserved for those disruptions of the reception of language stimuli where the transmission function of the central nervous system is affected rather than the integrative function which produces the symbolic formulation of language. The agnosias are seen as being very specific to modalities; that is, a disruption of a particular transmission pathway is not necessarily related to disruption of input along any other modality. The effect on total language of an agnosia is largely on the reception of stimuli along the modality concerned, but may be more than that. The ability to formulate symbols at the conceptual level is, to a large degree, dependent upon stimulation from external transmission of new stimuli. When this process is lacking, the organism tends to express only internalized states, and to that degree fails to relate to his environment. When a major modality of input is entirely blocked, such patients act as though deafened or blinded. The basic capacity to formulate symbols, however, is most often found to be unaffected.

Specific islands of ability are often retained; that is, a patient with a severe generalized visual agnosia may still retain the ability to function with visually presented numbers. In other patients only one or more of the visual transmissive processes may be affected. Thus, a patient may be able to respond to geometric forms but not to common life forms; to words and not to letters; or to sentences he hears but not to specific single words along the same pathway. Patients have been observed who retain the ability to imitate or copy stimuli received along a disrupted pathway, even though they cannot recognize or conceptualize stimuli along the same pathway.

It is essential, then, in the diagnostic description of an agnosia, to qualify the term by modality, by type of loss within the modality, and by the degree of loss within each type.

The great majority of brain-injured, language-disturbed adults will show some type or degree of agnosia. It is important to differentiate these problems from the symbolic ones, not only in type but also in degree of language disturbance. The therapy for the agnosias is most often directly related to the disorder, while for the symbolic problems the therapy choice is usually one of language stimulation rather than direct training. The transmissive problems also seem to affect most patients differently than do the symbolic ones. Commonly, the patient with visual agnosia of any type will complain of poor vision and a desire for ocular examination and even more directly for glasses. The patient with auditory agnosia very often will ask to have stimuli repeated more loudly and even ask for audiometric examination or hearing aid amplification. These ideas of peripheral loss, if not resolved satisfactorily, tend to become fixed and may obviate language therapy.

Apraxia. Apraxia is the disruption of or inability to transmit a motor pattern along a specific modality; difficulty in the articulation of speech or the formulation of letters in writing or the movements of gesture or pantomime.

The apraxias, as the term is used here, include all of the specific motor defects, from the most central disorders where the actual recall of motor positioning and sequencing of tongue, lips, palate, etc., is affected, to the various levels and degrees of dysarthria and agraphia.

Verbal apraxia is the loss of ability to produce at will the motor acts of articulation. Verbal apraxia often blocks any diagnosis of aphasia, yet it can be demonstrated that apraxias are independent of the symbolic process. It can be shown in an apraxic patient, for example, that he understands what is said to him, formulates symbols in his mind, has available the syntax of the language, but cannot recall or control the motor act of articulation. In the writing act, the same independence of disability is not uncommonly seen. Patients have been observed who can speak adequately and read orally, and yet have difficulty forming letters in graphic production. Frequently, the apraxic dysfunction in oral acts is accompanied by apraxic agraphia, but this is thought to be the existence of two separate problems since each can function independently.

The *dysarthrias* are seen as lower levels of verbal apraxia dependent for their type upon location of the neural disability. The more central a problem of articulation is, the more it seems like a true apraxia. Thus, central dysarthria affects articulation not only in speed of movement and consequent elision and omission of sounds produced or attempted (due to dysdiadochokinesis) but also produces reversals of sounds and syllables within words and between words as well as substitution of phonetic patterns.

The more distal disturbances in articulation, the peripheral dysarthrias, show only the problem of speed of articulation without the reversals and substitutions. Consequently, the peripheral dysarthrias typically show elongated vowels and slow articulation. They reveal dysdiadochokinesis or the inability to make rapid alternating movements of the speech musculature as their basic disorder.

Apraxia, like its input counterpart, agnosia, is a purely transmissive dysfunction independent of the symbolic formulation process, but affecting it through dysarthric or apraxic distortion which fails to communicate to the listener (the basic purpose of language) and often produces a lack of closure and a sense of failure for the speaker.

Following are some common terms used in describing various language disorders:

Anomia: inability to formulate names or nouns (not felt to be a distinguishable disorder in this schema, but part of semantic aphasia).

Paraphasia: difficulty with syntax and grammatical expression (seen as a type of aphasia; see syntactic aphasia).

Paragrammatism: the reversal or elision of sounds and syllables in words (an apraxic dysfunction in this schema; see central dysarthria).

Agrammatism: so-called telegraphic speech—without grammar (seen here as a type of aphasia; see syntactic aphasia).

COMMON PHYSICAL CONCOMITANTS

It is often necessary to recall that aphasia and other language disorders occur only as the result of brain impairment. It must be remembered that the aphasic patient may be subject to all of the ills that beset any brain-injured person. Certain physical disabilities and psychological aftereffects, in fact, may play an important role in the total recovery plan for any patient. Most prominent of the physical handicaps present in the great majority of adult aphasic patients are the hemiplegias or hemipareses. Not only are these major hurdles which the patient must overcome, but often they are unresolvable and adaptations must be developed to reduce their debilitating physical effects. Since aphasia occurs most often as the result of left cortical disturbance, the paralyses most often effect the previously dominant right side of the body. When this paralysis or paresis remains the patient must acquire the ability to shift his major muscular activities to the left side—he must become left-handed. Too often this shift is accomplished with little or no therapeutic attention whereas it is believed it should always receive some primary attention. Techniques are available for teaching left-handed writing, and they should be utilized. Very few patients can make the shift efficiently without assistance. Actually this is one of the few instances where new practices can be instituted by each member of the rehabilitation team. The patient needs to become more than a left-handed writer, he must become a left-sider for all motoric activity. Writing, of course, is where the language and physical debilities come together. Often a patient cannot express himself graphically, not because of an agraphia—a central disorder of writing—but because he has lost control over his dominant hand and when assisted can express himself adequately using his left hand. Every physical-motoric act he learns with his left hand will make writing with that hand easier for him.

A second relatively common physical disability found in some aphasic patients are limitations in function of the visual fields. This is called hemianopia. Homonymous hemianopia, in which the parallel quadrant of each eye loses its function, is the most common type encountered. The effect on reading is sometimes quite dramatic. The eyes retain their normal visual acuity but are limited in their cone of vision. Patients are observed who read quite adequately until the printed page goes beyond their visual field. Until they are taught to do otherwise, many adults fail to recognize the problem and act as though the print had stopped two or three words from the end of the page.

This loss of lateral vision extends itself to every act of life; such patients need to learn to turn their heads to the right or they collide with people or things. Driving a car may be difficult for them until they learn to adjust to the visual limitations. There are no known treatments for the hemianopias. Usually they are permanent, although changes in their completeness seem to occur in some instances. Adaptation and adjustment therapy usually is successful. It should, however, never be considered as an automatic occurrence even though the logic of adaption is so simple. Man is an animal conditioned throughout his life to look straight ahead. He can see whatever there is to see within his cone of vision. When that cone is reduced or flattened on one side, he needs to be taught to turn his head. The cone of vision will be reduced but in almost every instance remains sufficient for most activities.

Vertigo, tinnitus, optic atrophy, diplopia, localized headaches, and tremors are physical conditions not uncommonly seen as aftereffects of brain damage. For the most part they disappear as symptoms with time. Epileptiform seizures, both petit and grand mal, are also relatively common physical aftereffects of brain trauma, especially where head injury is involved. Grand mal seizures—where complete unconsciousness occurs—are not only physically debilitating but are also psychologically most disturbing to patients. Fortunately, most seizures are controllable with medication. Often a full seizure is indistinguishable in a behavioral sense from that of a stroke. Whenever a brain-injured patient becomes unconscious, medical assistance should be sought. Frequently, the distinction between the two—seizure or stroke—can be best understood in retrospect. A stroke is the product of an alteration in the cerebrovascular system which serves to obliterate the source of blood supply to the brain with its consequent loss of useful neural tissue. A seizure, on the other hand, is a momentary interruption of the flow of energy within the nervous system. Both may include unconsciousness but only the "stroke" leaves permanent residuals. Because it is possible to obviate seizures by medication, every brain-impaired adult should be under the care of a competent physician. The seizures may in this way be minimized; without such care, however, the patient who may be subject to seizures may have real vocational and avocational limitations. These should be understood in the over-all planning of therapy and of living. (A fuller discussion of the physiological factors commonly effecting aphasic adults can be found in Wepman, 1968.)

COMMON PSYCHOLOGICAL CHARACTERISTICS

As in the case of the contributing physical disabilities, the aphasic brain-injured adult may demonstrate a wide variety of common behavioral manifestations. Some of these effect his language; almost all of them effect his day-to-day living. Rehabilitation therapists as well as those most closely related to the patient in everyday living should be aware of these factors and the role they may play in recovery.

The list below includes some of those behavior patterns most commonly seen after brain impairment. None are pathognomonic, however; and while their presence may indicate the extent of a disordered thought process, their absence is in no sense to be interpreted as an indication of a lesser damage.

BEHAVIOR INDICATORS COMMONLY SEEN AFTER BRAIN IMPAIRMENT *

Egocentricity: The tendency to turn inward.

Euphoria: A state of well-being; usually an early behavioral sign which disappears after the acute stage of recovery. When it does not disappear, the prognosis for recovery is very limited.

Emotional Lability: The tendency to cry under almost any or all conditions. Also a common early post-traumatic sign which tends to disappear after the acute post-traumatic period. Also, when and if it does not disappear, the prognosis is limited.

Perseveration: In thought, word, and action. As though the cognitive and linguistic processes once undertaken cannot be voluntarily stopped.

Reduced Initiative: As though it takes a greater effort to perform any act than the individual seems able to put forth.

Increased Fatigability: Especially during the early post-traumatic period, as though the body and mind needed more rest for recovery to ensue, which it probably does. If this sign continues for a long time, the prognosis for recovery is poor.

Increased Irritability: Especially to be noted after the acute stage is over. Every frustration leads to discomfort and a tendency toward immediate overreaction.

Memory Loss: Especially noticed as immediate failure to recall specific items: faces, people, ideas, etc. Less of a tendency for old personal recall to be effected.

Widely Fluctuating Behavior: As though a well-regulated plan for action was difficult to follow. Even in language usage certain situations may result in exaggerated behavior at one moment and what appears to be apathy the next. Usually these wide discrepancies disappear with time.

It has been widely noted that the effect of brain damage upon personality in general is to be seen as an exacerbation of the typical behavioral patterns of the individual. Dependent people become more dependent; aggressive people, more aggressive. Rarely does a person change from one type to another. In fact, if such a change is noted, the usual conclusion is that this changed behavior was the underlying personality of the premorbid state which is thought to have been controlled or repressed for psychological reasons.

*Adapted from Garrett and Levine, 1962.

PRINCIPLES OF RECOVERY

The rehabilitation team as well as the family should recognize certain principles about recovery from aphasia—certain of the communication problems generally besetting the individual patient. While these principles are generalizations and therefore may not apply to any given patient, they have been formulated after experiences with many patients and may be found extremely useful.

First, recovery of the ability to communicate is based on three factors: stimulation, facilitation, and motivation (Wepman, 1953). Briefly, these three mean the following: stimulation is what is done to and with the patient by any outside agent; facilitation is the degree to which the impaired nervous system is capable of reacting; motivation is the patient's internal drive to get better.

Every contact the patient has can be thought of as a form of stimulation, but it must be constantly remembered that communication exists in literally every act of life, not just in an aspect of it called language or aphasia therapy. In fact, a patient may be better able to accept language stimulation in physical therapy or occupational therapy, for example, than he can in a directed-speech or language-therapy program.

Stimulation, then, can be thought of as formal when what is involved is directly related to training toward improvement of the language act and as informal when it makes use of life situations in which language usage is incidental. In both forms the specific stimuli used or the method employed to secure verbal response is unimportant. What is important is that the patient be stimulated at his level of comprehension and function.

Facilitation of the existing nervous system means simply that it is recognized that the physical effects of stroke or trauma limit the residual activity of the nervous system. This impaired system, it is hoped, will, through restabilization and reorganization, be able to take over most or all of the functions impaired by the damage. It must be recognized, however, that this is rarely completely true. Approximate function and adaptation does occur but almost always with some limitation; that is, the end product, the newly constituted nervous system, is not in every way as successful as the previously unimpaired system was before the trauma occurred. Perhaps the best example of this is the almost universally recognized sign following brain injury of a slowing down of reaction time. Even when patients seem to recover both their physical and linguistic abilities, they still most often show slower reaction time. Of course, when recovery is incomplete the slowing down of both sensory processing and motor behavior is quite apparent. Every member of the rehabilitation team or family must both recognize this and act upon it. The impaired patient needs more time—more time to process what he sees and hears, more time to integrate it and associate to it, more time to react and, in the reaction, more time to complete the muscular action.

Facilitation is another way of saying how the impaired system works. Because it is impaired, it can only work at some slower speed or it may only be able to repeat things or imitate things seen or heard. Facilitation is the limitation on recovery placed by the impairment of the organic structure. It is most important that the patient not be constantly approached with tasks beyond his capacity to perform, nor reproached for not performing as the observer believes he should. The limitations are real ones. A gross example would be that one never asks a hemiplegic patient to run; his musculature, being paralyzed, will obviously not support him. Similarly, one doesn't expect an unintelligible aphasic, a jargon speaker, to pronounce carefully; he is unable to pronounce words because of his neurological disability. Facilitation is how much a patient can do with what he has left, so all stimulation must be in terms of how facilitatable the patient is.

Motivation, the third aspect of recovery, relates to the internal state or drive of the patient. Families or therapists only stimulate; the patient is motivated. One doesn't externally motivate a patient. Rather, a climate conducive to change in a desired direction is provided. Within this environment the patient can be maximally stimulated, both formally and informally, but the motivation factor is the patient's level of aspiration, his drive to succeed, to get better.

The first principle of recovery, then, is that patients should be stimulated to the level of their facilitation ability and within the expectancy of their motivation. For some this will mean that the entire therapy is designed to give maximal external support to very minimal efforts.

Stimulation may need to take the form of total acceptance if the facilitating factor is low and the motivating factor equally so. On the other hand, with high motivation even a severely impaired, therefore poorly facilitated, patient can be favorably stimulated. Again, what is done for and with the patient is not so important; but that something is being done is most important.

The second principle of recovery relates to the capacity of the patient to recognize and correct his own errors. In other words, to use or develop his feedback and monitoring system. It is aphoristic to say that if a patient can recognize his errors he can be helped to correct them and will likely improve; if he cannot recognize his own errors, however, the prognosis for recovery is poor. Change occurs in behavior if our actions are negatively regarded or positively rewarded; if neither the rejection nor the affirmation is recognized, no change will occur (Wepman, 1958).

The third general principle of recovery relates to the recognition that not only is the aphasic a language-disturbed patient but that he has also suffered an impairment to his central nervous system, as noted earlier. This is often overlooked. The communication problem appears so pervasive that other effects are often minimized. yet they may be at the very core of the patient's problem as he struggles to readapt himself to society.

Some of these behavior characteristics directly affecting recovery should be recalled because of their day-by-day importance in the life pattern of the recovering patient. For example, poor auditory and visual immediate memory, poor productivity, slower reaction time, and a tendency toward concrete rather than abstract behavior affect much more than language behavior. Poor memory means there may need to be a repetition of requests and demands made on the patient. Poor productivity may mean that his attempts to complete projects are minimal. An earlier section dealt with the reaction speed. Any task, verbal or otherwise, may take the patient longer to comprehend and longer to react to than one would expect. One study of aphasic subjects showed that their general comprehension was improved significantly, for example, whenever a pause was inserted between each word of a request. Finally, there is a widely recognized tendency in many brain-injured adults to revert to a simpler, less abstract mode of existence. All disciplines working with the rehabilitation of the aphasic patient as well as their families should bear these principles in mind and see the recovering patients in terms of their ability to be intelligible when they try to communicate. Nothing known about language recovery for the aphasic adult is more productive than the forming of close interpersonal relations with people, professional and nonprofessional alike. It should be the role of every member of the team to assist the patient in making these meaningful human contacts.

For the rehabilitation worker it might be important to understand the aphasic patient not in linguistic terms, which are essential for the language therapist, but in terms of the patient's functional ability to communicate. A suggested form for such a classification system which some centers have found useful is shown below.

A SIX-POINT SCALE OF COMPREHENSION AND INTELLIGIBILITY

1) Fluent speech with good intelligibility, although occasional errors of articulation and word-finding may be common. Frequently self-corrects many of his own errors.
2) Little fluency, but transmits meanings by single words. Syntax may be garbled, word endings omitted, but comprehension and intelligibility is generally good.
3) Some fluency and intelligibility apparent but word-finding, especially for nominal speech, may make over-all pattern circumlocutious. Difficulty in being specific in speech may lead to a wide overuse of pronouns and reduction of nouns.
4) Speech sounds intact; often with fluency but little meaning is conveyed to the listener. May revert to neologistic substitutions at the most telling part of a statement. Rarely recognizes this tendency or substitutions of inappropriate words. Because of inadequate feedback, the patient acts as though what he has said is meaningful.
5) Talks with great fluency but little or nothing of what he says is intelligible. No self-recognition of lack of intelligibility, therefore, no self-correction.
6) Unable to comprehend or communicate verbally except for occasional automatic words or phrases.

By recognizing the level of communicability the therapist or family can judge how much or little one can use verbal behavior in working with the patient. It is necessary to use caution in any assumption about what a given patient intends by what he says. Both verbal and nonverbal behavior must be understood as part of the communication act. While research fails to find a meaningful correlation between retained intelligence and ability to speak, it must be understood that probably more goes on internally in every patient than he is able to express. Do not underestimate a patient's ability to understand what is being said to or about him. Communication is not limited to words and nonverbal clues; facial expressions, stress patterns, and gestures play a most important role. It is better to assume that the patient understands whatever he hears and sees in at least a general way. Probably the most consistent negative reaction of patients to therapists and families comes about when this is overlooked and the patient is talked about in his presence as though he were not there (Buck, 1963).

PSYCHOSOCIAL ASPECTS OF REHABILITATION

Aphasia is most often described as a neurologic or linguistic event. To this must be added the impelling role of the society or milieu in which the patient must live.

In 1951 the present writer pointed out the unlikelihood of aphasia recovery in a milieu which infantilizes the patient, increases his dependency, and limits his social environment (Garrett and Levine, 1962). In common with other brain-impaired subjects, the aphasic patient is known to show what have come to be called typical "organic" signs in his nonlanguage behavior. He is, after all, a brain-injured patient; that is, he has lost some part of his previously intact cortex. His readaption to life often takes a form recognizably like that of others with impaired cortical ability. Such behavioral manifestations, some directly due to trauma, others to the mode of adaptation, and still others to the constraints of the environment, force the often unspoken and too often unrecognized perspective in which the patient is seen.

These psychosocial aspects of aphasia have been only briefly noted in the literature, as though language impairment could be resolved in a vacuum. The self-concept of the patient has been of less concern than his vocabulary or the location of his neural lesion. Hodgins, in his insightful book on aphasia *Episode* (1964), makes much of this. He relates how professionals in different medical and adjunctive disciplines treat the patient as an object rather than as a person. He points out persuasively how self-pity invades the patient's mind. This behavior is often rewarded by professional staff in the hospital and family and friends in the post-hospital experience.

Literally no studies have investigated the effect of the environment on such patients. Illustrative case histories, however, are growing in number. Both self-revealing reports and the collected comments of aphasic patients have attested in the literature to the psychological and psychosocial effects of aphasia (Buck, 1963; Ritchie, 1961; Sies and Butler, 1963; Hodgins, 1964; and Rolnik and Hoops, 1969).

The stress placed upon such factors as the milieu and climate of therapy; the recognition of both long- and short-term goals leading to renewed interpersonal relations; the specific role of the family of the aphasic patient in the recovery process, and the reintroduction of the patient into an interpersonal world have been shown to be most important factors (Wepman, 1968).

The family of the aphasic subject can be helpful, or they can hinder. Making family members helpful is one of the most difficult yet most essential tasks of rehabilitation. If from the onset of the disorder the family sees the patient as a convalescing person striving toward independence and the useful life patterns of a human being, if they see him as one who needs help but is not helpless, one who needs understanding, but not cloying sympathy, then a climate can be molded maximizing recovery. Otherwise, over-dependence, invalidism, and hopelessness surround the patient. Withdrawal rather than self-seeking is a common result.

One patient had a bad experience; in fact, he had a series of them in just this factor of the milieu of his rehabilitative effort. After a good hospital stay of four weeks duration, where many active processes of the milieu were generated toward recovery, and where speech, occupational, and physical therapists had worked with the medical specialists toward recognizable goals, he went home to an atmosphere of despondency. His wife saw no future for him or for herself. Although indoctrinated by the hospital staff, she permitted her earlier conditioning to overtake her new instruction. Sick people need a darkened room; one talks and walks softly in the presence of illness. The children were hushed, the house more the anteroom to a morgue than a recovery room; the atmosphere was one of anxiety. After all, he had suffered a debilitating stroke; his heart had been affected. She, his wife, needed to assume the decisionmaking role he had not permitted her when he was healthy. She foresaw no good result.

Her anxiety and her hopelessness transmitted themselves to him. His decline, after a good start, was evident. The climate was the worst possible for getting better. The language therapist, the occupational therapist, and the physical therapist tried, on home visits, to offset this climate but with no effect. The wife's attitude, twenty-four hours a day, denied their efforts. The patient's withdrawal was complete. It was not his aphasia which discouraged therapy, it was the climate of a recovery space which denied him recovery.

THE GOALS OF REHABILITATION

Important as the milieu and climate of therapy are, they will be found of little value without properly established goals. These must be understandable from the viewpoints of the patient, his family, and his therapists. He must not only function in a space continuum, but in a temporal continuum as well. He must see himself recovering; where he has been is as important as where he is going; yesterday is as important as tomorrow, for the perspective of recovery must be the baseline for his change.

During the early postmorbid stage patients are most often unable, because of their egocentricity, state of shock, and self-concern, to visualize goals. Therapy must establish day-by-day achievements; "movement toward effective living" is the phrase adopted by certain therapists. The sooner these small steps can be undertaken, and their accomplishment recognized, the more rapidly can the over-all therapeutic results be placed in a useful perspective. Where one has been is important, not as a goal, but as a recognition of movement from whatever nadir of achievement. The ghost of the past often denies achievement. The day-by-day recognition of change, the sense of accomplishment to balance the sense of futility and failure, the knowledge of progress—for the patient, these are all important; for the family they are equally so.

Early stages of recovery must be visualized in terms of these small steps toward effectiveness; most importantly, not in terms of *words* but in terms of acts. Language is the substitute for action. It can more easily follow action but often cannot precede it. If the family can see this, soon the patient will be able to do so. Only after the readjustment to life that follows a thing as devastating as a stroke with aphasia can real progress toward future goals be achieved.

Long-term goals are useful as the patient becomes capable of differentiating what he does today in a larger frame of reference. With an increased ability to be self-critical, there comes a need to be self-critical toward some recognizable end.

The rehabilitation worker's and the family's ability to work in this frame of reference, to see the small-term goals as being productive of steps toward the larger life goals, being accepting of the changes that occur in the small specific functions of daily living, seeing them as steppingstones vital to progress, not attempting to equate each day's failures with the larger needs, but counting the blessings as they occur—these are the attitudes that the therapist must have and transmit to the family and to the patient when he can encompass them.

Timing is very important here. Unrealistic long-term goals, when established too early, produce frustration, futility, anxiety, and withdrawal; when properly timed, they serve as stimulating forces leading to increased motivation. Without goals, therapy is doomed to endless exercises without hope of real recovery—exercises for exercise sake, or for the therapist's sake. With goals that are clear, the family, with all of its collective feelings of incompetence and inadequacy, can function helpfully and provide the climate and milieu so vital to recovery. The effect of a negative and negating, hopeless attitude on the climate and milieu has been briefly mentioned. This attitude is most often the product of inadequately trained families whose goal behavior is confused because of a failure to visualize changes, potential as well as achieved. But beyond this assumed attitude, due to lack of background and knowledge, are the basic personalities of the people involved.

Some wives, husbands, and children make excellent therapists by the very nature of their ability to assume roles requiring independence of function and decisionmaking in their contacts with the patient, while still providing room for him to re-establish his ego and achieve effectiveness in living.

Lifelong patterns of dependence upon the dominant male must be reversed with his incapacitation, reversed but not rigidly held, possessed but not totally exercised. These are the needs. To become the independent member of the patient's family and to maintain that role, often not permitting the psychological growth of the patient as he strives to recapture his ego-status, is the often-encountered process.

Wives, especially, have been observed who, for the first time enjoying comparative freedom of control, will not willingly release it to a husband attempting to re-establish himself. Temporary acceptance is a difficult psychological position; the patient, in his early stages of recovery, is necessarily dependent. Only through the acceptance of another's lead can he grope through the daily living problems. If this stage satisfies some well-hidden maternal instinct in his wife (or his therapist) to keep him dependent so that they are needed, recovery becomes a chimera, a talked-of but unrealizable goal. Often, with even the best of psychotherapy, the yielding of dominance by the wife is unrealizable.

Older children of aphasic patients often out of mistaken kindliness keep their parents hopelessly enmeshed in their dependencies. Therapists who are unable to give up emotionalized although unrecognized dominance over their patients keep them from recovering. So do wives verbalizing their goodness to the patient, their understanding of his needs before he expresses them, helping the patient before he needs their help. They are fulfilling his desires *before* he can even realize what he wants, and certainly before he can express them, in the mistaken view that they are doing *everything* they can for their husbands, patients, or parents.

From examples such as these comes the conviction that rehabilitation should be thought of in terms of an expanded use of previously learned behavior. Not learning how to talk, but the re-establishment of language usage. Not stimulus-response behavior, but spontaneous use of verbal expressions.

Goals for aphasic adults must of necessity be limited by their recovered ability to communicate. Vocational counseling with this limitation in mind may have to change for each subject over time as the recovery progresses. Initial planning for vocational futures may be as direct as establishing a self-care program with the aid of the patient's family. This may be as far as rehabilitative practices go if the patient remains in a global or noncommunicative state. With progressive recovery of language usage broader horizons can be envisioned. It is most important that such planning, however, be undertaken slowly, even piecemeal. Self-care in a physical sense, the ability to maintain personal hygiene, to dress oneself, to eat independently, etc. can be supplemented by language-directed self-care; by exercise of simple verbal communication substitutes for the actions implied. This stage of rehabilitation can be a most important first step. Psychologically the aphasic patient is most likely to evidence a marked negative reaction to recovery, especially where premorbid vocations and avocations were highly verbal in nature. The ghost of the past often becomes a burden which is overwhelming to the patient. New goals, usually short-term therapeutically oriented ones, must be identified and recognized as they are met.

A most common reaction pattern is the acceptance of a state of debility in communication—a failure to try if the result is largely unrewarding. Such passive dependency must be worked with quite specifically. Thus, a patient of previously good but not aggressive verbal ability is likely to appear to stay on a plateau in treatment if the recovery appears to him to be insubstantial and at his introspective level literally impossible. One such patient failed to respond to any therapy or counseling even though it was thought by those around him that his potential was greater than the effort he was making. Only the introduction of very explicit short-term goals, such as helping around the house, making his own bed, talking as he could to his children about their work, putting away the daily marketing, succeeded in acting as a catalyst for further and broader explorations of things to do. From the negative-passive-nontalking state, this patient was able to move ahead to more elaborate efforts using both returning language and physical abilities. A place was developed for him running a cigar and newspaper counter in an office building. His speech improved with increasing use. This may be the most important lesson to learn. Recovery of language is not the product of direct therapy alone, but rather of the daily use of verbal behavior in a natural situation.

One patient, a trial lawyer of some note, who might be described as an aggressive speaker, recovered the ability to read and write, but in a realistic sense he never again became fluent in command of spoken language. Semantic wordfinding characterized his slow and halting speech.

Nevertheless, he was again able to research a legal brief and even prepare a written outline of a court presentation quite successfully. This was a change for him, but a useful and practical one which he came to recognize as being worthwhile.

Another patient, who prior to his stroke had been a brilliant advertising man but in recovery had plateaued at a level of telegraphic, asyntactic speech, found that applying his new level of verbal ability, which permitted only substantive word-concepts, made a better copywriter out of him. He thought only in terms of direct, specific interests. His words were largely concrete expressions rather than abstractions. He was able to work again in his own field, which had been his goal throughout the recovery process.

Still another source of much difficulty relates to the manner in which therapists in general tend to overlook the psychosocial aspects of aphasia, especially in patients whose recovery programs are limited to the artificiality of the clinic. Comments have been made previously on the need to understand a patient's pretraumatic vocational and avocational drives in order to foster a therapy in keeping with his life expectation. The patient who rather violently attacked a therapist when he was introduced to a preprimer as his source material for a day's word-finding illustrates this. A patient is entitled to be treated other than as a deficient child. If programs for recovery are to be used they should be carefully constructed to meet not only the therapist's concern but also the patient's needs.

Yet, even more than our imperfect knowledge of and reference to the patient's personality is the tendency to treat a patient as though he lived alone, in a nonspeaking, nonthinking, nonacting world. The effect on therapy of the personality of the people in the patient's environment is readily seen.

One patient, for example, following his stroke had a severe, global type aphasia. In the course of time, his understanding of what was said to him improved, as did his ability to secure some meaning from the printed page. He could copy most things he saw, but could not write spontaneously. His condition improved while he was hospitalized during the first three poststroke months. However, his home environment had changed. His most amenable and accepting wife (while he was hospitalized) became completely over-protective of every act he attempted as soon as he came home. She resented the therapist's provision of increasingly difficult material. She infantilized the patient to such a degree that he fell back upon gesture rather than attempt verbalization when she stressed the need for him to be "perfect" in whatever he tried. She acted as though she had lost a husband but gained a baby son. Her maternalism gave him succor, and his behavior relapsed into complete infantlike withdrawal. No ordinary, directed therapy could cope with this situation. It took the combined psychotherapeutic efforts of a team of therapists including a psychologist to reduce the burden of the assumed parent-child relationship before any rehabilitation goal could be achieved.

This case history not only illustrates the environmental aspects so essential in rehabilitation but it also introduces the concept that aphasia, while the direct product of neurological impairment, evidences its linguistic process alteration by the stages of dependency through which a patient must pass in achieving a satisfactory state of rehabilitation. Most patients return to their homes from relatively brief absences in the hospital during the acute stages of their neurological and linguistic disturbances. In those instances where physical recovery is necessary, some rehabilitative efforts are made, just as when speech and reading are still affected some language therapy is or can be provided. What is so often overlooked, however, is the role of the patient as a convalescent in his family, the attitudes and personality of the people closest to him, and their ability to turn the world, not just their homes, into a therapeutic agency.

A common expression of affect on the part of hemiplegic adult aphasic patients is their demand for dependency. Too often they become autocratic manipulators of home and hearth. Latent dominant needs that had been suppressed pretraumatically become evident as aphasic patients "rule" their wives or husbands. They demand attention, show little inner resources for self-care, demonstrate their inadequate emotional control by utilizing every means to obtain their regressed needs. The therapist in such a situation must be cautious about becoming "involved" in the domestic inequities that are evident, yet must work toward the establishment of an equitable relationship. Otherwise, therapy for language will be meaningless. It will exist in the vacuum of therapist-patient, stimulus-response behavior, out of context with the reality of the patient's life pattern.

The behavior of a wife toward her husband who was recovering from a stroke is one example, as shown above. It is only fair to point out that husbands of wives who are aphasic most often err even more. Almost invariably they try to do too much for the patient. Their guilt for needing to leave their wives each day becomes overwhelming, so when they are at home they outdo themselves. They not only offer their assistance, they insist on their right to provide it. While they may not infantilize their wives, they quite openly increase their dependency. They sometimes almost openly refuse to let them get better.

Therapy when offered via the husband or the wife of the types illustrated is usually resolved by being reduced to childlike repetition. They run their lives and their spouses' lives entirely from the heart and almost never from the head. There is a great danger that outside direct-language therapy will feed into this type of situation. The materials of therapy—the vocabulary, the pictures, the books, etc., are often selected for their utter simplicity. The patient is rarely provided with the stuff of which abstractions are made.

To overcome this climate of good will the patient must develop outgoing behavior almost in spite of well-meaning but misguided mates. The therapist in this situation who is limited to educational learning techniques is often helpless. His basic role should be to create a climate for recovery, one in which change and frustration can provide the opportunity for the restoration of function. What is done in such therapy is less important than the fact of its being done. The family's role in recovery must be turned into an active, seeking mutual program. Most of all, it is up to the rehabilitation worker to create this family role. The group dynamic is more important than the individual's use of verbal symbols.

More attention must be paid to the psychosocial environment, the interpsychic and intrapsychic life of the patient. He will not nor can he be expected to redevelop verbal communication where therapy is conducted in a vacuum apart from life. The patient must readjust to life and to its changing processes. Admittedly, the cases presented here are somewhat unusual. Not every individual changes personality in the face of opportunity, but enough do to make the psychosocial aspects of aphasia as important in the rehabilitation picture as the physiological or the psycholinguistic aspects, wherever they occur.

The language disorders complicate rehabilitation for the brain-injured adult. Yet, it is most important to recognize that such patients are amenable to therapy. For the most part, they can be helped to recover to a state of usefulness. This must be the goal of rehabilitation practices —the development of a useful existence for every patient.

REFERENCES

Buck, M. 1963. The language disorders. J. Rehab. 29:37–38.

Garrett, J. and E. S. Levine, eds. 1962. Psychological practices with the physically disabled. New York, Columbia University Press.

Head, H. 1926. Aphasia and kindred disorders of speech. 2 vols. New York, Macmillan.

Hodgins, E. 1964. Episode. New York, Atheneum.

Morris, C. W. 1938. Foundation of the theory of signs, in O. Neurath, ed., International encylcopedia of unified science, Vol. 1, No. 2. Chicago, University of Chicago Press.

Ritchie, D. 1961. Stroke. New York, Doubleday.

Rolnik, M. and H. R. Hoops. 1969. Aphasia as seen by the aphasic. J. Speech Hear. Dis. 34:48–53.

Sies, L. F. and R. Butler. 1963. A personal account of dysphasia. J. Speech Hear. Dis. 28:261–66.

Wepman, J. M. 1953. A conceptual model for the processes involved in recovery from aphasia. J. Speech Hear. Dis. 18:4–13.

—— 1958. The relationship between self-correction and recovery from aphasia. J. Speech Hear. Dis. 23:302–5.

—— 1965. Aphasia and the family. American Heart Association pamphlet.

—— 1968. Mental disorders: organic aspects, in David L. Sills, ed., International encyclopedia of the social sciences, II, 133–39. New York, Macmillan and Free Press.

Wepman, J. M. and L. V. Jones. 1967. The language modalities test for Aphasia. Chicago, University of Chicago Education-Industry Service.

—— 1969. Five aphasias: a commentary on aphasia as a regressive linguistic phenomenon, in M. O. Rioch and E. A. Weinstein, eds., Disorders of communication. Baltimore, Williams and Wilkins.

—— 1956. Studies in aphasia: psycholinguistic methods and a case study, in V. E. Hall, ed., Brain function. Los Angeles and Berkeley, University of California Press.

ADDITIONAL READINGS

Adler, E. 1969. Stroke in Israel. Jerusalem, Polypress Ltd.

American Speech and Hearing Association. 1968. A guide to clinical services in speech pathology and audiology. Washington, D.C.

Archibald, Yvonne M., L. V. Jones, and J. M. Wepman. 1967. Nonverbal cognitive performance in aphasic and nonbrain damaged patients. Cortex 3:275–94.

—— 1967. Performance on nonverbal cognitive tests following unilateral cortical injury to the right and left hemisphere. J. Nerv. Ment. Dis. 145:25–36.

Archibald, Yvonne M. and J. M. Wepman. 1968. Language disturbance and nonverbal cognitive performance in eight patients following injury to the right hemisphere. Brain 91:117–30.

Bauer, R. W. and J. M. Wepman. 1955. Lateralization of cerebral functions. J. Speech Hear. Dis. 20:171–77.

Benson, D. F. 1967. Fluency in aphasia correlation with radioactive scan localization. Cortex 3:373–94.

Benton, A. 1964. Contributions to aphasia before Broca. Cortex 1:314–27.

Benton, A. and R. J. Joynt. 1960. Early description of aphasia. A. M. A. Arch. Neurol. 3:205–21.

Broca, P. 1861. Remarques sur le siège de la faculté du langage: articule suivé d'une observation d'aphémie. Bull. Société Anatomique de Paris 36:331.

Carson, D. H., R. S. Carson, and R. S. Tikofsky. 1968. On learning characteristics of the adult aphasic. Cortex 4:92–112.

Critchley, M. 1953. The Parietal Lobes. London, Arnold.

Doktor, Marjorie and O. L. Taylor. 1968. (Personal communication).

Eisenson, J., J. J. Auer, and J. V. Irwin. 1963. The psychology of communication. New York, Appleton-Century-Crofts.

Fitzhugh, K. B., L. Fitzhugh, and R. M. Reitan. 1962. Wechsler-Bellevue comparisons in groups with "chronic" and "current" lateralized and diffuse brain lesions. J. Consult. Psychol. 26:306–10.

Freedman, Marion, and Dahlia Bar David. 1959. A study of the bilingual and polyglot adult aphasic patient in Israel. Rambam Government Hospital, Haifa, Israel.

Geschwind, N. 1964. The paradoxical position of Kurt Goldstein in the history of aphasia. Cortex 1:213–24.

—— 1965. Disconnexion syndromes in animals and man. Brain 88:237–94.

Goldstein, K. 1939. The organism. New York, American Book.

—— 1948. Language and language disturbances. New York, Grune and Stratton.

Goodglass, H. and J. Berko. 1960. Agrammatism and inflectional morphology in English. J. Speech Hear. Res. 3:257–67.

Goodglass, H., B. Klein, P. Carey, and K. Jones. 1966. Specific semantic word categories in aphasia. Cortex 2:74–89.

Goodglass, H. and J. Mayer. 1958. Agrammatism in aphasia. J. Speech Hear. Dis. 23:99–111.

Goodglass, H. and F. A. Quadfasel. 1954. Language laterality in left-handed aphasics. Brain 77:521–48.

Goodglass, H., F. A. Quadfasel, and W. H. Timberlake. 1964. Phrase length and the type and severity of aphasia. Cortex 2:133–53.

Holmes, J. E., and R. L. Sadoff. 1966. Aphasia due to a right hemisphere tumor in a right-handed man. Neurology 16:392–97.

Howes, D. 1966. A word count of spoken English. J. Verbal Learning and Verbal Behav. 6:572–606.

Jakobson, R. 1964. Towards a linguistic typology of aphasic impairments, in A. V. S. de Reuck and M. O'Connor, eds., Disorders of language. Boston, Little Brown, pp. 21–40.

Jakobson, R. and M. Halle. 1956. Fundamentals of language. The Hague, Mouton.

Jones, L. V. and J. M. Wepman. 1966. A spoken word count. Chicago, Language Research Associates.

Konorski, J. 1961. Pathophysiological analysis of various forms of speech disorders and an attempt of their classification. Rozprowy Wydziata Nauk Medycznyck, R. VI-T-11, 9–32, Warsaw, Poland.

Kreindler, A. and A. Fradis. 1968. Performances in aphasia. Paris, Gauthier-Villars.

Luria, A. R. 1964. Factors and forms of aphasia, in A. V. S. de Reuck and M. O'Connor, eds., Disorders of language. Boston, Little Brown, pp. 143–60.

McBride, Carmen. 1969. Silent victory. Chicago, Nelson-Hall.

Marx, O. M. 1966. Aphasia studies and language theory in the 19th century. Bull. Hist. Med. 40:328–49.

Mead, G. H. 1934. Mind, Self and Society. Chicago, University of Chicago Press.

Milner, B., C. Branch, and T. Rasmussen. 1964. Observations on cerebral dominance, in A. V. S. de Rueck and M. O'Connor, eds., Disorders of language. Boston, Little Brown.

Nielson, J. M. 1946. Agnosia, apraxia, aphasia. New York, Hoeber and Co.

Osgood, C. E., and M. S. Miron. 1963. Approaches to the study of aphasia. Urbana, University of Illinois Press.

Penfield, W. and L. Roberts. 1959. Speech and brain mechanisms. Princeton, Princeton University Press.

Pribram, K. H. 1960. A review of theory in physiological psychology. Annu. Rev. Psychol. 11:1–40.

Quarton, G. C. 1968. Neural communications: experiment and theory. Science 159:335–52.

Reitan, R. M. 1966. Problems and prospects in studying the psychological correlates of brain lesions. Cortex 2:127–254.

Russell, W. R. and M. L. E. Espir. 1961. Traumatic aphasia. London, Oxford University Press.

Sarno, Martha. 1968. Preliminary report: a study of recovery in severe aphasia using programmed instruction, in John Black, ed., Proceedings of Conference on Language Retraining for Aphasics. Columbus, Ohio State University.

Schuell, H., J. Jenkins, and E. Jimenez-Pabon. 1964. Aphasia in adults. New York, Hoeber.

Sefer, Joyce and E. H. Henrickson. 1966. The relationship between word association and grammatical classes in aphasia. J. Speech Hear. Res. 9:529–41.

Taylor, O. and C. B. Anderson. 1968. Neuropsycholinguistics and language retraining, in John Black, ed., Proceedings of Conference on Language Retraining for Aphasics. Columbus, Ohio State University.

Tikofsky, R. S. 1966. Language problems in adults, in R. W. Rieber and R. S. Brubaker, eds., Speech pathology. Amsterdam, North-Holland Publishing Company, pp. 261–84.

Weisenburg, T. and K. McBride. 1935. Aphasia. New York, Commonwealth Fund.

Wepman, J. M. 1951. Recovery from aphasia. New York, Ronald.

—— 1958. Aphasia and the "whole-person" concept. Ann. Arch. rehab. Ther. 6:1–7.

Wepman, J. M. and L. V. Jones. 1965. Language: a perspective from the study of aphasia, in S. Rosenberg, ed., Directions in psycholinguistics. New York, Macmillan.

—— 1966. Studies in aphasia: classification of aphasic speech by the noun-pronoun ratio. Brit. J. Dis. Communication 1:46–54.

—— 1967. Grammatical indicants of speaking style in normal and aphasic speakers, in K. Salzinger and Suzanne Salzinger, eds., Research in verbal behavior and some neurophysiological implications. New York, Academic Press.

Wepman, J. M., L. V. Jones, R. D. Bock, and Doris Van Pelt. October, 1960. Studies in aphasia: background and theoretical formulations. J. Speech Hear. Dis. 25:225–34.

Wepman, J. M. and Anne Morency. 1963. Film strips as an adjunct to aphasia therapy. J. Speech Hear. Dis. 28:191–94.

Wernicke, C. 1874. Der aphasische symptomencomplex. Breslau.

Zangwill, O. L. 1961. Asymmetry of cerebral hemisphere function, in H. Garland, ed., Scientific aspects of neurology. London.

B. BERTHOLD WOLFF

ARTHRITIS AND RHEUMATISM

ARTHRITIS AND RHEUMATISM are umbrella terms covering a large variety of diverse diseases primarily affecting joints and connective tissues. Arthritis literally means inflammation of a joint, while rheumatism is derived from the word "rheum," which denotes a watery discharge from mucous membranes. In modern usage, however, rheumatism refers to joint and muscle inflammation and pain. Some of these diseases are very common, such as osteoarthritis and rheumatoid arthritis, while others, such as scleroderma, are only rarely encountered. The more common forms of arthritis tend to be chronic and progressive but are seldom fatal. However, a few less common types do have serious prognostic implications, and in some patients may even lead to death, largely because of secondary involvement of other organs and tissues.

Arthritis and rheumatism have always been among the most disabling and crippling of diseases. Signs of arthritis have been found in skeletons of early man. Some forms of arthritis have been observed in animals, and occasionally animal models are used experimentally in order to learn more about arthritis in man.

INCIDENCE

On the basis of the National Health Education Committee survey of 1971 the following statistics pertaining to the incidence of arthritis and

B. BERTHOLD WOLFF, PH.D., is Research Associate Professor of Clinical Psychology, New York University School of Medicine, Past President of the Allied Health Professions Section, and former Medical Council Director of The Arthritis Foundation.

rheumatism in the United States have been published. There are currently about 17 million people who are afflicted with arthritis severe enough to require medical attention, roughly one out of every eleven Americans. Furthermore, it is estimated that at least 50 million Americans have some form of arthritis, although many do not need treatment and others do not seek medical care. These statistics are indeed very striking because they imply that only about one out of every three arthritis sufferers receives medical and professional care for his condition.

Arthritis and rheumatism are second only to heart and vascular diseases as the most widespread chronic illness in the United States today. It is stated by The Arthritis Foundation that the leading causes of activity limitation in the United States today are 16.4 per cent for heart conditions and 14.8 per cent for arthritis and rheumatism. Similarly, arthritis and rheumatism are ranked second among the chronic conditions which prevent people from performing their major activities, such as work, keeping a home, or attending school, with 24.9 per cent reporting heart conditions as cause, and 16.5 per cent reporting arthritis and rheumatism. Furthermore, it is estimated that 3.25 million arthritis victims are disabled, which means that they are limited in their usual activities at any given time. Of these, 331,000 are under forty-five years of age. In addition, 639,000, or 15.8 per cent of these disabled individuals, are unable to carry on their major activities because of their disease.

These statistics indicate that arthritis and rheumatism are a serious economic problem to this nation. It is estimated that arthritis and rheumatism produce 205 million days of restricted activity annually, and that 12.2 million days are lost from work (that is, regular jobs) annually. It is quite apparent that the economic loss in terms of dollar value is tremendous, probably around 3.6 billion dollars per year. Of this, about 1.7 billion dollars are lost in income by individuals unable to work, and approximately 1 billion dollars is required annually for medical care, treatment, and drugs.

It is also of interest that some occupations are more usually affected by arthritis and rheumatism than others. It has been noted that individuals who work outdoors or do manual work appear to suffer more from the rheumatic diseases than those in sedentary occupations. Thus, more farmers are stricken with arthritis and rheumatism than individuals in any other occupational field, while factory workers make up the second largest occupational group. There is also an interesting sex difference, as approximately three times as many women as men suffer from arthritis and rheumatism.

The prevalence of the rheumatic diseases in many countries led to the establishment in 1928 of a professional organization, the International League Against Rheumatism, which holds meetings every four years. The League has three subdivisions, the European, the Pan American, and the Southeast Asian and Pacific Leagues, which comprise the various national professional societies in each of these areas. In the United States, the American Rheumatism Association was founded in 1934 and is a member of the Pan American League. It is a purely professional organization comprising physicians and other scientists working in the general area of the rheumatic and connective tissue diseases, and currently has a membership of over 2,100. As such it is the largest professional society of its kind in the world. In addition to this professional organization, the Arthritis and Rheumatism Foundation was founded in 1948 as a voluntary health organization with the primary aim of raising funds for both research and clinical care in the field of arthritis. These two organizations amalgamated in 1965 to become The Arthritis Foundation. Currently, The Arthritis Foundation consists of a lay division, comprising nonprofessional volunteers who raise money to further the fight against arthritis, and a professional division, known as the Medical Council, composed of the American Rheumatism Association Section and a new Allied Health Professions Section. The latter's membership includes many allied health professionals, such as physical therapists, occupational therapists, nurses, rehabilitation counselors, social workers, and psychologists, as well as physicians. These two professional sections provide media of communication for the professional workers in the field, usually consisting of two national meetings per year as well as frequent clinical and scientific workshops.

There are some seventy-five local chapters of The Arthritis Foundation distributed across the United States. The local chapter is primarily concerned with fund raising in its home area, and a percentage of such income is paid to the national organization, thus yielding two major lines of attack on arthritis. On the national level, the money raised is awarded either in the form of research grants to arthritis centers or fellowships to individuals wishing to do clinical work or research in arthritis. At the local level, the chapters distribute funds available to them to clinics, hospitals, and other institutions, as well as to some professional individuals. All work together to try and conquer these widespread diseases.

Federal, state, and local government agencies also supply funds for research, training, and clinical services in arthritis. At a federal level, the National Institute of Arthritis and Metabolic Diseases, which supports research in a large variety of diseases, allocates approximately 9 per cent of its budget for arthritis. The Social and Rehabilitation Service has supported research and demonstration projects in the field of arthritis, particularly those related to the rehabilitation of the chronic arthritis patient. The Veterans' Administration also has funds available for arthritis, especially as in 1968 there were over 300,000 veterans receiving compensation for arthritis and the rheumatic diseases. Regional medical programs and health manpower agencies also include arthritis. Some funds are also available at state and local government levels, such as the Division of Vocational Rehabilitation. On the whole, however, here as in many other health areas, there is an acute shortage of funds for the delivery of required health care and research for arthritis.

DIAGNOSTIC CLASSIFICATIONS

There are over eighty different kinds of rheumatic diseases that attack the joints and/or other connective tissues, and of these the three major ones are osteoarthritis, rheumatoid arthritis, and gout. There are several other rheumatic diseases which are not as common as these three, but which should be mentioned since they are seen sufficiently frequently to be included here. These are rheumatic fever, ankylosing spondylitis, scleroderma, and systemic lupus erythematosus. There are many other syndromes and diseases, such as psoriatic arthritis, Reiter's syndrome, and fibrositis, which are occasionally encountered by the rehabilitation worker but do not warrant discussion here since their incidence is small compared to the major forms of arthritis.

The following diagnostic classification, definitions, and descriptions are based largely on the 1964 and 1972 editions of the "Primer on the

Rheumatic Diseases" (1964, 1972), prepared by Committees of the American Rheumatism Association. The interested reader is referred to them for more thorough and detailed discussions of the various rheumatic and connective tissue diseases.

OSTEOARTHRITIS (DEGENERATIVE JOINT DISEASE)

About 10 million Americans have osteoarthritis severe enough to cause pain. Osteoarthritis is associated with aging and degeneration of joint tissues. Pathologically, it is basically a deterioration of articular cartilage and overgrowth of juxta-articular bone. The disease is most common in the elderly, but may occur at any age as a sequel to joint injury or dysplasia. The most frequently affected sites are the distal interphalangeal joints, particularly in women after the menopause, but of more clinical importance are similar pathological changes occurring primarily in weight-bearing joints of older individuals of both sexes. There are no systemic manifestations. It is of interest to observe that only a small proportion of patients with the pathological lesions of osteoarthritis have clinical symptoms, and these symptoms do not necessarily correlate with x-ray changes. Joint pain, particularly on motion and weight bearing, stiffness after periods of rest, and aching at times of inclement weather are the most common clinical manifestations. Usually these symptoms begin insidiously and progress somewhat irregularly. Disability may be negligible or may become total, particularly if hips or knees are involved.

RHEUMATOID ARTHRITIS

Rheumatoid arthritis affects about 5 million people in the United States today and may be considered the most devastating and crippling form of arthritis. It is a systemic disease primarily affecting connective tissue. Although there may be many lesions, joint inflammation is the dominant clinical manifestation. The course is variable but tends to be chronic and progressive, leading to rather characteristic deformities and disabilities. The majority of its victims are young and middle-aged adults, usually in their most productive years between the ages of twenty and forty-five, although it may begin both earlier and at later ages.

Most of the pathological changes of rheumatoid arthritis tend to be nonspecific. Inflammation is important, and usually the synovial membrane demonstrates changes such as edema, congestion, and cellular infiltration. A thickening of the articular soft tissue is rather characteristic. As this inflammatory and thickening process progresses, the synovial tissue grows from the margin of the joint over the surface of the articular cartilage or it may erode between it and the bone. This erosion of both articular cartilage and bone may progress to a total destruction of the original joint surfaces. Adhesions between the opposing layers of such diseased tissue (pannus) can lead to ankylosis of the joint, the fibrous tissue being replaced by bone, completely obliterating the original joint. Another characteristic lesion is a rheumatoid or subcutaneous nodule which most commonly occurs over the extensor surfaces of the forearms.

There is no single characteristic clinical picture of rheumatoid arthritis. In the majority of patients the onset tends to be insidious, with ill-defined aching and stiffness, often only poorly localized in joints, followed by the gradual appearance of the articular disease in the form of inflammation, swelling, warmth, and tenderness. In adults, most patients tend to have a polyarticular involvement affecting the small joints of the hands and feet. There is a tendency for the involvement to be symmetrical, that is, affecting the same joints on both sides.

A very important characteristic of rheumatoid arthritis is the occurrence of remissions and exacerbations of the disease. This has important implications for rehabilitation. Only in a small number of patients, about 20 per cent, is full remission achieved.

The primary cause of rheumatoid arthritis is still unknown. There is also no specific cure, but it is often possible to successfully control the disease or to ameliorate its associated suffering.

JUVENILE RHEUMATOID ARTHRITIS

This condition occurs in children under the age of fourteen years. While it is considered to be a part of a continuum involving adult rheumatoid arthritis, the involvement of joints, the greater frequency of assymmetry, changes in the growth pattern secondary to the disease, and the absence of rheumatoid factor from the serum are the major features which distinguish adult rheumatoid arthritis from juvenile rheumatoid arthritis. The disease may appear at any age, including infancy, but generally it begins between eighteen months and three years of age, with girls more frequently affected than boys. The joint inflammations and deformities which occur in children resemble those in adults, but many children may deny pain. However, growth is also affected, particularly near the epiphyses of the affected joint due to the destruction of ossification centers or premature epiphyseal closure. A rather characteristic sign of this disease is a receding chin due to temporomandibular joint lesions.

GOUT

About 1 million Americans suffer from gout, a disease which most often affects the joints of the feet, especially the big toe. Gout is a metabolic disease characterized biochemically by an increased serum uric acid concentration and clinically by recurrent episodes of acute arthritis and by the deposits of urate salts as tophi. Men constitute by far the largest proportion of gout patients. It is very rare in childhood but begins to appear following puberty. The incidence rises in males during early middle age, while in women it is rarely manifested prior to the menopause. A susceptibility to gout may be inherited. An attack of this disease may last for days or weeks and is usually accompanied by severe pain. Fortunately, gout can now be controlled by drugs and treatment which reduce the uric acid level in the blood and tissues.

RHEUMATIC FEVER

Rheumatic fever is an acute systemic disease associated with inflammation, fever, and painful joints. While its name emphasizes the joint involvement, its importance lies in the fact that it affects and frequently damages the heart. Heart damage can be fatal during the acute stage of the disease or can lead to chronic damage of the heart valves. Rheumatic fever follows a streptococcus infection, and repeated attacks are common. It may occur at any age, but is rare in infancy and most frequently observed between the ages of five and fifteen. Fortunately, the judicious use of antibiotics, especially penicillin, can prevent streptococcus infection, and thus in turn prevent flare-ups of rheumatic fever.

ANKYLOSING SPONDYLITIS

Ankylosing spondylitis, occasionally referred to as rheumatoid spondylitis or Marie-Strumpell disease in older literature, is a chronic progressive polyarthritis. It is characterized by involvement of the sacroiliac joints, the spinal apophyseal or synovial joints, and the adjacent soft tissues. An early symptom is frequently low back pain which is not alleviated by rest. Morning stiffness of the back is common. The patient may awake early with back pain and may obtain some relief by walking about. As the disease progresses gradual fusion of the hips, spine, and neck may occur, and in severe cases the patient may look somewhat like a "pretzel." About three to five times as many men as women are liable to get ankylosing spondylitis, and onset is most often in the late teens and before thirty years of age. The severe deformities of this disease present a challenge for rehabilitation, and long-term physiatric and orthopedic measures are often required.

SCLERODERMA

Scleroderma (progressive systemic sclerosis) is a chronic disease of unknown etiology, characterized by fibrous thickening of the skin and diffuse sclerosis of internal organs, especially the gastrointestinal tract, kidneys, heart, and lungs. Onset is insidious, with Raynaud's phenomenon and/or stiffness of fingers. Skin changes usually occur first on the hands. The disease is progressive and gradual and may lead to death from uremia, cardiac dysfunction, hypertension, pulmonary involvement, or malnutrition. It usually begins between thirty to fifty years of age, and about twice as many women as men are attacked by the disease. There is no specific treatment.

SYSTEMIC LUPUS ERYTHEMATOSUS

Systemic lupus erythematosus is an inflammatory connective tissue disorder which involves various organs. There is no characteristic pattern of the disease, although severe joint pain with little evidence of arthritis is common, and many clinical features are similar to rheumatoid arthritis. Diagnosis is facilitated if a positive LE cell test, which is a serological reaction, is present. Lupus nephritis is a serious complication. While lupus may have a benign course over many years it may also cause death, especially from renal involvement, in a few weeks. Usually, however, the patient may live for several years, especially if treated judiciously with corticosteroids. The "butterfly rash" over the cheekbones is diagnostically significant, but observed only in a minority of patients. Neurotic or psychotic behavior patterns, usually manifesting themselves as depression or paranoia, are common, and tend to be associated with very active disease. These behavior patterns, however, are reversible when the patient is treated with corticosteroids. Systemic lupus erythematosus is chiefly a disease of young women in their child-bearing years, but may begin at any age in either sex. A small, private, voluntary health organization, the Lupus Foundation, exists, which supports clinical services and research.

MEDICAL-PHYSICAL ASPECTS

While the large variety of rheumatic and connective tissue diseases prevents generalizations as to the physical symptoms and disability, it is possible to present some of the broad medical-physical aspects of arthritis. However, it must be emphasized that there are certain marked differences between diagnostic groups. The following general description is more appropriate to osteoarthritis and rheumatoid arthritis than to rheumatic fever or systemic lupus erythematosus.

In general, the onset of arthritis tends to be somewhat insidious. It may occasionally be acute in rheumatoid arthritis, while in osteoarthritis x-ray changes of the joint may often be observed prior to the presence of such clinical manifestations as stiffness, pain, and deformity. Many patients first complain of "morning stiffness," literally characterized by stiffness in the involved joint in the early morning. It takes a considerable amount of moving the affected joint before it becomes more functional. Thus, many of these patients require several hours to get up, wash, dress, and make breakfast before they are functionally ready to start work. Consequently, the patient has difficulty in holding a job which requires starting at normal working hours, such as 8 or 9 A.M. However, the patient usually becomes less stiff during the late morning and can then often manage to perform his work. Unfortunately, the patient fatigues easily and by late afternoon or early evening must rest again. It becomes difficult for him to work an eight-hour shift, even if he starts later in the day. This has serious economic implications for the wage earner who may be unable to hold a job or may be restricted to only part-time work. The arthritic housewife with an active family has similar problems. In the early morning she may not be able to dress and provide breakfast for her family, although she may cope with her household chores later in the day. In the evening she may again be too fatigued to prepare dinner for the family.

Fortunately, while the above description is fairly typical, a large number of patients with arthritis, where the number of joints involved is minimal or where the disease is mild or in an early or a chronic inactive stage, are capable of coping with their work. However, in acute stages, multiple joint involvement, or severe deformity, the above symptoms result in serious functional impairment. On the other hand, it should be mentioned that in ankylosing spondylitis, even if there is severe joint involvement of the spine and hips and major crippling, many of the patients are able to work a full day. The arthritis of ankylosing spondylitis thus often differs in this functional aspect from rheumatoid or osteoarthritis.

In terms of the patient's suffering, the single most serious problem in arthritis is pain. While morning stiffness, deformity, and fatigue are all potentially disabling, the presence of pain is the worst and most disabling handicap. Pain may not be present in early, mild, or chronic inactive stages of arthritis, but it is usually found in acute, advanced, and chronic active phases. Pain, especially in weight-bearing joints, can restrict a patient's activities most severely and seriously interfere with his physical rehabilitation regimen. Fortunately, under good medical care and supervision, the pain due to arthritis can often be controlled fairly adequately.

OSTEOARTHRITIS

While the most frequently affected joints are the distal interphalangeal joints (the joints nearest the tips of fingers and toes), involvement of the weight-bearing joints, especially hips and knees, and particularly in older individuals, is much more seriously disabling to the patient. Trauma due to occupational stress may lead to arthritis in relevant joints, such as the elbow, wrist, and knees. Involvement of the distal interphalangeal joints may lead to lesions, called Heberden's nodes, which are deforming bony protuberances which may result in flexion and angulation, although usually not painful. Unlike rheumatoid arthritis, in osteoarthritis the involvement of joints tends to be restricted to a few rather than many. Furthermore, again in contrast to rheumatoid arthritis, there is no systemic disease, and many laboratory tests, such as the erythrocyte (red cell) sedimentation rate, are within normal limits.

RHEUMATOID ARTHRITIS

Rheumatoid arthritis is a systemic disease (unlike osteoarthritis), and in its acute stages is associated with inflammation, fever, malaise, anemia, and other symptoms of systemic involvement in addition to arthritis. Various laboratory tests, such as the sedimentation rate, demonstrate abnormal changes. Rheumatoid factors, which are macroglobulins, are found in the serum of many patients, and with certain chemical compounds (for example, latex) yield characteristic agglutinations. The patient tends to be quite sick during the acute phase. However, there is no characteristic clinical picture of rheumatoid arthritis, its variations are numerous, and many patients never show the acute condition.

In rheumatoid arthritis the affected joint tends to become inflamed, red, swollen, and painful. There is a tendency for symmetrical joints to be involved. Furthermore, unlike osteoarthritis, the arthritis tends to affect many different joints at different times. Pain, morning stiffness, and fatigue are common.

The course of rheumatoid arthritis is often characterized by phases of remissions and exacerbations, although there is usually a progression of the disease toward crippling and deformity. Involvement and disability of a given joint may be followed by remission, which in turn may be followed by exacerbation affecting other joints. However, whereas a few patients may remain in an essentially active stage most of their lives others may never be active. There are tremendous differences both within and between patients in terms of acute, subacute, and chronic stages of the disease, although many patients demonstrate alternation between chronic active and inactive stages. It should be emphasized that, although remissions are common, once a joint has become damaged by the disease processes leading to destruction of tissue and deformity, such changes are not reversible during the remission phase, although pain, inflammation, and swelling, may disappear.

The etiology of rheumatoid arthritis is as yet unknown. Currently, there are two major theories as to the primary cause of rheumatoid arthritis, both having a body of support. One postulates some triggering action by a latent virus while the other suggests an autoimmune reaction.

In the preceding diagnostic classification section, some of the medical-physical aspects of common rheumatic and connective tissue diseases were briefly described. This generalized discussion of arthritis is applicable to a greater or lesser extent to some of the other rheumatic diseases. The similarity between adult and juvenile rheumatoid arthritis has already been mentioned, but monoarticular disease is more common in the juvenile form. In children, care must be taken that the affected joint is not traumatized by vigorous physical activities, particularly if there are no complaints of pain. The adaptability and versatility of the developing child and adolescent permit better adjustment to the disease and deformity, with generally better rehabilitative outcome than in older individuals with adult rheumatoid arthritis.

About 90 per cent of gout patients are men. While the great toe is most commonly affected, other joints may also be involved. In acute gout, pain tends to be very severe and is accompanied by chills and shivers. The patient cannot bear the weight of bedsheets or the jarring of another person walking in the room. In chronic gout, formation of tophi (nodular urate deposits) at various body loci are common.

Rheumatic fever is a sequel of streptococcal infections, but the development of antibiotic drugs, especially penicillin, has greatly decreased its incidence. While acute migratory polyarthritis, usually affecting the large joints of the extremities, is observed in typical attacks of rheumatic fever, the subsequent involvement of the heart, which may be fatal, is much more important. Consequently, the rehabilitation worker is more likely to encounter a rheumatic fever patient with chronic heart damage than with arthritis.

The arthritis of ankylosing spondylitis is in many ways similar to that described for rheumatoid arthritis, but there tends to be back and hip involvement. The ankylosis (or bony fusion) of the spine tends to be progressive until some or many vertebrae are fused and motion is completely lost, leading to the poker-back type of deformity or cervicodorsal kyphosis with an inability to see the horizon. Consequently, the patient must be very posture conscious. Pain control is important, as it will usually permit the patient to pursue his occupation.

In systemic lupus erythematosus the arthritis may resemble that of rheumatoid arthritis, or there may be severe joint pain with little or no evidence of arthritis. Deformities, if they occur, tend to be less severe than in rheumatoid arthritis. The more important systemic and other aspects of the disease have already been discussed. In scleroderma the arthritis, usually stiffness of the fingers, is also less important than the skin lesions and other organ involvement, which eventually may lead to death.

TREATMENT

MANAGEMENT AND THERAPIES

Osteoarthritis. There is no specific treatment or cure for osteoarthritis. Treatment tends to be symptomatic, and the main objectives of therapy are directed toward relief of pain and prevention of avoidable disability or progression of the disease processes.

Drug treatment is primarily restricted to analgesics, such as aspirin, to relieve pain. In some patients, phenylbutazone or indomethacin are helpful, but potent analgesics, especially narcotics, should be eschewed. Corticosteroids should *not* be given, although intra-articular injections of hydrocortisone, when used sparingly, may yield temporary relief.

Physical therapy plays an important role in treatment. Therapeutic exercises and appropriate rest are of value. Physical stress on the involved joint should be avoided. The patient should be trained to walk properly with a cane or crutches when required. Local heat may give temporary relief from pain.

Orthopedic surgery can be of considerable help. Reconstructive or corrective surgery to one or more joints can alleviate pain, increase stability, and improve function. However, prophylactic surgery is even more important to prevent progression of disability or deformity in the involved joint.

Rheumatoid Arthritis. There is no cure as yet for rheumatoid arthritis, and there are no specific treatments. Each patient's therapy has to be fitted to his individual symptoms and needs. In general, treatment is directed at reducing inflammation, controlling pain, and preventing disability.

Drug treatment is perhaps the most important form of therapy for rheumatoid arthritis. A wide variety of drugs are used, all of which have certain advantages and disadvantages. While there is considerable agreement among rheumatologists as to the use of some drugs, there is also a considerable diversity of opinion as to the value of others.

Aspirin has been widely used for many years for the treatment of rheumatoid arthritis, and most rheumatologists agree as to its value. However, it must be given in adequate doses, which implies fairly large amounts varying from about twelve to twenty-four tablets daily. Aspirin is one of the most effective as well as least dangerous of drugs in relieving certain symptoms, such as pain and stiffness, and possibly in reducing inflammation. Unfortunately, massive dosages of aspirin over a long time span frequently cause gastrointestinal distress such as bleeding and stomach ulcers. Various forms of aspirin, such as buffered and enteric-coated aspirin, are available to overcome such gastrointestinal problems.

Injections of gold salts have been used effectively for many years in treatment of rheumatoid arthritis. Gold seems to restrict the disease activity and also suppresses many of the inflammatory changes. However, rheumatologists differ as to the value of gold injections. Furthermore, while gold injections seem to be beneficial in about half the patients, one-third of all patients develop toxic and other undesirable side reactions.

Phenylbutazone is a synthetic anti-inflammatory drug and an effective pain reliever for many patients with arthritis. Unfortunately, quite a few patients do not seem to benefit from it, and some develop undesirable side reactions. Indomethacin is a new anti-inflammatory agent which may relieve certain symptoms of rheumatoid arthritis. It can be used for a long period and has relatively minor side effects.

Corticosteroids were considered "miracle" drugs fifteen or twenty years ago, but more recently they are less frequently prescribed. While these steroids are effective anti-inflammatory and pain-relieving agents, they are also highly potent, do not alter the course of the disease, and may lead to serious toxic and other side effects. Therefore, they tend to be used now only for severe and special cases. Similarly, anti-malarial drugs, such as chloroquine, are no longer used by most rheumatologists because of their toxic side effects and serious long-term threat to vision, leading to blindness.

Physical therapy, combined with adequate and appropriate drug treatment, is important in the management of patients with chronic rheumatoid arthritis. Supervised physical exercises and rest can be very helpful, and are directed primarily at preventing greater disability in affected joints. Orthopedic surgical measures also play a role in the management of the patient. While there has been a tendency for many physicians to wait until a patient has developed deformity in and destruction of an affected joint before referral to the orthopedic surgeon, it should be emphasized that prophylactic surgery can be of considerable help before the involved joint has been seriously damaged. Splinting of affected joints is also employed, although the benefits of such treatment are equivocal.

Other Rheumatic and Connective Tissue Diseases. Much relating to rheumatoid arthritis is also applicable to the treatment and management of other types of rheumatic and connective tissue diseases. Drug treatment is very important. Colchicine, phenylbutazone, and indomethacin can control acute and painful attacks of gout, while allopurinol, probenecid, and other medications are prescribed to prevent the excessive accumulation of uric acid. Rheumatic fever is controlled by the administration of antibiotics, especially penicillin, to prevent streptococcal infections. Aspirin and indomethacin are useful for ankylosing spondylitis. The latter disease may also require long-term physical and surgical treatments, involving exercises, traction, and surgery. Corticosteroids are prescribed during acute phases of systemic lupus erythematosus, but must be administered with great caution, particularly as fairly high doses are usually required. Aspirin is of benefit during milder attacks or between attacks and reduces joint pain. Lupus patients are also warned to avoid excessive exposure to the sun and to use any drug very sparingly because of frequent adverse reactions. More recently, because immune mechanisms are known to be involved in systemic lupus, a new class of drugs, immunosuppressives, are also more commonly being used.

THE MULTIDISCIPLINARY APPROACH

The emphasis on the multidisciplinary treatment team approach for chronic diseases has recently become somewhat passé. Nevertheless, the value of such a team approach in the management of chronic arthritis is great. While the primary *medical* management of the patient should, in this writer's opinion, always be in the hands of a competent rheumatologist, other medical and allied health specialists play important roles as well. The following multidisciplinary team model is considered in my opinion to exemplify good patient care for chronic arthritis and is followed by some of the existing clinical arthritis centers in the United States.

Excluding research activities, a comprehensive clinical arthritis unit may be divided into five components. There must be a *medical* section, which delivers medical care, such as physical examinations, drug treatment, diagnostic work-ups, etc., and which should consist of a rheumatologist (a physician specializing in internal medicine with rheumatology as the subspecialty), a pediatrician, nurse, medical laboratory technician, radiologist and X-ray technician, and medical photographer. (X-rays and photographs are important records to indicate the degree of involvement, structural damage, and deformity of affected joints at various stages of the disease.) Second, a *rehabilitation medicine* section directs its efforts at the physical management of the patient. It should consist of a physiatrist (a physician specializing in physical and rehabilitation medicine), physical therapist, and occupational therapist. Third, a *surgical* section provides orthopedic procedures for the management of chronic arthritis and consists of the orthopedic surgeon. Fourth, a *pathology* section examines material from biopsies and surgery, primarily for diagnostic purposes and consists of a pathologist and technician. And fifth, a *behavioral sciences* section provides psychosocial support and vocational assistance to the patient and his family. It should consist of a medical social worker, a vocational rehabilitation counselor, a clinical psychologist and/or a clinical psychiatrist, and—in wealthy units —a social or cultural anthropologist. In addition, such an arthritis team should also have the services of other medical and allied health specialists available, such as dentists, immunologists, dermatologists, etc., on a consultant basis.

Obviously, such services can usually be provided only by large medical centers. On the basis of my own experience, gained from familiarity with a large and comprehensive arthritis group and from numerous site visits to many of the clinical arthritis centers in the United States, the best patient care is delivered when each member of the multidisciplinary treatment team is an integral part of the whole arthritis unit, and thus feels that he or she "belongs" to the group. In other words, while each team member may have a primary appointment in a specialized academic or hospital department, the team member should be assigned on a permanent basis to the arthritis group and participate in the various clinical and professional activities (grand rounds, conferences, seminars) of the unit. In contrast, staff members who are assigned only for a given period, on a rotating basis, to the arthritis unit often fail to identify with the team, are not integrated in it, and often lose interest in arthritis.

CHARLATANISM

The fact that there is as yet no known cure for arthritis, combined with the very unfortunate negative attitude toward arthritis on the part of many busy physicians, leads many patients to turn to folklore, unscrupulous advertisement, and charlatans. Thus, they waste their money on purchasing copper bracelets, consuming strange elixirs which allegedly "cure" arthritis, eating special diets, and the like. None of these so-called treatments are of scientific value, although occasionally (but usually only very temporarily) placebo effects may occur. It has been estimated that arthritis patients waste millions of dollars annually on such useless treatments, medications, diets, and charlatans.

PSYCHOLOGICAL IMPLICATIONS

Historically, the psychological implications of arthritis have been emphasized or de-emphasized. Alexander's contribution to psychosomatic medicine (1952) raised the question as to whether or not rheumatoid arthritis was a psychosomatic disease. Consequently, many psychiatrists and some rheumatologists believed that rheumatoid arthritis was indeed one of the psychosomatic diseases, and the concept of a "rheumatoid personality" arose. In recent years this concept has been de-emphasized, and there are probably only a few rheumatologists who now believe in the existence of a "rheumatoid personality," although many psychiatrists, psychologists, and other health professionals still cling to this belief.

Some years ago the diagnostic classification of the rheumatic and connective tissue diseases contained a category called "psychogenic rheumatism" (Hollander, 1966). The 1953 edition of the "Primer on the Rheumatic Diseases" (American Rheumatism Association) contained such a category, but the following edition of 1964 (The Arthritis Foundation) omitted this category, and instead discussed musculoskeletal symptoms related to psychological processes. This change is subtle, but instead of discussing psychogenic rheumatism, which implies psychological mechanisms for the disease, it is merely mentioned that such psychological conditions as conversion reactions may have physical concomitants involving the musculoskeletal structures. The current concept in rheumatological circles tends to be that, while there are individuals with musculoskeletal symptoms without "organic" cause, such symptoms are secondary to the primary psychiatric disorder, and should thus be placed in a psychiatric and not rheumatologic taxonomy. It is also possible that certain psychophysiological mechanisms yield stress which may involve the musculature (The Arthritis Foundation, 1972).

It is considered that no generalizations as to psychological implications can be made in view of the wide variety of these diseases. On the other hand, some interesting psychosocial findings are available for certain of the disease entities, particularly rheumatoid arthritis. It thus seems logical to consider psychological implications under the different diagnostic headings.

OSTEOARTHRITIS

This common crippling disease, which affects so many millions of Americans, does not present a typical or specific psychological picture. I definitely believe that there is *no* objective scientific evidence indicating or suggesting that there is a specific personality type or constellation of psychosocial variables which make one individual more prone to osteoarthritis than another. There is some evidence that the disease may be associated with genetic factors, judged by the familial incidence of the disease. Sex also plays a role. However, psychosocial variables do not appear to be important in the etiology of the disease, unless one considers certain occupations which involve physical stress to the affected joint as falling within this category.

Many patients with osteoarthritis tend to become depressed. This should be regarded as an adjustive reaction to a real problem. It is important to inform and reassure the patient as to the generally good prognosis in regard to a lack of involvement of other joints in an attempt to prevent the depression from becoming chronic. Unfortunately, since many of the patients tend to belong to older age groups, they may find it very hard to adjust to the physical trauma and limitations of a painful and disabled joint, and may become irritable as well as depressed. However, the psychological management of such patients should be similar to that rendered in other chronic diseases where there is pain and/or functional limitation.

RHEUMATOID ARTHRITIS

Most of the psychosocial studies and research in the general area of the connective tissue diseases have focused on rheumatoid arthritis. There are probably several reasons for this. While osteoarthritis claims the largest number of victims in the field of arthritis, it is a degenerative joint disease to which "anybody" is liable. Thus, to postulate special psychosocial variables or personality characteristics seems senseless. Furthermore, patients with osteoarthritis appear to demonstrate less "aberrant" behavior than those with rheumatoid arthritis. On the other hand, the patient with rheumatoid arthritis has often been observed to display certain behavior patterns which he seems to share with other rheumatoid patients. He is also often regarded as being more "difficult" than many other diagnostic groups by physicians and allied health professionals. Furthermore, rheumatoid arthritis also affects so many people that such alleged difficult behavior patterns have attracted attention and stimulated research. In addition, as the etiology of rheumatoid arthritis is still unknown, the work of Alexander (1952), Halliday (1937), Ludwig (1952), and others, implying a psychosomatic basis for rheumatoid arthritis, encouraged studies of psychosocial variables associated with arthritis.

King (1955) published an excellent review in which he summarized the results of some fifty earlier papers. On the basis of these earlier studies, King described the typical rheumatoid arthritis patient as possessing subconscious hostility with sadistic and destructive fantasies that are associated with an inability to express anger or aggression openly. This characteristic was termed "contained hostility" by Cobb (1959). Furthermore, the typical rheumatoid arthritis patient appeared to have marked difficulties in forming close interpersonal relationships and seemed to lack sexual identification. Many studies also suggested that severe emotional stress preceded the onset of rheumatoid arthritis. This constellation of psychosocial variables was labeled "rheumatoid personality" by some workers. King concluded that most of the earlier studies were scientifically poor and lacked controls. More recent reviews, notably those by Scotch and Geiger (1962) and by Moos (1964), underscored the scientific poverty of the earlier investigations.

Fortunately, during the last decade a number of scientifically more adequate studies dealing with psychosocial variables in rheumatoid arthritis have been published. These studies were recently reviewed by Wolff (1971), who also asked four basic questions. (1) Is it correct that a *majority* of rheumatoid arthritis patients demonstrate some common or typical personality and psychosocial characteristics? (2) If such common characteristics do exist, are they *specific* to rheumatoid arthritis? (3) If such specific characteristics do exist, are they *primary* personality traits and constellations or are they *secondary* to the physical disease? (4) If there are specific personality and psychosocial characteristics, what are the behavioral mechanisms by which they precipitate or affect the onset or course of the physical disease?

Wolff concluded: (1) There are some personality characteristics which are often observed in rheumatoid arthritis, such as neurotic response patterns, especially reactive depression, dependency, poor ego strength, hostility, rigidity, and overconcern with bodily functions. It is these factors which tend to impress the physician and allied health professional and which give rise to the label of "difficult" patient. However, I would like to emphasize here that while some of these characteristics are indeed common they are far from universal and a large number of rheumatoid arthritis patients do not evidence such characteristics. The reactive depression is probably the most widespread psychological symptom and is almost invariably found in studies utilizing personality tests, such as the Minnesota Multiphasic Personality Inventory; (2) It is fairly obvious that many of these common personality characteristics are also observed in other diseases or other disability groups and thus they are not specific to rheumatoid arthritis; (3) It is my considered opinion that most of the available evidence suggests that these common characteristics are secondary to the physical disease and not premorbid or primary traits. However, there exists some controversy in this area (Solomon, 1970). The behavioral mechanisms responsible for the above common psychological characteristics would seem to be related to pain, disability, and generalized malaise.

In terms of rehabilitation there is evidence that psychological and social factors do play a role and influence outcome of treatment, especially physical and orthopedic rehabilitation.

JUVENILE RHEUMATOID ARTHRITIS

I have observed some rather interesting psychological differences between adults with juvenile rheumatoid arthritis (individuals in which the physical disease started in infancy, childhood, or early adolescence) and those with rheumatoid arthritis (persons in which the physical disease started after adulthood was reached). In general, the grown-up juvenile rheumatoid arthritis patient superficially appears to be better adjusted to his physical illness and disability than the rheumatoid arthritis patient who suffered the onset of the disease later in life. Juvenile rheumatoid arthritis patients seem to relate better to the health professionals and evidence less depression.

This may be due to the fact that the physical disease coexists with the psychological maturation of the child with juvenile rheumatoid arthritis and thus enables him to adjust better to the disease. The adult rheumatoid arthritis patient, on the other hand, has a fully developed personality and suddenly is faced by the trauma of the physical disease. Thus, adjustment is more difficult.

A second interesting difference appears to be that, although the adult juvenile rheumatoid arthritis patient seems superficially better adjusted to the disease, he tends to possess some deeper personality problems, especially in the psychosexual area. Many of the adult patients with juvenile rheumatoid arthritis who were seen by me in my work appeared to be unable to form normal heterosexual relationships, while the majority of rheumatoid arthritis patients observed did form more or less "normal" heterosexual relationships. The latter observation is in contrast to some earlier published papers which emphasized the poor sexual adjustment of rheumatoid arthritis patients and their allegedly greater incidence of divorce. In over 500 rheumatoid arthritis patients studied by me and my associates, heterosexual or marital maladjustment greater than normal was simply not found.

ANKYLOSING SPONDYLITIS

I have long been impressed by the fact that in a series of over 100 adult ankylosing spondylitis patients, many of whom had very severe deformities, vocational adjustment was superior to that of the rheumatoid arthritis patient. Most of the ankylosing spondylitis patients (the large majority of whom were young men) were able to hold full-time competitive jobs in spite of severe crippling. This may in part be due to the fact that there is little generalized malaise present in comparison to rheumatoid arthritis, and as bony fusion becomes more complete in joints the pain tends to decrease or disappear. It may also be a function of sex and age. Spondylitis patients are generally younger than rheumatoid arthritis patients and thus more likely to seek and find employment, and as most are men there may be greater social stress upon them to have a job.

Psychological problems are present, but these seem to be related to the physical deformity and cosmetic reasons. These young men and women are prevented by their disability from participating in many of the usual social activities, and in addition some look quite grotesque. These psychological problems are probably similar to those observed in other physical disabilities.

GOUT

While gout is the third most common of the rheumatic and connective tissue diseases, comparatively little has been published about the psychosocial components of the disease. Recent advances in drug treatment of gout, which permit effective control of excess uric acid in the blood and tissues, probably pose a smaller threat by the disease to the individual's personality structure than, say, rheumatoid arthritis. Excruciating pain is the most disabling symptom of gout and patients obviously differ in their response to pain. This topic will be more fully discussed later. However, it appears that there are no typical or specific gout personality or psychosocial characteristics.

SYSTEMIC LUPUS ERYTHEMATOSUS

This serious disease mainly affecting young women has grave personality and psychosocial implications. Such psychosocial characteristics must, however, be considered as a reaction to the physical disease rather than as basic personality variables. While many patients live for many years with the disease, the generally poor prognosis poses a major psychological threat to the individual. The physical symptoms, such as fever, arthritis, skin lesions, organ involvement, etc., are obviously very distressful. Emotional disturbances are often observed and may reflect an inability to cope with the physical threat and trauma of the disease. Depression is very common. Occasionally, psychotic behavior is noted, which may be functional in origin, but probably more frequently has an organic basis due to involvement of the central nervous system by the disease processes or it may be drug induced. Some patients receive very high doses of corticosteroids, which may lead to "steroid" psychosis. This is reversible when the drugs are decreased. It has also been observed that lupus patients with an organic psychosis due to central nervous system involvement may show an improvement in their psychotic behavior patterns when adequate medication is given. Diagnostically, it is of interest to attempt to distinguish between these two types of organic psychosis by means of psychological or psychiatric evaluations, as the drug-induced psychosis has more benign prognostic implications than have those with central nervous system involvement. Such differentiation is not easy. The interested reader is referred to Stern and Robbins (1960) for a discussion of psychosis associated with lupus.

SPECIAL CONSIDERATIONS IN PSYCHOSOCIAL
AND VOCATIONAL REHABILITATION

The diversity of the rheumatic and connective tissue diseases requires once again separate discussions of implications for rehabilitation. However, two components, pain and disability (that is, crippling and deformity), are common to many of the types of arthritis and deserve consideration on their own.

PAIN

Psychologically, pain is probably the most important symptom of the rheumatic and connective tissue diseases. Pain is not always present, but it does occur so frequently in arthritis, especially during active phases of the disease, that it is a major cause of functional disability.

The behavioral and physiological mechanisms of pain in general are as yet poorly understood. We have neither a generally accepted scientific definition of pain nor do we know what constitutes the adequate stimulus for pain. We do know that a given physical stimulus may cause pain in a given individual on one occasion and the very same stimulus may not induce pain in the same person on another occasion. It is generally accepted that psychosocial and cultural factors greatly modify the pain response.

While there have been several important physiological theories of pain during the past century, there has been a paucity of psychological theories. The most important recent neurophysiological theory is that of Melzack and Wall (1965), who postulated that pain is the result of a dynamic interaction of stimulus patterns mediated by slow and fast conducting nerve fibers involved in peripheral input *to* compared to feedback *from* the brain and controlled by certain groups of nerve cells likened to a "gate." Pain results when the "gate" is pushed open by the force of "messages" transmitted by incoming slow-conducting fibers which overcome the inhibitory feedback from the brain. Coexisting with this neurophysiological theory and not necessarily mutually exclusive are chemical theories of pain, which claim that the "painful" stimulus is a chemical substance, such as histamine, bradykinin, other polypeptides, etc.

Philosophical theories of pain have, of course, existed for thousands of years. Plato considered pain and pleasure as passions of the soul. These hedonistic philosophical approaches are reflected in modern times in the psychoanalytic pleasure-pain principle and in Christian ethics. However, these fundamentally philosophical approaches stand apart from and do not contribute to our scientific knowledge of human pain behavior. There are really no comprehensive psychological theories based on good and valid experimental studies. Petrie (1960) recently put forth an interesting theory, based on some experimental work. She suggested that individuals can be classified on the basis of their internal handling of sensory material. Some increase their sensory input subjectively—the augmenters—and these individuals thus can tolerate pain poorly but suffer less from sensory deprivation. In contrast, others decrease their sensory input subjectively—the reducers—and thus tolerate pain better but sensory deprivation more poorly.

In most human analgesic assays it is a common observation that usually about one third of the patients are "placebo reactors." Attempts to define the personality characteristics of such placebo reactors have been relatively unsuccessful. It is doubtful if it actually is a meaningful category since the same individuals may react to placebo in some but not in other conditions. There is considerable evidence that anxiety reduces tolerance to pain while direct control of noxious stimulation enhances it. Tolerance to pain appears to increase with age; in homogeneous groups women tend to be more sensitive to pain than men; the nondominant side is usually less tolerant than the dominant side; and sociocultural factors greatly influence the response to pain.

This immense variety of biological, psychosocial, and cultural factors influencing the response to pain makes it extremely difficult to discuss pain in arthritis or in other diseases in a meaningful manner. Very severe pain, irrespective of cause (whether arthritis, cancer, kidney stones, angina, etc.), tends to be a leveler of personality differences. The patient in severe pain generally seeks only relief from pain and has no interest in and usually is incapable of focusing on other matters, such as rehabilitation in the form of exercises. Individual differences become more important when pain is moderate, and it is possible to discriminate between poor and better tolerators of this moderate pain. Some patients are receptive to other interests and activities (including rehabilitation) when in moderate pain, while some are not and remain overwhelmed by even moderate pain. It is in mild pain that most of the previously discussed factors emerge most forcefully, and large individual differences can be observed. Some patients remain intolerant of mild pain (even if subjectively recognized as "mild") while others can function reasonably adequately.

It would be very useful if it were possible to predict a given patient's tolerance to pain. The standard psychological and projective tests have not been found very useful in this area. Furthermore, in my own experience, a patient's subjective description of his ability (or inability) to tolerate pain while being interviewed (when the patient usually has no or only minimal pain) is greatly distorted by the patient's self-image and lack of "norms," and, generally, bears little relationship to his actual behavior during moderate or severe pain. Several investigators have developed laboratory pain-inducing techniques and have attempted to utilize the response to experimentally produced pain as a predictor of response to clinical pain. However, there is as yet no universally accepted standard laboratory pain technique which permits such predictions. Wolff (1971) has developed a battery of different laboratory pain-inducing methods, involving both cutaneous and deep somatic (that is, intramuscular) stimulation, and subjected the various types of pain responses to factor analysis. One of the obtained factors was strongly suggestive of representing "pure" pain endurance, and if validated may permit the development of an objective experimental battery of tests for the prediction of pain.

In arthritis, pain has two major but opposing psychological implications for the patient. The first is that the pain due to arthritis is usually perceived as not life-threatening (in contrast to, say, the pain suffered by cancer or heart patients). Consequently, the pain itself is not as anxiety provoking as in some other chronic diseases, although the severity per se of the pain obviously causes suffering and distress. Second, the pain tends to impose functional limitations, especially in terms of locomotion or manual manipulation, and thus tends to be perceived as severely restricting or confining to the patient. This in turn may become anxiety provoking. Therefore, while the pain itself is stressful, the anxiety tends to be less than for some other diseases. On the other hand, the secondary results of the pain (in terms of motion) tend to evoke anxiety.

There is an interesting comment which should be made. The arthritis patient often has to carry out therapeutic exercises of his involved and painful joints, which in turn increases the pain. Usually, the patient is given relatively mild oral analgesics rather than potent drugs to ameliorate the pain without making him "dopey." Such mild analgesics usually help the patient and tend to lower the level of his suffering during rest, but while he is actually doing his exercises such drugs may have little effect on the pain. Therefore, tolerance to pain is still an important factor even with medication.

DISABILITY

A progressive crippling of one or more joints is a frequent accompaniment of arthritis. While the functional limitation imposed by pain is reversible the crippling due to the disease processes tends to be irreversible because of the tissue destruction and changes. However, surgery can often improve the disabled joint. In any event, the crippling of a joint in arthritis poses problems for the rehabilitation counselor which differ somewhat from those produced by static crippling due to other diseases or injury. In a disease or injury producing a static (that is, nonprogressive physical disability), the rehabilitation worker can obtain a good idea as to both the limitation and potential function of the involved body locus. On the other hand, the progressive and changeable nature of arthritis makes it very difficult for the rehabilitation worker to envisage what potential function of the involved joint will be available, say, in six months' time. The disease processes may have caused additional crippling in the same joint or alternately the inflammation and destruction may have subsided but other joints may have become involved.

The locus of the involved joint is of major importance. Involvement of the finger joints of the dominant hand are of greater concern and pose greater rehabilitative problems than similar involvement of joints of the nondominant hand. There are some differences between the major types of arthritis which will be discussed next, but in general the rehabilitation worker would be well advised to bear in mind the possibility that function of an involved joint is likely to deteriorate. However, no hard and fast rules can be made. Often excellent results can be achieved with appropriate therapeutic measures or during remission of the disease.

In general, cosmetic implications of deformity in arthritis are often of less concern to both the patient and the physician than in some other conditions. Usually, prophylactic or reconstructive orthopedic surgery of an involved arthritis joint also achieves a cosmetic improvement. In this writer's experience with over a thousand arthritis patients it was very rare for a patient to request purely cosmetic without functional improvement, although, naturally, many patients hope for cosmetic improvement secondary to the functional improvement.

OSTEOARTHRITIS

Implications for rehabilitation in osteoarthritis are probably less difficult and serious than those for some of the other rheumatic and connective tissue diseases. In osteoarthritis, if the joint destruction is due to physical trauma, implications are fairly simple. Stress to the involved joint should be avoided, and thus if the arthritis contraindicates a given vocation, the counselor should either consider alternative activities within the same occupation involving less stress or the use of healthy joints. If this is not possible, as for a laborer whose activity consists of digging, then vocational training in some other type of occupation less stressful to the upper joints is indicated. Unfortunately, as is often so with the manual laborer, he may be unskilled, suffer from marked educational deprivation, and occasionally have cognitive limitations. Thus, retraining in some other occupation becomes difficult.

Osteoarthritis due to trauma may be seen in adults of all ages, but is less common than that due to degenerative changes accompanying aging processes. Fortunately, fewer joints are usually involved than in rheumatoid arthritis, and thus healthy joints can often be substituted for the involved joint.

Psychological implications of osteoarthritis are usually less significant than for many of the other rheumatic diseases and most patients seem to adjust better to their disease than in other forms of arthritis. Depression, especially in the elderly, is common, but can be treated fairly readily.

RHEUMATOID ARTHRITIS

Rehabilitation in rheumatoid arthritis is a great challenge. There are three major sources of difficulty, namely pain, progressive disability, and remission and exacerbation of the disease. These present an ever-changing picture of the patient's condition. In a static disability, the counselor knows the patient's disability limits, while in rheumatoid arthritis the variable and progressive nature of the disability constantly alters the functional baseline of the patient. During the inactive remission phase a patient may be able to do many things, while during an acute exacerbation of the disease the patient may be too sick to do anything. There is a tendency for an involved joint to become progressively more limited functionally following each acute attack. Morning stiffness, discussed previously, is another complication for vocational adjustment.

During acute phases of rheumatoid arthritis, long-term rehabilitative plans should be deferred until the physician has obtained some control of pain and inflammation by means of drugs. As there is multiple-joint involvement, it is not easy to substitute a noninvolved joint for an involved joint. As a matter of fact, as a patient starts to use a noninvolved joint more heavily to protect an involved joint, more stress is placed on the previously healthy joint and frequently arthritis also develops in that joint. A major requirement for rehabilitation thus becomes stress reduction on joints. The patient must be trained to avoid stress on the joint by appropriate physical and occupational therapy, such as periods of controlled exercises with proper rest, judicious use of a cane or crutches, splinting, and other therapeutic approaches. No patient should be permitted to stay at home and "rest" without supervision, as uncontrolled rest (that is, inactivity of an arthritic joint) over a period of time without exercises can lead to rapid and serious deterioration of the involved joint. This is not to say that rest should be avoided. Periods of rest are most important, but they must be therapeutically controlled.

I am sure I will never forget seeing an eighteen-year-old girl with rheumatoid arthritis who had consulted her family doctor and was told to go home and rest and subsequently stayed in bed for a year without medical supervision. When she was finally brought to the hospital all her joints were fused in the fetal position, no motion was left, and some of her teeth had to be removed for tube feeding. While this admittedly is an extreme example, it is unfortunately a common event for rheumatologists to see patients with many fused joints simply because the patient stayed at home in bed without proper medical or nursing care.

On the positive side, there is the example of a young woman in her early twenties with involvement of nearly all the joints of her upper and lower extremities, including the hips, who also could hardly move and whose hair had fallen out. Under proper medical and nursing care the acute phase of her rheumatoid arthritis was quickly controlled, and, fortunately, destruction of most of her joints had not yet occurred. When she was seen again several months later following intensive physical rehabilitation she had so greatly improved that she walked unassisted, her hair had grown, and she was again an attractive young woman able to function as a wife and mother.

In chronic rheumatoid arthritis, rehabilitation is usually a life-long task. Each rehabilitative approach must be tailored to the individual patient's needs and often changed to meet each new challenge brought about by the progression of the disease. Unfortunately, many rehabilitation counselors unfamiliar with arthritis are misled by the patient's appearance when he is first referred for counseling (usually at a time when the patient is feeling and functioning better). The counselor sets up unrealistic vocational programs, and, later, when faced with failure, projects his own professional mismanagement on the patient, calling him "uncooperative" or "not motivated." These are harsh words, but they should *not* be construed as implying bad faith on the part of the counselor. They are, rather, indicative of a lack of training, knowledge, and experience with the problems, particularly the ups and downs, of rheumatoid arthritis.

Physicians and allied health professionals treating the chronic rheumatoid arthritis patient frequently remark that the patient is difficult to work with, tends to be hostile, and is uncooperative. There seems to be little doubt that indeed many of the chronic rheumatoid arthritis patients do display some common personality characteristics, such as described before, including depression, latent hostility, and inability to form close interpersonal relationships. It has also been suggested that emotional stress precedes the onset of rheumatoid arthritis. However, as previously stated, it is my opinion that most of these personality characteristics are probably secondary to the physical disease processes and reflect difficulties in coping with an impairment of movement and pain. Many of these symptoms may be noticed in other disability groups, and furthermore, many chronic rheumatoid arthritis patients do not display these characteristics. More objective and controlled studies are required to elicit better and more valid information about the primary and/or secondary nature of these psychosocial characteristics.

In any event, since many patients do demonstrate this type of behavior, it is not infrequent for the health professional to be repulsed by it. Unfortunately, much of American medical and health practices are still based on Anglo-Saxon, somewhat puritanical and middle-class cultural patterns and value systems, in which to be tolerant of pain and cooperative with the health professional is "good" and complaining about pain and displaying a negative attitude to rehabilitation are "bad." These implicit prejudices of the medical and allied health professional have to be overcome in order to render good health care to the patient. It is particularly in this area that the experienced social worker, psychologist, and psychiatrist can offer important services to both the patient and other health professionals. The rehabilitation worker must be sensitive to the patient's sociocultural milieu and attempt to view the disease and disability from that standpoint. The behavioral scientist should also explain to his colleagues why the patient seems to respond in an apparent hostile and uncooperative fashion.

Finally, it must again be said that the common exacerbations and remissions—the ups and downs—of chronic rheumatoid arthritis create uncertainty as to tomorrow. The patient never knows if in a week's time he will be able to function or if he will be incapacitated and in pain. It is this uncertainty which produces fear and anxiety counteracting rehabilitation. Other consequences may be that the patient loses any real interest in his rehabilitation program. It is here that again the good medical management of the patient must be emphasized. Sensitive drug treatment, physical therapy, and appropriate rest can greatly minimize the arthritic symptoms and help the patient to function at a more even level.

JUVENILE RHEUMATOID ARTHRITIS

It has already been suggested that the adult patient with early juvenile rheumatoid arthritis may be more receptive to rehabilitation than the generally older adult with rheumatoid arthritis. The early juvenile arthritic patient incorporated some adjustment to the disease processes in his formative years, and thus superficially may cope better with his problems than the rheumatoid arthritis patient. On the other hand, some of the deeper psychological problems occasionally seen in juvenile rheumatoid arthritis require professional psychotherapy.

The implications for rehabilitation discussed for rheumatoid arthritis apply also to juvenile rheumatoid arthritis, except for the above possible personality differences.

ANKYLOSING SPONDYLITIS

The professional worker treating patients with ankylosing spondylitis may notice some interesting psychosocial and vocational differences between these patients and those with rheumatoid arthritis. While often the spondylitic patient is more crippled he, nevertheless, appears to lead a more "normal" psychosocial life and is able to function more effectively in an occupational setting. The spondylitic patient frequently has severe involvement of his hip (sacroiliac) joints and spine but his hands tend to be less affected compared to patients with rheumatoid arthritis. Thus, it is important to ensure that accessibility to his place of employment is possible in terms of transportation, avoidance of stairs, etc. Special chairs may have to be provided, and if certain parts of the spine are fused occasionally special glasses (such as prisms) may have to be obtained to enable the patient to see his work on a table or bench in front of him. Unlike rheumatoid arthritis, the disability is more fixed on certain joints, and thus rehabilitation becomes simplified, the disease not generally jumping from one set of joints in one body locus to another.

In view of the fact that the majority of patients with ankylosing spondylitis are young men rather than women (in contrast with rheumatoid arthritis in which more women than men are affected) the proportionally greater number of spondylitic patients usefully employed may reflect in part social pressures rather than disease processes. However, most of the spondylitic women observed by me also had fairly good work records. Thus, both the physical condition and sociocultural factors appear to lend themselves to satisfactory vocational adjustment.

GOUT

Recent advances in the more effective treatment of gout make this disease of less concern to rehabilitation workers than some of the other rheumatic and connective tissue diseases. Furthermore, the greater frequency of involvement of the toes rather than the other joints also lessens the threatening impact of the disease on the patient. During acute stages of gout medical treatment rather than rehabilitation is indicated. While the number of patients with gout is large, it is probably correct to state that proportionally fewer gout than rheumatoid arthritis patients are seen in rehabilitation departments.

SYSTEMIC LUPUS ERYTHEMATOSUS

Generally, fairly intensive rehabilitation efforts are required for patients with systemic lupus erythematosus. However, it is most important that these efforts be closely coordinated with the medical management of the patients. Frequently, prognosis has to be guarded and the rehabilitation regimen has to be geared to the individual patient's condition, prognosis, and psychological state. Supportive or more intensive psychotherapy is often indicated.

CONCLUSIONS

It cannot be emphasized too strongly that individual patients within the same disease category differ from one another. There are millions of individuals with arthritis who manage to function effectively without any rehabilitation services and who will ordinarily never be seen in a rehabilitation department. Those patients referred to rehabilitation departments tend to represent the most severely disabled individuals and thus may produce a rather slanted and biased perception of arthritis in the rehabilitation worker. In view of the generally progressive nature of arthritis in these more disabled patients, the challenge to the rehabilitation worker is different from that posed by other more static conditions, such as paraplegia, amputation, or cerebral palsy. The best suggestion which can be offered is that the interested rehabilitation worker familiarize himself with the more common forms of the rheumatic and connective tissue diseases, such as those discussed in this chapter, by reading pertinent sections of the "Primer on the Rheumatic Diseases" (1972), and the various free pamphlets on rheumatoid arthritis, osteoarthritis, gout, and related diseases published by The Arthritis Foundation. Two other useful publications by The Arthritis Foundation are *Home Care Programs for Arthritis* (Rosengarten, *et al.,* 1970) and *A Manual on Arthritis for Allied Health Professionals* (Coyne, *et al.,* 1972).

REFERENCES

Alexander, F. 1952. Psychosomatic medicine. London, England, Allen & Unwin, pp. 201–9.

American Rheumatism Association. May–June, 1953. Primer on the rheumatic diseases. Journal of the American Medical Association 152:323–31, 405–14, 522–31.

The Arthritis Foundation. October–November, 1964. Primer on the rheumatic diseases. Journal of the American Medical Association 190:127–40, 425–44, 509–30, 741–51.

—— 1972. Primer on the rheumatic diseases. Journal of the American Medical Association. In press.

Cobb, S. October, 1959. Contained hostility in rheumatoid arthritis. Arthritis and Rheumatism, 2:419–25.

Coyne, N., J. Iley, J. Klinger, V. Lanyi, M. Morrow, R. Rosengarten, A. Williams, and B. B. Wolff. 1972. A manual on arthritis for allied health professionals. New York, The Arthritis Foundation.

Halliday, J. L. January–February, 1937. Psychological factors in rheumatism. The British Medical Journal, 1:213–17, 264–69.

Hollander, J. L., ed. 1966. Arthritis and allied conditions. 7th ed. A textbook of rheumatology. Philadelphia, Lea and Febiger.

King, S. H. September, 1955. Psychosocial factors associated with rheumatoid arthritis. Journal of Chronic Diseases, 2:287–302.

Ludwig, A. O. April, 1952. Psychogenic factors in rheumatoid arthritis. Bulletin on Rheumatic Diseases 2:15–16.

Melzack, R. and P. D. Wall. November, 1965. Pain mechanisms: a new theory. Science 150:971–79.

Moos, R. H. 1964. Personality factors associated with rheumatoid arthritis: a review. Journal of Chronic Diseases 17:41–55.

National Health Education Committee. 1971. Facts on arthritis. New York, The Arthritis Foundation.

Petrie, A. 1960. Some psychological aspects of pain and the relief of suffering. Annals of the New York Academy of Sciences 86:13–27.

Rosengarten, R., N. Coyne, J. Klinger, M. Morrow, E. Terry, and B. B. Wolff. 1970. Home care programs in arthritis. A manual for patients. New York, The Arthritis Foundation.

Scotch, N. A. and H. J. Geiger. 1962. The epidemiology of rheumatoid arthritis: a review with special attention to social factors. Journal of Chronic Diseases 15:1037–67.

Solomon, G. F. 1970. Psychophysiological aspects of rheumatoid arthritis and auto-immune disease, in O. W. Hill, ed., Modern trends in psychosomatic medicine. London, Appleton-Century-Crofts, II, 189–216.

Stern, M. and E. S. Robbins. August, 1960. Psychoses in systemic lupus erythematosus. A. M. A. Archives of General Psychiatry 3:206–12.

Wolff, B. B. 1971. Current psychosocial concepts in rheumatoid arthritis. Bulletin on the Rheumatic Diseases 22:656–61.

Wolff, B. B. December, 1971. Factor analysis of human pain responses: pain endurance as a specific pain factor. Journal of Abnormal Psychology 78:292–98.

THE AMPUTEE

ALTHOUGH ALL AMPUTEES are identical in that they have suffered the loss of a whole limb or of a segment of a limb or limbs, certain related factors exert a critically important differential influence upon how these people must be treated in a rehabilitation setting. Obviously, the factors that influence the care and treatment of a child born with a missing limb are considerably different from those that affect the management of an adult with an amputation resulting from accident, or of an elderly person whose amputation in the later life-years was necessitated by diabetes.

In 1961 Dr. Allen Russek proposed that the treatment goals and therefore rehabilitation practices with amputees be viewed in terms of the rehabilitation potential of each individual patient, with the implication that any series of invariant procedures which tend to treat all amputees alike are of little value. He chose to classify the adult amputee population in terms of five levels of functional potential: Class I—Full Restoration; Class II—Partial Restoration; Class III—Self-care plus; Class IV—Self-care minus; Class V—Cosmetic plus.

The significance of Russek's formulation is immediately recognizable. It clearly calls for an elucidation of the criteria upon which each individual amputee patient is to be categorized. It requires an identification of the specific considerations which reliably affect each patient's potential as well as the rehabilitation program. The major concern of the present chapter is with such factors and influences.

SIDNEY FISHMAN, Ph.D., is Adjunct Professor and Senior Research Scientist, School of Education and Post-Graduate Medical School, New York University.

TERMINOLOGY,   ETIOLOGY,   AND   INCIDENCE

Consideration of the incidence and etiology of amputations is best approached in terms of three broad age groups: (a) the juvenile group
(birth to adolescence); (b) the adult group (adolescence to fifty-five
years); (c) the geriatric group (age fifty-six years and upward). Of
course, these age categories are quite arbitrary since amputee problems
are not completely separated on the basis of age groupings as indicated.
The fluctuating relationship between a person's physiological and psychological functioning and chronological age is always a complicating
factor. One nine-year-old may be comparable in physical and psychological maturity to another twelve-year-old. One person may be as old
at the age of sixty as another is at seventy. Consequently, these age categories are usable only as guides.

A graphic indication of the increase of the occurrence of amputations
with age is presented in Figure 1. An explanation of these statistics lies

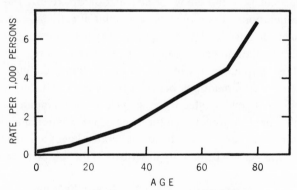

FIGURE 1. Incidence of Major Amputations

in the three major causes of amputation: (a) congenital (present at birth
and occasionally involving surgery when stump revisions are required);
(b) traumatic (resulting from accidents and injuries and usually requiring surgical ablations and revisions of the stump); and (c) disease (involving elective surgical removal of diseased extremities).

It is interesting to note from the table on page 402 that the large incidence of upper extremity amputations occurs among younger people and that, as age increases, the rate of lower-extremity amputations becomes predominant. This trend is due to the fact that congenital and traumatic amputations which affect younger people are frequently of the upper extremity, whereas the elective amputations of the lower extremities associated with disease are far more common in the older age groups.

Among the physical attributes affecting the treatment and functional rehabilitation potential of an amputee, the "site of amputation" is fundamental. "Site" refers to the specific location of the amputation on the extremity(ies) that determines the effective length, strength, and mobility of the stump. Consequently, amputations are referred to in terms of the amount of physical loss which is sustained. As a rule, it is quite difficult to communicate with professional rehabilitation workers concerning amputees without an understanding of, and reference to, these amputation types. Figure 2, page 401 presents the usual sites of upper- and lower-extremity amputations (Berger, 1958).

All of the upper-extremity amputation types occurring between the wrist disarticulation and elbow disarticulation are referred to as below-elbow amputations, since they have similar functional characteristics. By the same token all of the amputation types occurring between the elbow disarticulation and shoulder disarticulation are referred to as above-elbow amputations. For the lower-extremity amputee, all of the individuals with amputations between the Syme's and knee disarticulation sites are known collectively as below-knee amputees, while all those with amputations between the knee disarticulation and the hip disarticulation sites are referred to as above-knee amputees. Consequently, amputees are commonly described in the following terms:

Upper Extremity	Lower Extremity
Partial Hand	Partial Foot
Wrist Disarticulation	Syme's
Below-Elbow	Below-Knee
Elbow Disarticulation	Knee Disarticulation
Above-Elbow	Above-Knee
Shoulder Disarticulation	Hip Disarticulation
Forequarter	Hemipelvectomy

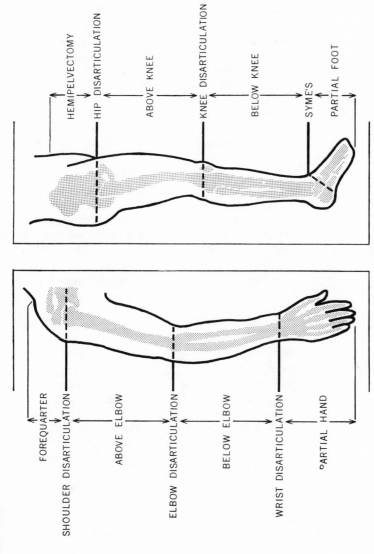

FIGURE 2. *Left*, Upper Extremity Amputations; *right*, Lower Extremity Amputations.

ETIOLOGY AND INCIDENCE OF MAJOR AMPUTATIONS

Category	Estimated Incidence *	Etiology
Juvenile (Birth to 16 years)	25,000 About equal numbers of males and females. Multiple amputees make up about 15 per cent of the group while the remaining 85 per cent are unilateral. More than twice as many upper extremity as lower extremity amputees.	Among child amputees up to 4 or 5 years of age practically all are congenital of unknown cause. From ages 6 to 16, approximately 65 per cent are congenital. This latter age group begins to be affected by injuries and there are also a very few surgical removals due to disease.
Adult (17 to 55 years)	175,000 Approximately 3 times as many male as female amputees. Bilateral and multiple amputees are less than 5 per cent of the entire group. Approximately 7 times as many lower extremity as upper extremity amputees.	The large majority (75 per cent) of amputations in this age group are due to injuries (accidents, war, etc.). A significant number are also due to diseases, particularly cancer.
Geriatric (Age 56 upward)	200,000 Better than 90 per cent lower extremity with a substantial majority being males. Perhaps 10–15 per cent are bilateral.	Practically all new amputations in this age category are due to disease (diabetes and cardiovascular conditions). Large numbers of patients whose limbs were amputated during their younger years also require treatment.
All ages	400,000	

* Estimates based on a liberal extrapolation of data from the United States Public Health Survey, the Rehabilitation Services Administration, the Veterans' Administration, and New York University Patient Censuses at Child Amputee Clinics (Bergholtz, 1970–71).

Depending upon the number of extremities that are affected, amputees are further described as unilateral (one arm or leg), bilateral (two arms or two legs), double (one leg and one arm), triple (three extremities), and quadrilateral (four extremities). The last three categories taken together are called multiple amputees.

FACTORS INFLUENCING AMPUTEE
REHABILITATION

The following factors represent the critically important differential influences mentioned above in the rehabilitation treatment of amputee patients:

Age: The status of the patient in regard to age has a critical influence on the nature of appropriate rehabilitation goals and procedures. In general terms, one can identify four life stages which call for markedly different rehabilitation practices, namely: the child, adolescent, mature adult, and geriatric client.

Amputation etiology and physical condition: Since the use of a prosthesis is dependent to a considerable degree upon the strength and coordination of the wearer, optimal utilization can be expected from young, athletic, and otherwise healthy individuals. Persons who suffer from physical disabilities frequently associated with amputation, such as coronary disease, diabetes, cancer, and the like, and which detract from strength and coordination, will be less capable of prosthetic use. Of special importance are the physical characteristics of the amputation stump which provide the major basis for suspension, control, and mobilization of the prosthesis. Consequently, stumps that are characterized by weakness, limited motion, redundant fatty tissue, sensitive neuroma, bony prominences, and/or scar tissue are less well suited for truly functional prosthetic wear.

Site and level of amputation(s): If the option should exist as to what level to amputate, the more of the natural extremity that remains the better the possibilities for prosthetic utilization and function, especially when a normal joint can be retained.* Therefore, when there is a choice,

---

* While generally true, this statement has a variety of technical exceptions which are beyond the scope of this paper.

in the area of lower-extremity amputations, the *below-knee* surgical procedure is far to be preferred in terms of rehabilitation potential to an *above-knee* procedure. Of course, where the necessity arises for two or more extremities to be amputated, the functional restoration possible with prosthetic use decreases substantially (Murdock, 1967).

Sex: In general, the physiological characteristics of the female (less muscular and more prone to fatty tissue) present special problems in the fitting of prostheses. If we also consider the unique cosmetic requirements of the female in regard to appearance, we find that special rehabilitation procedures are indicated to accommodate these needs.

Time since amputation surgery: The significance of this factor is discussed in some detail later in this chapter. The current trend is to utilize "early" if not "immediate" prosthetic fitting wherever possible.

Vocational status and functional goals: While acknowledging a variety of technical exceptions beyond the scope of this chapter, the activities that the amputee is expected to perform with the prosthesis in both the vocational and nonvocational setting have a very direct bearing on the nature of the device and treatment process. The proper selection of prosthetic devices and techniques must be directly related to anticipated vocational and functional uses.

Socioeconomic and demographic factors: Significant matters to be considered in rehabilitation planning relate to such matters as residence in urban versus rural areas, the availability of funds to pay for sophisticated devices possibly requiring relatively frequent maintenance, and the patient's motivation and interest in continuing follow-up and care. Each of these factors will frequently have an overriding influence on the rehabilitation goals and potentials of the patient and consequently on the management procedures to be employed.

MEDICAL AND PSYCHOLOGICAL
REHABILITATION

For ease of discussion, we may divide the rehabilitation process into two broad areas of concern: medical and health-related services; and psychological, social, and vocational services.

MEDICAL AND HEALTH-RELATED SERVICES

As regards the medical concerns in the rehabilitation of the amputee there appear to be four major responsibilities: (a) surgery; (b) prosthetic prescription and fabrication; (c) prosthetic training; and (d) evaluation.

Surgery. The goal of amputation surgery is, in the last analysis, an effort to provide the patient with a stump that is as pain-free as possible, and that has the strength and coordination necessary to act as the major motive power in controlling and moving any prosthetic device which may be utilized. It is therefore incumbent upon the surgeon to produce minimal surgical trauma and sequelae. This implies an optimal level for the surgery, a well-located, well-healed, nonsensitive scar, and remaining musculature which retains as much of its normal function as is possible (Burgess *et al.,* 1969).

Prosthetic Prescription and Fabrication. The only realistic hope of restoring a considerable measure of function and cosmesis to an individual with a lost extremity is to provide some sort of prosthetic appliance. An extraordinarily large variety of prosthetic devices, components, and techniques are available, and there exists a substantial body of knowledge dealing with the differential prescription of these items. In the prescription process legitimate alternatives range from "no prosthesis" to a "sophisticated intimately fitted cosmetic and functional device that closely simulates the normal." Here the rehabilitation treatment team is faced with an evaluation of the influencing factors mentioned earlier in order to select the most appropriate prosthesis and fitting procedure. A device incorporating the desired features is then fabricated (N.Y.U. Manuals for Prosthetists, 1971–1972.

Prosthetic Training. The third major step in the medical rehabilitation of the amputee is the process of teaching him to utilize the prosthetic device. This process, normally accomplished by the physical or occupational therapist, is highly variable and its length, complexity, and effectiveness are affected by the same influencing factors as mentioned previously. Therefore, it is not surprising that one patient learns all that he needs to know about using a prosthetic device in one hour while another needs weeks, if not months, of intensive instruction in order to achieve even mediocre function (N.Y.U. Manuals for Therapists, 1971).

Evaluation. The major problem involves the application of procedures for making judgments regarding the adequacy (or lack thereof) of the prosthetic device and/or treatment provided a given patient. These evaluation procedures must normally be applied several times during the period of the patient's rehabilitation and must take into account the changing medico-surgical, prosthetic, and psychological status of the patient in a reasonably objective way. These evaluation procedures are, in fact, our best indices of the achievement of rehabilitation goals (N.Y.U. Manuals for Physicians and Surgeons, 1971).

PSYCHOLOGICAL, SOCIAL, AND VOCATIONAL SERVICES

In regard to psychological matters in the rehabilitation of the amputee we may consider the following:

Amputee's Needs and Perceptions. It is quite clear that the rehabilitation procedures must also be influenced by the expressed and covert needs of the patient. The amputee's perception of his problem(s) may differ substantially from that of the physician, therapist, prosthetist, or counselor. It, therefore, becomes important to be able to comprehend the amputation experience in the patient's terms insofar as possible. This entire subject has been discussed in considerable detail in a prior publication by the author (Fishman, 1962). However, a brief recapitulation is called for here. Typically, there are five areas of concern that amputees reflect. They are:

1) *Restoration of Physical Function.* The patient faces the problem of adjusting to both permanent *limitations* in physical function resulting from the amputation and *intermittent, unpredictable failure* of the prosthetic device to provide available functions when desired.

2) *Restoration of Normal Appearance.* There are obvious real shortcomings to the cosmetic characteristics of a prosthetic device which are both visual and auditory in nature. The client will formulate his own opinions regarding the cosmetic adequacy of his prosthesis and these have to be handled in the rehabilitation process with as much care and attention as the objective realities of the cosmetic restoration itself.

3) *Minimization of Physical Discomfort.* There are a number of factors which detract from the physical comfort of the amputee, specifically phantom sensation and/or pain, weight of the prosthesis, weight-bearing by (pressure on) stump tissues marginally suited for this purpose,

lack of ventilation at the stump-prosthesis interface, lowered pain thresholds of the affected extremity, and the increased energy required to utilize a prosthesis. All of these considerations in terms of objective reality, as well as of psychological reality, must be dealt with during rehabilitation.

4) *Maximization of Vocational and Economic Potentials.* The premorbid educational, occupational, and socioeconomic status of the patient has a direct bearing upon the socially and economically productive activities in which he can hope to engage after rehabilitation. Consequently, the relationships between the physical loss and the functional demands of various occupations must also be thoroughly explored and understood.

In considering an appropriate vocation for an amputee client, two types of information are obviously required: (a) an understanding of the functional requirements of various occupations, and (b) an understanding of the functional limitations associated with amputation and prosthesis wear. In the first instance a distinction must be made between those occupations which primarily involve the *physical* resources of the worker (carrying, pushing, pulling, walking, lifting, loading, etc.) as contrasted with those occupations which primarily demand *intellectual and personality* characteristics (thinking, speaking, writing, persuasion, and decisionmaking). One can readily see that the suitability of any given employment for an amputee depends to a substantial degree on its *intellectual* versus *physical* requirements.

Viewing the problem from the vantage point of the client, the immediate questions that arise are: (a) Is the amputation of the upper or the lower extremity? (b) In each of these instances, is the amputation *above the knee* or *below the knee,* (or *above the elbow* or *below the elbow*)? (c) Are one or more extremities involved? As was pointed out earlier the unilateral *below* elbow and *below* knee amputee may expect to regain a maximum of functional capacities. Unilateral *above* knee and *above* elbow amputees will have substantially less in the way of functional potentials and patients with multilateral amputations even less.

In general those jobs which involve a substantial amount of upper-extremity activities, especially bilateral function, (assembly, drawing, manipulation, etc.) should be avoided by upper extremity amputees, while those involving substantial ambulation (walking, climbing, kneeling, etc.) should be avoided by lower extremity amputees. Unfortunately a precise cataloguing of jobs in relation to type and level of amputation is not possible since the performance potential of clients shows tremendous variation even after taking level and type of amputation into account. The situation, therefore, requires that the rehabilitation counselor be provided with substantial supervised clinical experience which will enable him to make meaningful judgments regarding the work potential of amputee clients, taking *all* cogent factors into consideration.

A last key question to be considered is the "retrainability" of the client which will control his ability to learn any new series of occupational tasks. To the degree that the client's age, prior education, work experience, economic status, and motivation permit him to learn these new activities, can the problem of vocational rehabilitation be solved, since this retrainability factor is often more important for a given person than the type, level, or multiplicity of amputations.

5) *Maximization of Psycho-Social Acceptance.* The self-concept and its effects on the client's ultimate motivation to be rehabilitated is intimately related with peer attitudes. The influence of environmental factors on the posthospitalization rehabilitation process is critical and, therefore, every effort must be made to provide the client with an appropriately supportive atmosphere rather than one catering to dependency and inactivity.

These personalized areas of concern noted above require the same degree of attention in the rehabilitation process as the more obvious factors outlined in the beginning of this chapter.

TEMPORAL CONSIDERATIONS

As mentioned previously, one critical factor in adjustment to a prosthesis is the length of time which has elapsed since the amputation surgery per se. Prosthetic techniques are now available which permit the fitting of a device immediately following surgery, while under other circumstances prostheses may not be fitted until months or even years have elapsed after the amputation. This straightforward matter of the elapsed time (between surgery and prosthetic fitting) and the amputee's experiences during this period have a significant bearing on the entire prosthetic restoration process.

During a period in which an individual is without the functional and cosmetic services of a prosthesis, it is necessary for him to develop a pattern of adjustment (both physiological and psychological) to enable him to function in spite of the loss of one or more extremities. It is possible for him to do this through the use of aids such as wheelchairs and crutches, performing tasks unimanually, avoiding a variety of activities, etc. If he is then, at a later date, provided with a prosthetic appliance he must undergo a second period of adjustment as he attempts to incorporate prosthetic function into his life pattern to a lesser or greater degree.

It is apparent, therefore, that if the postsurgical period of *nonprosthetic utilization* can be reduced or even eliminated, the need for the patient to undergo *two* rather separate and strenuous readjustments is alleviated. Since the period during which the patient is without a prosthesis is one in which he is ordinarily more functionally and cosmetically disabled (and presumably psychologically) than while wearing such a device, the desirability of avoiding this interim adjustment process is reinforced.

It is, therefore, now considered best practice to utilize the "immediate and early prosthetic fitting" procedure whenever possible (Burgess, *et al.,* 1969), implying that a prosthesis is provided as close to the time of surgery (or even at the time of surgery) as circumstances will permit (0 to 21 days postoperatively).

Regarding the temporal sequence of events and their relation to adjustment are the formulations of Fink (1967), who describes four sequential phases in the psychological adjustment process to serious physical disability, namely: (1) shock, (2) defensive retreat, (3) acknowledgment, and (4) adaptation. Each of the phases is summarized as follows:

1) *Shock.* Essentially shock is the patient's initial response to a threat to self-preservation, leaving the individual emotionally and intellectually numb and manifested by a disruption of organized thinking. The individual has no plan of action and is essentially without psychological resources. The reality of the situation is too much to handle, resulting in overall helplessness.

2) *Defensive Retreat.* As the patient's resources begin to mobilize, this phase of the adjustment process is prompted by the need for anxiety reduction, and energy is therefore invested in keeping circumstances

under control. The phase is characterized by a clinging to the past through the use of avoidance mechanisms (fantasy, denial, magical and rigid thinking). In Maslow's terms, the emphasis at this point is on "safety needs" and the patient resists any changes in his situation which might be considered threatening (Maslow, 1954).

3) *Acknowledgment.* This is a period of renewed psychological stress resulting from a breakdown of the prior defenses because of the lack of reinforcement of these avoidance mechanisms resulting from inadequate satisfactions. During this period, the patient usually recognizes changes in his physical self, thus provoking a period of stress characterized by depression and mourning. At the same time, there are the beginnings of intellectual and emotional reorganization which proceed in unique and variable patterns for each patient.

4) *Adaptation.* The extent to which the patient succeeds in this reorganization process depends on his "growth needs" to develop a renewed sense of self-respect, productivity, achievement, and social acceptance. This phase of adjustment is optimally characterized by the patient's willingness to take the necessary physical and psychological risks normally associated with the rehabilitation process.

It must be pointed out that not all patients are capable of proceeding successfully through this adjustment sequence and a number may not proceed beyond stage two or three. In the context of this formulation, immediate and early prosthetic fitting procedures have major psychological value in reducing the extent of the actual and perceived disability and consequently of the psychological trauma associated with it. This is possible since the patient is never (or for a very short period) without a limb (albeit an artificial one). The immediate availability and wear of a prosthesis may legitimately tend to reduce the initial shock, as well as the extent of the defensive reactions required. This in turn tends to facilitate the processes of acknowledgment and adaptation.

PSYCHOLOGICAL SUPPORTIVE PROCEDURES

In addition to the temporal considerations, there are a number of psychological procedures which are frequently suggested as being valuable in the management of the amputee as follows. These include the counseling relationship, substitution of goals, involvement in productive activities, and contact with previously rehabilitated amputees.

1) *Counseling relationship.* This relationship is designed to assist the patient in clarifying his perceptions of his disability by providing him with an acceptable setting for emotional release and accurate information and clarification regarding the functional and psychological consequences of his disability. This support will improve his ensuing attitudes toward prosthetic wear based upon realistic, factual information as opposed to inaccurate rumor or anxiety-provoked fears.

2) *Substitution of goals.* A second significant approach revolves about the introduction of substitute values and life goals in the place of those held prior to amputation and around the patient's ability to accept these new goals. For example, if the patient's occupation prior to amputation involved considerable use of the affected extremity, one can make significant psychological progress by discussing other occupations and activities that make significantly fewer demands on that extremity and yet hold satisfactions for the patient. As a substitute value or goal is offered and accepted, an important factor in developing frustration and conflict is thereby eliminated.

3) *Involvement in productive activity.* Since an amputee may be viewed as undergoing an emotional experience not dissimilar to those of people who suffer a catastrophe such as the death of a loved one, steps must be taken to gradually reinvolve the individual in a productive life-style. In both instances the emotional reactions of the bereaved operate in a circuitous fashion that must be interrupted at some point if the individual is to recover from the loss and re-enter normal life activities. These circumstances dictate the involvement of the amputee patient at the earliest psychologically suitable moment in some purposeful activity that will tend to divert him from a continuing preoccupation with his loss.

In this connection, prosthetic training procedures fulfill the extremely important function of involving the patient in challenging and important stimulation along these lines.

4) *Contact with previously rehabilitated amputees.* A technique that is sometimes helpful in motivating the amputee patient involves placing him in contact with previously rehabilitated amputees. This is a partic-

ularly important procedure to be used with those amputees who find it impossible to relate to or identify with the nonamputee professional worker. In fact, some are unable to profit from instruction or reassurance as a result of the attitude that no one who has not lost an extremity can really understand the amputee situation. In these instances, the involvement of suitably readjusted amputees as persons with whom the new patient may identify and from whom he may learn cannot be overestimated. A word of caution must be introduced, however, concerning the qualifications of the amputee to serve as "inspiration." An individual with similar physical impairments and of substantial personal adjustment must be selected so that the new amputee does not become an outlet for the mentor's own problems and anxieties.

There is no indication that professional psychological supportive procedures are necessary in every case. The need depends on the prior personality structure of the patient, the extent of his reaction to the disability, and on his capacity to cope with his disabled situation. A study of the individual's prior social, work, and family history will be useful in reflecting his ego strengths and the extent to which his behavior is dominated by the need to grow and be socially productive. In general, then, the most useful predictor of an individual's reaction to the amputation experience is his pattern of reactions to prior crises he may have encountered in life. An evaluation of these personality factors will determine whether special psychological intervention is indicated.

It is important to note that among amputees as a group there is no direct relationship between the extent of the physical loss and the patient's psychological difficulties. These difficulties are more dependent upon the personality attributes of the individual than the type of amputation. Therefore, one individual with a "limited" physical loss may present far greater adjustment problems than another with a "major" loss (Fishman, 1950).

For the overwhelming number of patients, treatment utilizing the resources of a prosthetic clinic team as discussed on the following pages should be quite satisfactory. It is of course implied that these professionals (physician or surgeon, therapist, prosthetist) will pursue their professional responsibilities with a reasonable degree of sensitivity to the patient's psychological needs.

PROSTHETIC REHABILITATION PROCEDURES

The prosthetic clinic may be viewed as a means of communication between specified health professions. It is essentially a method of organizing the activities and communications of a number of people and serves to provide necessary contact between the various specialists involved in prosthetic rehabilitation. The basic specialists concerned are the physician or surgeon, acting as "clinic chief"; the physical or occupational therapist; and the prosthetist.

Other personnel are often required, according to the special needs of the situation. In various clinics, the additional services of the rehabilitation counselor and social service worker have proven to be important (N.Y.U. Manual for Rehabilitation Counselors, 1972).

CLINIC GOALS

The major purposes and goals to be achieved by the prosthetic clinic are:

1) *Coordinated Pattern of Treatment.* In order to provide amputees with the best medical and prosthetic service, the contribution of each of the specialists must be made in coordination and conjunction with that of the others. It is becoming more infrequent, but certainly not unheard of, for a prosthetist or a physician to plan a prosthetic management program without acting in concert with the others.

When an individual is receiving treatment from more than one specialist and the anxieties of the situation provoke some degree of discontent, there is a noticeable tendency for some patients to distort the intentions and contributions of each profession in relation to the others. This is aggravated when the patient functions as a means of communication between the professionals concerned. Since there is always a certain degree of conscious and subconscious distortion of the patient's perceptions of the treatment processes, he should not be afforded the opportunity to complicate the process of communication among the various professionals concerned.

On another note, we may anticipate that the behavior and demeanor of the patient will differ when he is with the prosthetist as contrasted with the physician or therapist. These differences in overt behavior patterns may easily and logically suggest different patterns of treatment to each of the professions. It should be realized, though, that this varying behavior on the part of the patient may be transitory and that the best treatment lies in a uniform plan rather than in a number of discrete ones.

It is clear that prosthetic clinic procedures permit a more uniform evaluation of the patient and assist in circumventing some of the problems inherent in uncoordinated care.

2) *Staff and Patient Education.* It is true in prosthetics, as in other medical situations, that there are no standard procedures which apply with equal effectiveness to every patient. Moreover, prosthetics is a field in which the contribution of each specialist may only be partially understood by the others. Consequently, there is an important need for an interchange of ideas and a distillation of the best thinking through group discussion. In this sense, then, an important goal of the clinic is the mutual education of the treatment team members.

One aspect of this educational process is that the clinic serves as a vehicle which permits a limited, selected group of physicians and surgeons to specialize and become experts in the prosthetic field. There is not, ordinarily, a sufficient case load to keep very many physicians expertly conversant with prosthetic matters. However, there are assuredly sufficient cases to permit a small group of physicians and surgeons in each community to see appreciable numbers of amputee patients in the clinic situation. This fact encourages the establishment of groups with sufficient experience and education to make them competent both to prescribe and checkout prosthetic devices. Clearly this is a desirable goal since, not infrequently, physicians are called upon to pass judgment concerning prostheses who lack the necessary technical information and background to come to sound professional conclusions.

The role that the clinic must play in the education of the patient, his family, or both is equally important. Most patients and their families, arriving for prosthetic care, are subject to wide and varied misunderstandings and misinterpretations as to the ultimate use and value of a prosthesis. Consequently, clinic personnel must orient the patient concerning his goals and anticipations, as well as provide him with the best assistive device available.

3) *Professional Status of the Prosthetist.* It is probably true that a major factor in attaining patient satisfaction with the prosthetic service he receives is related to the personal attitudes and evaluations of the patient regarding the prosthetist. There are two considerations which may prompt a less-than-satisfactory attitude: the lack of status of the prosthetist as a part of an organized professional medical service; and the lack of training and experience of prosthetists in the proper handling of the psychological, interpersonal aspects of their vocation.

In the last analysis, the patient needs to adjust himself to and accept the product fabricated by the prosthetist, and there is substantial evidence that the patient's attitudes toward a *prosthesis* is closely related to his attitudes toward the *prosthetist.* It seems reasonable, therefore, that whatever can be done to improve the attitude of the patient toward the prosthetist will have a significant, positive bearing on the results of the treatment.

Although the ultimate solution of this problem involves long-range sociological and educational considerations, the prosthetic clinic helps on an interim basis by providing prosthetists with the opportunity to observe and participate in the professional medical care of patients. This cannot help but provide the beginnings of professional status which is sorely required.

PROSTHETIC CLINIC PROCEDURES

A pattern of prosthetic clinic operation has evolved which essentially includes the following steps:
1) Pre-Prescription Examination
2) Prescription
3) Pre-Fitting Treatment
4) Prosthetic Fabrication
5) Initial Checkout (Evaluation)
6) Prosthetic Training
7) Final Checkout (Evaluation)
8) Follow-Up

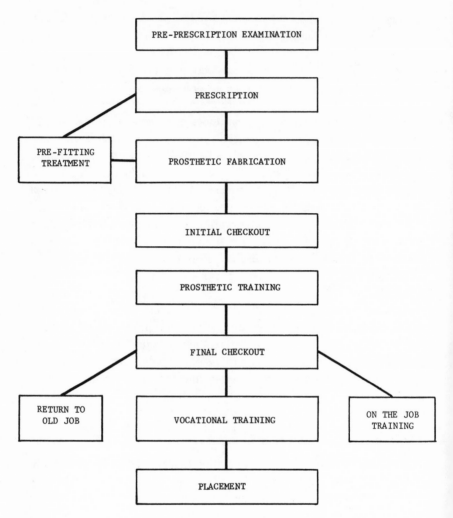

FIGURE 3. Prosthetic Clinic Procedures

1) *Pre-Prescription Examination.* It is recommended that the first meeting of the clinic, the so-called prescription meeting, be preceded by an appropriate physical and psychological examination of the patient so that pertinent information concerning the patient is available to the clinic members beforehand.

Forms are available to summarize the essentials of this examination of the amputee (see Medical Prosthetic Summary Form shown in Figure 4). Separate forms are available for the lower- and upper-extremity amputee. Study and analysis of this information provides a sound basis for determining the type and nature of the care required by the particular patient. The treatment may be medical, surgical, or prosthetic in nature, or a combination thereof.

2) *Prescription.* Ordinarily, the patient's first contact with the prosthetic clinic is for the purpose of developing an appropriate medical, surgical, or prosthetic prescription. At this point the pre-prescription examination results are evaluated, and those aspects of the patient's condition which have an immediate bearing on problems of prosthetic restoration are rechecked. This is followed by a *detailed* consideration of the appropriate treatment procedures for the patient in question. If the resulting prescription calls for medical care, the physician or the therapist, as indicated, would undertake its implementation. If the prescription is for further surgery, the surgeon would obviously take the necessary action. If the prescription is a prosthetic one, the prosthetist assumes the responsibility. In some instances, the prescription may involve several of these considerations but, usually, prosthetic treatment is deferred until medical and surgical care are sufficiently underway.

The prosthetic prescription should correctly be a detailed description of the device and services which a patient is to receive and should not merely be a series of generalized instructions. This is not in any real sense a "prescription." Vague instructions result in the prosthetist being unable to construct a definitive prosthesis with any assurance that his product will reflect the intent of the clinic or meet the needs of the patient.

The importance of a detailed prescription cannot be overemphasized. In the past, prosthetists have been placed in the position of planning complete appliances according to their own best judgment. After delivery of such appliances, the prosthetists have been subjected to criticism

MEDICAL PROSTHETIC SUMMARY FORM: LOWER EXTREMITY

A. PERSONAL FACTORS

1. Name_____ Date_____

2. Home address_____ Phone_____

3. Business address_____ Phone_____

4. Age_____ Height_____ Weight_____

5. (Circle items which apply)

   Male   Female   Veteran   Civilian   Single   Married

6. Present occupation (Give title and description of duties)

   _____

   _____

7. Future occupational plans_____

   _____

8. Hobbies and recreational interests_____

   _____

9. Is vocational guidance and training indicated? Yes_____ No_____

10. Financial arrangements_____

B. MEDICAL FACTORS

1. Date, cause, and site of amputation_____

   _____

2. Date(s) of revision(s), if any_____

   _____

3. Amputation: Right_____ Left_____

4. Length of stump:

   For below-knee:

   _____inches from medial tibial plateau to end of bone.

   _____inches from medial tibial plateau to end of flesh.

   For above-knee:

   _____inches from perineum to end of bone.

   _____inches from perineum to end of flesh.

Prosthetics and Orthotics
New York University
Post-Graduate Medical School

FIGURE 4

5. Length of sound side:

For below-knee _____ inches from medial tibial plateau to apex of medial malleolus.

For above-knee _____ inches from perineum to medial tibial plateau.

6. Percentage of stump length (Item 4 on page 1 divided by Item 5) _____ %

7. Amputation type:

Short: (10 per cent to 33 per cent of sound side length) _____

Medium: (34 per cent to 67 per cent of sound side length) _____

Long: (68 per cent to 100 per cent of sound side length) _____

8. Condition of hip:

a. Strength: Flexors_____   Extensors_____

   Abductors_____   Adductors_____

b. Range of motion: Flexion_____   Extension_____

   Abduction_____   Adduction_____

9. Condition of knee:

a. Strength: Flexors_____   Extensors_____

b. Range of motion: Flexion_____   Extension_____

c. Stability: Medio-lateral_____   Antero-posterior_____

d. Crepitation   _____

e. Recurvatum   _____

10. Condition of stump: (Check as many items as apply)

a. Shape: Cylindrical_____   Conical_____   Edematous_____

   Bony_____   Bulbous_____

b. Scar: Non-tender_____   Sensitive_____   Invaginated_____

   Well healed_____   Open_____   Adherent_____

c. Skin: Cold_____   Callus formation____   Abrasion_____

   Sensitive____   Discoloration_____   Dermatitis_____

d. Bones: Spurs_____   Fibula removed_____   Beveled_____

e. Musculature: Loose_____   Firm_____   Average_____

f. Special considerations: (flesh rolls, pressure sensitivity, muscle bunching, redundant tissue, neuromata, etc.)_____

_____

_____

C. PROSTHETIC FACTORS

1. How long has present prosthesis been worn?   Years_____ Months_____

2. Prosthesis is worn_____hours per day, _____days per week.

3. Description of present prosthesis: (Check as many items as apply)

For below-knee:

a. Socket type: Closed end_____ Open end_____ Soft_____

                         Hard_____ Other_____

b. Socket material: Plastic_____ Wood_____ Other_____

c. Suspension: Supra-condylar cuff_____ Waist belt____

                         Thigh corset and side joints_____ Other_____

d. Extension aid: Yes_____ .No_____

e. Check strap: Yes_____ No_____

f. Foot-ankle assembly: SACH_____ Single axis_____ Other_____

For above-knee:

a. Socket type: Ischio-gluteal bearing_____

                         Peripheral bearing_____ End-bearing___

                         Total contact____ Distal chamber_____

b. Socket material: Plastic_____ Wood_____ Other_____

c. Suspension: Suction_____ Silesian bandage_____

                         Pelvic belt_____ Other_____

d. Knee axes: Single_____ Polycentric____

       friction   High constant____ Low constant____ Hydraulic_____

                         Variable_____

       lock   Friction_____ Manual_____ None_____

       extension aid   Strap_____ Lever_____ None_____

e. Shank material: Wood_____ Other_____

       exterior   Plastic laminate_____ Enamel_____

f. Foot-ankle assembly: SACH_____ Single axis_____ Other_____

4. What is amputee's opinion of his present prosthesis and its components?

_____

_____

_____

5. Does amputee flex his knee when walking?   Yes_____ No_____

6. Assistive apparatus: Crutch(es)_____ Cane(s)_____ Walker_____

Under what circumstances is apparatus used?_____

_____

Examined by_____

concerning their choice of various components and their utilization of certain principles of fit and alignment. By obtaining a mutually acceptable, detailed prescription at the clinic session, such difficulties are minimized.

As a matter of practical clinic operation, it has been found desirable that the prosthetist contact the clinic chief if he wishes to recommend any significant change in the prescription during the course of fabrication. Such recommendations are often entirely legitimate, based on new evidence which comes to the fore during the fabrication and fitting procedure. However, the important requirement is that the clinic chief be familiarized and should concur with the contemplated changes before they are put into effect.

In prosthetics many judgments are calculated risks or best guesses. Since the prescription decisions reached should reflect the best judgment of all, it does not seem reasonable that the ethical and fiscal responsibilities of these judgments should be placed on the prosthetist alone but, rather, should be a joint responsibility of the clinic.

Experience in various clinics has shown that purchasers of prostheses prefer to place their trust and confidence in the clinic's judgment. Even in cases of failure, they are increasingly willing to tolerate the financial losses involved because they have become convinced that, through the clinic process, the best in professional judgment has been brought to bear on the problem. A typical form on which to record the "prescription" is presented in Figure 5.

3) *Pre-Fitting Treatment.* Where indicated, the patient is referred for appropriate physical therapy, which includes muscle strengthening and improvement of range of motion and muscular coordination, as well as procedures designed to encourage shrinkage of the stump and the relief of symptoms related to surgical trauma.

4) *Prosthetic Fabrication.* The fabrication of the prosthesis is completed by the prosthetist and essentially involves the implementation of the prescription written by the clinic.

5) *Initial Checkout (Evaluation).* After "prescription," the second major responsibility of the clinic is "initial checkout." There is some question as to whether the somewhat colloquial term "checkout" is the best word to describe this activity. However, since it has now become

PROSTHETIC PRESCRIPTION FORM: LOWER EXTREMITY

Patient's Name _____ Date _____

Amputation Type: Right_____   Left_____
    Hip Disarticulation_____   Short A/K_____   Medium A/K_____   Long A/K_____
    Knee Disarticulation_____   Short B/K_____   Medium B/K_____   Long B/K_____
    Syme's Amputation_____   Other_____

MEDICAL AND SURGICAL PRESCRIPTION

1. Is surgery indicated? Yes_____ No_____ If so, please specify condition and
   indicate treatment_____

   _____

2. Is preprosthetic therapy indicated? Yes_____ No_____ If so, please give
   detailed prescription and intended result_____

   _____

   _____

3. Should fitting be delayed for any reason? Yes_____ No_____ If so, why?

   _____

   _____

   _____

PROSTHETIC PRESCRIPTION   (Consider vocation, avocation, and patient preference, as
                            well as stump and general physical characteristics.)

1. Above-Knee
   a) Proximal Socket: Quadrilateral_____   Other*_____
   b) Distal Socket : Total Contact_____   Air Chamber_____
                        Hard End_____   Soft End_____
   c) Socket Material: Plastic_____   Wood_____   Other*_____

Prosthetics and Orthotics
New York University
Post-Graduate Medical School

FIGURE 5

d) Suspension : Suction_____ Pelvic Belt_____
                 Silesian Bandage_____ Other*_____
e) Knee Type : Single Axis_____ Other*_____
f) Knee Lock : None_____ Friction_____ Manual_____
g) Extension Aid: No_____ Yes_____ Indicate Type_____
h) Foot-Ankle : Single Axis_____ SACH_____ Other*_____

Indicate special modifications and reasons for any deviation from the basic prescription (plastic or wood quadrilateral socket, single axis knee, wood shank,
single axis ankle or SACH foot) _____

_____

_____

_____

2. Below-Knee
   a) Socket : Patellar Tendon Bearing_____ Other*_____
   b) Socket Material: Plastic_____ Other*_____
   c) Suspension : Cuff_____ Waist Belt_____ Thigh Lacer (Specify
                    intended function)_____ Other*_____
   d) Knee control : None_____ Fork Strap_____ Check Strap_____
                     Other*_____
   e) Foot-Ankle : SACH_____ Single Axis_____ Other*_____

Indicate special modifications and reasons for any deviation from the basic prescription (patellar tendon-bearing socket, cuff suspension, wood shank, SACH foot)

_____

_____

_____

_____

_____

*When prescribing "Other", please specify exactly what is intended.

                                                                        M.D.
                              _____

fairly well ingrained, it probably must be used until a better term presents itself.

Initial checkout is essentially the first evaluation of the prosthesis-amputee complex as a biomechanical entity. It may be defined as a systematic examination of the patient with the prosthesis. This is accomplished before training with the appliance is given and before the device is delivered to the patient. It is performed in some clinics with the appliance in the unfinished state, so that minor improvements may be introduced at a minimum cost. Initial checkout is important for two reasons: to provide assurance that the prescription developed by the clinic has been followed precisely; and to evaluate the biomechanical adequacy of the prosthetic device against set standards of quality, efficiency, and design.

It is most important that this latter purpose be accomplished by successful passing of initial checkout before permitting the patient to wear the device for any extended period. In this way, corrections can be introduced before the development of undesirable physical or psychological reactions. Learning to use even the best of prostheses is a difficult and arduous task for most patients. To ask them to attempt utilization of a device with discernible inadequacies seriously compounds the difficulties. It is, therefore, incumbent upon the clinic to assure itself that the prosthesis is as completely satisfactory as possible prior to approving it for wear, training, and delivery.

6) *Prosthetic Training.* Upon completion of a satisfactory evaluation of the prosthesis at initial checkout, the normal procedure calls for the referral of the patient to the therapist for appropriate prosthetic training. It is important to emphasize that the training properly occurs after all discernible shortcomings in the appliance have been remedied. This procedure permits a continuous, rational transition in the care of the patient from the prosthetist to the therapist.

The length, type, and intensity of training depend upon the nature of the disability, the characteristics of the patient, and on other lesser considerations. The therapist may permit the patient to wear the device at home at an appropriate point in the training program. When the therapist, by means of objective evaluations and clinical judgment, feels that the patient has profitably completed the training program, arrangements are made for the "final checkout."

7) *Final Checkout (Evaluation).* "Final Checkout" is perhaps best

defined as a procedure to assure the prosthetic clinic that the patient is not in immediate need of any further prosthetic, medical, or surgical attention.

At this checkout, which is the third major responsibility of the clinic, the extent and effectiveness of the patient's use of the prosthesis is evaluated, the biomechanical adequacy of the device is reviewed, and the physical and psychological status of the individual is confirmed. Upon ascertaining that these three factors are all satisfactory and that the patient would not profit from any further immediate prosthetic, medical, or surgical care, the patient may be considered to have completed the necessary treatment.

A typical form for recording the results of checkout (both initial and final) is presented in Figure 6. Detailed instructions for the implementation of checkout are beyond the scope of this paper but are available in the literature (N. Y. U. Manuals for Physicians and Surgeons, 1971).

8) *Follow-Up.* Since the prosthesis is subject to mechanical changes and the patient is frequently subject to physical alterations, the optimal patient-prosthesis relationship may be thought of as transitory. Consequently, the maximum in prosthetic function is obtainable only when the patient is available for follow-up examinations over an indefinite period.

One suggested pattern for such follow-up visits is one visit every six months. Others have recommended a graduated schedule of visits. In either case, the purpose of these visits is to determine that no changes have taken place in the physical characteristics of the patient (especially the stump) which adversely affect the fit and alignment of the appliance and that no mechanical deficiencies have developed which tend to make the operation of the device less efficient. Some of the changes which take place are such that the patient himself may not be aware of them, whereas the clinic, utilizing more expert observation and objective measures, is able to uncover such shortcomings.

The three fundamental steps in the prosthetic clinic process, prescription, initial checkout, and final checkout, are viewed as a basic minimum in the care of any individual requiring a prosthesis for the first time. In the case of a patient who is being seen solely for the replacement of his appliance, the initial and final checkouts are conveniently

PROSTHETIC CHECKOUT: ABOVE-KNEE

Date _____

Name of Patient _____

Type of Amputation _____

_____

_____

Initial Checkout ( )   Final Checkout ( )

        Pass ( )   Provisional Pass ( )   Fail ( )

If the patient needs further attention, please indicate the type of
treatment required:

Medical-Surgical _____ ( )   Training _____ ( )

Prosthetic _____ ( )   Other _____ ( )
                                    (Vocational, Psychological, etc.)

Recommendations and Comments _____

_____

_____

_____

_____

                                    _____
                                         Clinic Chief
FIGURE 6

PROSTHETIC CHECKOUT: ABOVE-KNEE

_____ 1. Is the prosthesis as prescribed?
If a recheck, have previous recommendations been accomplished?

Check with the Patient Standing

Fit and Alignment

_____ 2. Is the patient comfortable while standing with the midlines of the heels not more than 6 inches apart?

_____ 3. Is the adductor longus tendon properly located in its channel and is the patient free from excessive pressure in the antero-medial aspect of the socket?

_____ 4. Does the ischial tuberosity rest properly on the ischial seat?

_____ 5. Is the prosthesis the correct length?

_____ 6. Is the knee stable on weight-bearing? (without the patient using excessive effort in pressing backward with his stump)

_____ 7. Is the brim of the posterior wall approximately parallel to the ground?

_____ 8. Is the patient free from vertical pressure in the area of the perineum?

_____ 9. When the valve of a total contact socket is removed, does stump tissue protrude slightly into the valve hole and have satisfactory consistency? (approximately that of the thenar eminence)

Suspension

_____ 10. Are the lateral and anterior attachments of the Silesian bandage correctly located?

_____ 11. Does the pelvic band accurately fit the contours of the body?

_____ 12. Is the center of the pelvic joint set slightly above and ahead of the promontory of the greater trochanter?

_____ 13. Is the valve located to facilitate pulling out the stump socket and the manual release of pressure?

Check with the Patient Sitting

_____ 14. Does the socket remain securely on the stump?

_____ 15. Does the shank remain in good alignment?

_____ 16. Is the center of the knee bolt 1/2 to 3/4 inch above the level of the medial tibial plateau?

_____ 17. Can the patient remain seated without a burning sensation in the hamstring area?

_____ 18. Can the patient rise to a standing position without objectionable air noise?

PROSTHETIC CHECKOUT: ABOVE-KNEE

Check with the Patient Walking

Performance

_____ 19. Is the patient's performance in level walking satisfactory?
Indicate below the gait deviations that require attention.

a) Abducted Gait ( )	g) Uneven Heel Rise ( )	
b) Lateral Bending	h) Terminal Swing Impact ( )	
of Trunk ( )	i) Foot Slap ( )	
c) Circumduction ( )	j) Uneven Length of	
d) Medial Whip ( )	Steps ( )	
e) Lateral Whip ( )	k) Lumbar Lordosis ( )	
f) Rotation of Foot	l) Vaulting ( )	
on Heel Strike ( )	m) Other ( )	

Comments and Recommendations:_____
_____

_____ 20. Is suction maintained during walking?

_____ 21. With a total contact socket, does the patient have the sensation of continued contact between the stump and socket in
both swing and stance phases?

_____ 22. Does the patient go up and down inclines satisfactorily?

_____ 23. Does the patient go up and down stairs satisfactorily?

Socket

(Check these items after the performance evaluation has been done.)

_____ 24. Does the ischial tuberosity maintain its position on the
ischial seat?

_____ 25. Is any flesh roll above the socket minimal?

_____ 26. Does the lateral wall of the socket maintain firm and even
contact with the lateral aspect of the stump?

Miscellaneous

_____ 27. Does the prosthesis operate quietly?

_____ 28. Are the size, contours, and color of the prosthesis approximately the same as those of the sound limb?

_____ 29. Does the patient consider the prosthesis satisfactory as to
comfort, function, and appearance?

Check with the Prosthesis Off the Patient

Examination of the Stump

_____ 30. Is the patient's stump free from abrasions, discoloration,
and excessive perspiration immediately after the prosthesis
is removed?

PROSTHETIC CHECKOUT: ABOVE-KNEE

Examination of the Prosthesis

_____ 31. Are the anterior and lateral walls at least 2 inches higher than the posterior wall?

_____ 32. Does the inside of the socket have a smooth finish?

_____ 33. Is there satisfactory clearance at knee and ankle articulations?

_____ 34. Are the posterior surfaces of the thigh and shank shaped so that there is minimal concentration of pressure when the knee is fully flexed?

_____ 35. With the prosthesis in the kneeling position, can the thigh piece be brought to at least the vertical position?

_____ 36. In the total contact socket, is the bottom of the valve hole at the level of the bottom of the socket? (It may be lower, particularly with a soft insert.)

_____ 37. Is a back pad attached to the posterior wall of the socket?

_____ 38. Is the general workmanship satisfactory?

_____ 39. Do the components function properly?

combined into a single step, assuming satisfactory follow-up procedures are in effect. On the other hand, when conditions are less than ideal, both the initial and final checkouts may require several repetitions before they are satisfactorily completed. In rare cases, a new prescription may be indicated (N.Y.U. Manual for Rehabilitation Counselors, 1972).

OTHER CLINIC CONSIDERATIONS

There are several additional considerations which are neither medical nor prosthetic in the strictly technical sense and yet seriously affect clinic operations. It seems appropriate that some attention be given to these factors. They include the following:

1) *Clinic Administration or Coordination.* In order to keep the natural confusion which a patient experiences in appearing before a clinic at a minimum, it is important that such considerations as schedules for patients, the proper preparation of forms, the care of checkout equipment, the reduction of waiting time for patients, and the availability of a single person on whom the patient can always rely for counsel, be taken into account in the organization of a smoothly functioning clinic.

2) *Physical Arrangements.* It is sometimes overlooked that a quiet, large, well-lighted room for the clinic meeting, with both the waiting and dressing areas appropriately separated from the clinic operations per se, as well as a reasonable scheme for the control of visitors, are important requirements. The use of sample prostheses, pictures, charts, and other material of an audio-visual nature is helpful in the orientation of the patients.

3) *Interaction Among Clinic Members.* One not-infrequent problem is the domination of the clinic activities by one of its members, usually the physician or the prosthetist. Some clinic chiefs, perhaps because of status considerations, do not ask questions nor draw sufficiently upon the knowledge of the other clinic members. Rather, they resolve what may be to them an embarrassing situation in a manner which curtails the potential contribution of other members of the group.

On the other hand, the prosthetist may, at times, control the clinic. In this instance, no discussions evolve concerning controversial prosthetic issues and, in effect, the clinic becomes a stage for the prosthetist. From time to time, this problem arises when there is a lack of interest on the part of the physician, or when he is burdened with responsibilities which do not permit sufficient time for attention to prosthetic work. The ideal situation exists, of course, when each member's experience is fully utilized in solving the problem at hand. It is the responsibility of the clinic chief to set the tone for this interaction and, ordinarily, the physician's experience and status are required to set a desirable pattern to these meetings. Consequently, in a very real sense, the effective prosthetic clinic is an exercise in medical leadership.

4) *Psychological Effects on Patients.* There can be no gainsaying the importance of the psychological factors which make up good prosthetic adjustment. This process, although complex, seems to involve at least two important considerations for clinic operation. They consist of providing the patient with a clear-cut understanding of the treatment process and of the prosthetic equipment which he is expected to wear, as well as a sense of friendly interest, psychological support, and personal concern.

In conclusion, clinics which overlook any of the above factors, regardless of the degree of technical competence exercised by the members of the rehabilitation team, find results of their treatment are less satisfactory. The prosthetic clinic is an integral part of the process of psychological rehabilitation and must provide a personal type of support, as well as appropriate technical service.

REFERENCES

Berger, N. Spring, 1958. Studies of the upper-extremity amputee II, the population (1953–55). Artificial Limbs 5:1:57–72.

Bergholtz, S. G. 1970–71. Patient census at child amputee clinics. Prosthetics and Orthotics. New York, NYU Post-Graduate Medical School.

Burgess, E. M., R. L. Romano, and J. H. Zettl. August, 1969. The management of lower-extremity amputations. TR 10–6, Veterans Administration. Washington, D. C., Superintendent of Documents, U.S. Government Printing Office.

Fink, S. L. November, 1967. Crisis and motivation: a theoretical model. Archives of Physical Medicine & Rehabilitation 48:11:592–97.

Fishman, S. 1950. Some facts and opinions concerning amputees: a questionnaire survey. New York, New York University.

—— 1962. Amputation, in J. F. Garrett and E. S. Levine, eds., Psychological practices with the physically disabled. New York, Columbia University Press, pp. 1–50.

Maslow, A. H. 1954. Motivation and personality. New York, Harper.

Murdoch, G. April, 1967. Levels of amputation and limiting factors. Annals of the Royal College of Surgeons of England 40:204–16.

New York University Manuals. Prosthetics and Orthotics. New York, NYU Post-Graduate Medical School.

> *For Physicians and Surgeons*
> a. Lower-Extremity Prosthetics, 1971.
> b. Upper-Extremity Prosthetics, 1971.
>
> *For Therapists*
> a. Lower-Extremity Prosthetics, 1971.
> b. Upper-Extremity Prosthetics, 1971.
>
> *For Prosthetists*
> a. Lower-Extremity Prosthetics, 1972.
> b. Upper-Extremity Prosthetics, 1971.
>
> *For Rehabilitation Counselors*
> a. Prosthetics and Orthotics, 1972.

Russek, A. S. October, 1961. Management of lower extremity amputees. Archives of Physical Medicine & Rehabilitation 42:10:687–703.

THE BLIND AND THE
VISUALLY IMPAIRED

No ONE WOULD ARGUE with the premise that restoration of vision is the best possible kind of rehabilitation for the visually disabled. In this regard, the surgical area of rehabilitation in particular has assumed a significant role in the total process. New surgical techniques and developments in the field of optics during the past twenty-five years have greatly expanded the horizons of physical restoration.

However, the focus of this chapter is on youths and adults for whom surgery is impractical as well as on those who suffer a major visual loss even with best correction. These two groups include individuals defined as legally blind and those with severe visual limitations. These are the visually disabled persons who need the most extensive social and/or rehabilitation services in order to carry on reasonably normal lives.

DEFINITIONS, INCIDENCE,
PRINCIPAL GROUPS

As defined in the Social Security Act of 1967,

An individual shall be considered to be blind if he has central visual acuity of 20/200 or less in the better eye with the use of a correcting lens. An eye

DOUGLAS C. MAC FARLAND, ph.d., is Director, Office for the Blind and Visually Handicapped, Rehabilitation Services Administration, Social and Rehabilitation Service, Department of Health, Education and Welfare, Washington, D.C.

which is accompanied by a limitation in the fields of vision such that the widest diameter of the visual field subtends an angle no greater than 20 degrees shall be considered for purposes of the first sentence of this subsection as having a central visual acuity of 20/200 or less.

Persons with "severe visual limitations" are broadly defined by the National Center for Health Statistics (Wilson, 1963–1964) as those with both eyes involved who cannot read newsprint even with best correction.

Based on these definitions, the most recently published figures of the National Society for the Prevention of Blindness (1969) indicate that there are approximately 435,000 blind persons in the United States today. The National Center for Health Statistics (Wilson, 1963–1964) estimates the number of persons with severe visual limitations at 969,-000 throughout the country. The total number of Americans suffering to a greater or lesser extent from a visual disability that requires corrective lenses is estimated by Duane (1965) as 90 million.

It is generally agreed that in the severely handicapped groups, more than 50 per cent and perhaps in excess of 60 per cent are in the age range of sixty to sixty-five years and older. A review of the chronological tabulation published by the National Society for the Prevention of Blindness (1966, 1969) indicates a significant increase of blindness with advancing age. It follows, therefore, that a program of rehabilitation services is as essential for the geriatric blind population as for the young adults and the middle-aged group. Significant pioneering efforts have been instituted along these lines during the past several years (MacFarland, 1968). But although many of the techniques now applied in vocational rehabilitation are applicable for such persons, much research is still necessary to determine how the techniques can be adapted to be more effective for the geriatric blind and how much of the process is reasonable and necessary. A modicum of social services has already been introduced as part of the Social Security legislation. But until a total system of social service delivery is available, work for this group will progress at a snail's pace.

At the other end of the age range, we have the school-age and preschool groups of blind and severely visually impaired individuals. According to the statistics compiled by the American Printing House for the Blind (1970), there are 12,812 blind children attending the public schools, and 7,951 children enrolled in residential schools for the blind. As to the severely visually disabled children, two estimates are generally accepted in establishing incidence. One is that one out of every 500 school children in the United States has a visual impairment severe enough to warrant special consideration (National Society for the Prevention of Blindness, 1966, 1969). The other estimate (Lesowitz, 1970) indicates that there are approximately one and one-half times as many severely visually impaired persons as those falling within the definition of blindness. According to Scott (1969), blind and visually handicapped children have both public and private resources available in sufficient supply to provide them with an adequate education; and, in fact, a disproportionate amount of public and private funds is spent on this smaller group to the detriment of older blind persons. That this is true in certain instances is indisputable. But whether it is universally true is open to question. Relevant discussions are presented by Kohn (1970), Werntz (1970), and Bledsoe (1970).

Of greatest current concern is still another group of blind and severely visually impaired individuals. This is the multiply handicapped group. Suffering from severely disabling conditions in addition to blindness, this group is posing new problems for the educator and rehabilitation worker who deal with the visually impaired. As a result of the rubella epidemics of 1963 and 1965, approximately 30,000 babies were seriously affected by this seemingly mild disease whose effect on the foetus in the first trimester of pregnancy can cause such devastating results as deafness, blindness, deaf-blindness, mental retardation, and other deviate conditions (Wagner, 1967). It is anticipated that thousands of blind and deaf-blind children will be applying for educational services as a result of rubella epidemics (Waterhouse, 1967). Perhaps the most comprehensive study of multiply handicapped blind youngsters was that conducted by Lowenfeld (1968) covering all blind children in California. Among the many startling findings was the fact that more than 50 per cent of the 1,900 blind children surveyed were definitely classified as multiply handicapped. If these data are applied on a percentage basis across the nation, it soon becomes evident that what was thought to be a sound educational program for blind children in the past will be woefully inadequate for those enrolling for educational services in the next several decades.

VOCATIONAL REHABILITATION:
BACKGROUND AND SETTINGS

PROGRAM DEVELOPMENT

Vocational rehabilitation for the blind, and for all practical purposes for the severely visually limited, began with the passage of P. L. 113, The Bardon-LaFollette Act, in 1943 (The Bardon-LaFollette Act, 78th Congress). Legislation and funding of vocational rehabilitation services for the severely disabled were particularly fortuitous at this time because of the tremendously expanded employment opportunities made possible by war production. Employment opportunities were further spearheaded by the intense interest in the blinded veterans of World War II, and by their high motivation to overcome some of the traditional prejudices toward the blind as well as to dispel myths which seem to lock all but the most capable blind persons in stereotype occupations.

The program has grown enormously with the increase of state and federal interest and support, as evidenced by the passage of P. L. 565 in 1954 (The Vocational Rehabilitation Act of 1954, 83rd Congress), P. L. 333 in 1965 (The Vocational Rehabilitation Act Ammendments of 1965, 89th Congress), and other legislative improvements enacted during the late 1960s.

The growth of vocational rehabilitation and its consequent effects on the visually disabled can be graphically illustrated in the following comparisons. In 1943 fewer than 1,000 blind persons were considered rehabilitated. In 1965 this number had risen to 5,450 (Magers, 1966); in 1970, to approximately 8,000, with a total of 24,000 blind and severely visually impaired persons rehabilitated in this period (Magers, 1971).

At present, extensive vocational rehabilitation services are available to a blind person in every state. In 1969 there were thirty-four separate agencies as well as special units in fifty-four states and jurisdictions (Magers, 1969). A number of reorganizations have occurred since that time. An exact list is available from the Office for the Blind and Visually Handicapped, Rehabilitation Services Administration.

SETTINGS

In considering the rehabilitation needs and problems of the blind and the visually handicapped, it is difficult to avoid discussing a philosophical argument that has raged for a number of decades. Put in its simplest form, the question is whether a newly blinded person needs the services of a special agency for the blind or might better profit from the services of a professional organization developed to meet the needs of disabled persons. A sharper way to bring the argument into focus is to say "specialist versus generalist." Papers have been presented on these topics in many professional meetings. Perhaps the subject was best placed in perspective in an article by Seward (1968) in *Blindness Annual.*

Special rehabilitation adjustment centers for the blind have been established throughout the country. They are of greatest assistance to those who have been adventitiously blinded. They are, however, also used to a considerable extent as habilitation centers for those who are congenitally blind and have not yet been taught some of the techniques vital to an independent life.

The major subjects taught at such centers are mobility, communication skills (including braille, typing, the use of talking books, tape recorders, the telephone), activities of daily living (such as good grooming, table etiquette, the social graces), physical conditioning, and prevocational skills designed to improve manual dexterity and body coordination.

For many years these centers concentrated on the totally blind. Their belief was that much of the training was inapplicable to those who had some remaining sight. The limitations of this practice, however, have been recognized within the past few years, and efforts are now being made to incorporate necessary adjustive techniques for the severely visually impaired as well as for the totally blind. In this connection, rehabilitation adjustment training should not be confused with the usual concept of vocational rehabilitation training. Where rehabilitation training is most effective, adjustment services are given prior to and separated from intensive training for a vocational objective.

In addition to the comprehensive services tendered by public agencies, there are those provided by hundreds of private organizations. The most recent publication of the American Foundation for the Blind

(1969) lists approximately 800 separate agencies. However, perhaps fewer than half of these provide comprehensive services. The problem that is understood by some but must be differentiated for all is to help the agency determine what services are necessary, how to provide them quickly, and then return the individual to the community. The extent of successful rehabilitation depends, in large measure, on how well the blind person integrates with the community and to what extent the agency has assisted him to do so.

KEY REHABILITATION NEEDS
AND PROBLEMS

The greatest need of the blind rehabilitant is for an understanding and acceptance of his disability. The ramifications of blindness are severe and varied, and should never be underestimated. For some individuals, the period of psychological trauma and subsequent adjustment is long; for others, relatively short. Whatever the duration, it is a period of significant stress. Reverend Thomas J. Carroll (1961) termed it "the period of mourning." It is a time when the best-trained professional workers are needed to help the individual along the road back to normalcy.

Contrary to the belief of many, deep psychiatric upsets and psychological maladjustments occur no more frequently in the blind person than in his sighted peer. What is needed here is not a special brand of psychiatry/psychology, but a professional who understands the whole person and recognizes the implications that blindness may have when superimposed on emotional upset. Cholden (1958) was perhaps the first to explain the emotional implications of blindness, and how true psychiatric problems of a blind person should be managed. It cannot be emphasized too strongly that blindness in and of itself does not cause deep-seated emotional problems unless the symptoms of emotional upset go unrecognized and untreated.

FAMILY ATTITUDES

Of crucial importance in adjustment to blindness and rehabilitation is an acceptance of both the disability and the disabled individual by the family. There are countless documentations of case histories where a great deal of time, effort, and money was spent in helping a client overcome his visual disability and achieve independence in travel and other necessary activities, only to find that when he returned home the family was not prepared for the independence displayed, and systematically went about destroying it. The following is an example.

Mr. B had just returned home from a rehabilitation adjustment center, where he learned communicative skills, activities of daily living, mobility, and other precursors to vocational training. Everyone who worked with him was enthusiastic about his vocational potential, and the plan was that after a short stay at home he would go on to an intensive period of vocational training. However, during his stay at home his wife made it quite apparent that his use of a long cane, whether white or colored, was embarrassing to her and a source of pity and gossip among the neighbors. A little propaganda of this kind can quickly undo the self-confidence that has been instilled in a client. In Mr. B.'s case, it became virtually impossible for him to take the next big step in his rehabilitation program.

Another example of family pressure is the blind person who is provided with adjustment as well as vocational training and is now ready to take a job. During the initial stages of trauma caused by blindness, his wife accepts outside employment to increase the meager family budget. However, she soon finds that this reversal of roles is for her a pleasant experience. She does not care to relinquish it and raises obstructions to any threat to her new role.

It is easy to see even from these brief illustrations how family pressures and attitudes can militate against successful rehabilitation. In the author's opinion, a rehabilitant's achievements are directly proportional to the understanding of and participation in the rehabilitation process by the family. Here lies a major source of the motivation necessary for success in rehabilitation. Unless the counselor and his close collaborator, the family social worker, are able to explain the rehabilitation goals to the satisfaction of the family and have them assist in helping the client attain his maximum potential, rehabilitation, if not doomed to failure, is working against overwhelming odds.

COMMUNITY ATTITUDES

Community acceptance of blindness as a disability has been slow. Investigations (Duane, 1965) indicate that blindness engenders a universal and profound feeling of fear on the part of most of our citizenry. In one study (Duane, 1967) it was found that blindness is exceeded only by cancer as the disabling condition most feared by the public. The need for community acceptance is, however, essential to rehabilitation, and much work has gone into creating public understanding and acceptance. Better programs of public education are being carried out, the number of volunteers working in behalf of the blind is exceeding by far the number working with other disability groups, and the number of blind and visually impaired persons who are successfully returned to the community is steadily increasing. Fears are gradually being overcome. However, the battle is not yet won. In the author's opinion, it could take half a century and more before blind persons are accepted by all sectors of society without special intervention by counselors or other professional personnel.

MOBILITY

Perhaps the greatest loss a blind person experiences is that of mobility, of freedom of movement from place to place, the ability to go from here to there unhampered by not seeing. Two methods of travel training for blind and visually handicapped persons that are most universally accepted employ the long cane and the guide dog. These provide the blind person with the travel skills that are essential to his vocational as well as social success.

The guide dog movement started after World War I in Germany. It was introduced in the United States in 1929 by Dorothy Eustice Harrison when she began the Seeing Eye, Incorporated (Ebeling, 1950). Today, there are many institutions throughout the country that train seeing-eye dogs for blind persons.

According to one study (Finestone, 1960), less than 2 per cent of the blind population can make use of a guide dog. For the others, a practical and popular solution to the mobility problem is the use of the long cane. A technique for using the long cane was developed by Richard Hoover as a result of his work with blinded veterans at Valley Forge during the latter part of World War II (Hoover, 1968). Many refinements have since been added to the "Hoover technique."

In 1960 "mobility" became the core of a graduate study program, and Boston College began to offer a master's degree in peripatology (Switzer and Bledsoe, 1967). A year later a similar course was initiated at Western Michigan University, and another was later added at Los Angeles State College. All were supported in part by the Social and Rehabilitation Service of the United States Department of Health, Education and Welfare. Support has also been provided by the United States Office of Education for mobility instructors to be used in the education of blind children. At present, there are both graduate and undergraduate programs supported by the Office of Education for this purpose.

OTHER "SIGHT SUBSTITUTES"

It is important to recognize that the application of rehabilitation services to the visually disabled population does not mean increasing sight. It means, rather, the improvement of visual function for the person who has residual vision and the provision of sight substitutes for those who are totally blind or who have only light projection or light perception.

Mobility instruction is a sight-substitute technique. For a totally blind person, mobility instruction makes it possible to overcome the hazardous obstacles encountered in extensive travel either through proper application of cane techniques or the use of a guide dog. These are his sight substitutes.

Another example of sight substitute is to be found in the area of communications, specifically reading, in which the totally blind are taught to use braille, talking books, and tape recordings. All of these serve as a blind person's sight substitutes in competing with seeing peers in schools and colleges, and also in making better use of leisure time.

For the partially sighted, large-type print or special microscopic lenses are provided which permit reading the printed page through enlarging or magnifying the letters. But, as with other sight substitute techniques, it is an adaptive technique (especially in the use of subnormal vision aids) that broadens the use of limited vision but does not improve visual acuity.

In this respect, rehabilitation of the visually disabled differs markedly from rehabilitation techniques applied to other disability groups. Provision of sight substitutes and proper adjustment to the disability bear, in the author's opinion, a direct and measurable correlation to the degree of success that a blind or visually disabled person can expect to achieve.

NEEDED PERSONNEL

In the opinion of many educational experts (Howe, *Blindness Annual* 1965), most learning takes place through visual observation. When a person has just lost his sight, special personnel are needed to teach him skills in such activities of daily living as grooming, table etiquette, social graces, and the use of sight substitutes. These would include, but not be limited to, highly skilled mobility instructors who teach the blind person independent travel through the use of the cane or a dog guide.

Rehabilitation teachers also play a very important role in such instruction as the use of braille, talking books, and tape recordings, as well as writing, typing, and other communication skills. In an adequately staffed rehabilitation adjustment center, ancillary personnel must also be available to provide training in the techniques of daily living, in teaching the newly blinded person methods necessary to develop good grooming habits and table etiquette, such as cutting meat and eating in a socially acceptable manner.

Special assistance is also necessary in training the individual to accept and utilize new approaches to recreation and to instruct in a number of prevocational areas in order to assess the blind person's innate ability with respect to hand coordination and finger dexterity, and to improve these skills wherever possible.

These few examples by no means exhaust the types of specialists required to assist a newly blinded person in adapting to his disability. As previously noted, for specialists such as mobility instructors and rehabilitation teachers total preparation may include completion of a degree at the graduate level. However, rapidly expanding demands for personnel in this area have led to training efforts for the preparation of aide personnel.

Many of the routine tasks performed by the graduate-degree personnel can be included in training programs for paraprofessionals. Trained aides working under the direction of professionals with supervisory experience can greatly expand the number of blind persons served annually. This is a particularly important advantage as we move toward providing rehabilitative services for older blind persons without the necessity for a vocational objective.

In connection with needed personnel, it is also important to note that many of the services required to rehabilitate a blind person are generic in character, and the same specialist who provides these services for the sighted can with very little assistance provide the same services for the blind or severely visually impaired. For example, marriage counseling, assistance with financial planning, psychotherapy, child management for the blind parent, and counseling for integration in community activities are but a few of the generic services which can and should be provided to blind citizens by the same practitioner who serves the nondisabled population.

THE REHABILITATION PROCESS:
SPECIAL CONSIDERATIONS

It is important to recognize at the outset that there is no special "psychology of the blind" or "blindness personality." This is the opinion held by the vast majority of experts in the field. On occasion it might appear, superficially, that the nature of the disability has produced profound personality changes. But in each instance where this seems to be the case, a careful study of the circumstances leading to the disability will indicate glaring gaps in the rehabilitation process. There may be lack of proper training, untreated emotional upsets, inadequacy of adjustment techniques applied to the problem, and undesirable family and community relationships. The blind individual reacts more to inadequacies of treatment than to blindess per se. Blind persons are, first and foremost, individuals who are no different from their sighted peers. What differences exist lie in special considerations that must be applied in order to reach a satisfactory rehabilitation goal. A number are reviewed in this section.

OPHTHALMOLOGICAL INFORMATION

It is imperative for counselors of the visually handicapped to be familiar with ophthalmological conditions and their impact on training, placement, and job satisfaction. Limitations of space preclude a comprehensive review at this time of the restrictions that might result from specific ophthalmological conditions. For this, the reader is referred to Vail's (1959) publication on the subject. For present purposes, a few examples must suffice to illustrate the point.

An individual who is subject to detached retinas must avoid work that requires stooping, bending, lifting weights, or work that might precipitate sudden jarring. While these restrictions may not rule out many occupations, both the counselor and the client must be aware of them in planning practical training and placement.

Examples of other eye conditions that affect type of employment are: aniridia, or light sensitivity; retinitis pigmentosa, which in its early and progressive stages causes severe curtailment of vision under twilight and night conditions and which is often termed night blindness; and diabetic retinopathy, which involves frequent hemorrhages of the eye. In this latter condition, since blood in the eye must be absorbed by osmosis it is very possible for an individual to have a visual acuity nearly approaching normal sight one day, and to be close to total blindness the next.

The counselor must also be familiar with ophthalmological conditions in order to recognize whether a client can profit from the use of subnormal vision aids, either microscopic or telescopic lenses, and to what extent benefit from such aids can be anticipated. In making such determination, it is the counselor's responsibility to maintain the interest and desire of the client without stimulating him to get a goal that is unrealistic and unattainable.

AUDIOLOGICAL INFORMATION

Perhaps the single most important piece of medical information in counseling the blind or visually handicapped individual is auditory perception: the type and amount of hearing loss, if any, whether the condition is monaural or binaural, and what the recommended otological treatment might be. The reasons for this are obvious. Hearing is a blind person's major sight substitute. It is critical for communication, for orientation by sound-location, and for determining the extent to which a blind person can become a proficient traveler. Dallenbach, Supa, and Cotzin (1944) call hearing "facial vision." In later studies (Worchel and Dallenbach, 1947) it was found that the ability to perceive objects was directly related to keenness of auditory perception. Obviously, for a counselor to be effective in work with the visually handicapped, he must have not only basic knowledge of ophthalmological conditions but of otological and audiological conditions as well.

OTHER MEDICAL INFORMATION

Diabetes is now the third largest cause of blindness in the United States (National Society for the Prevention of Blindness, 1966, 1969). In developing a program for an individual blinded or visually impaired from diabetic retinopathy, the counselor must build into the adjustment training program techniques that will permit the client to administer insulin without assistance. The counselor should also be aware of and test for possible nerve damage that would cause a lack of the special sensitivity in the fingers and in touch that is so necessary to a blind person wishing to learn braille or needing top finger dexterity to perform the major aspects of an industrial task. In addition, the counselor must be familiar with the ordinary precautionary measures that must be observed by the average diabetic. For example, a diabetic should not perform tasks for which he must come in contact with equipment that could cause burns. Care should also be exercised in selecting work so that the visually impaired diabetic is not placed in close proximity to moving machinery. Even the slightest possibility of a diabetic coma could place the client in a very perilous situation.

Other medical factors of importance to the counselor are neurological and orthopedic disabilities that affect balance and gait, both of which are critically important in determining proficiency in mobility. Also of importance is information concerning conditions which affect the normal function of the olfactory nerve. Identifications through smell are of great importance to blind persons, over and above supplying environmental orientation in mobility.

THE INTERVIEW

In an initial counseling interview with a blind person, the same basic information is required as for anyone undergoing the rehabilitation process. This includes medical reports, personal history, family relationships, socioeconomic circumstances, and so forth. In addition, as just discussed, the results of a complete ophthalmological examination must be known to the counselor, who must possess an awareness of the special problems that might result from a variety of medical complications.

In regard to the interview proper, when dealing with the blind or the near blind, it is necessary to recognize the importance of complete privacy during the interview. It is not possible for the severely visually disabled person to determine when others have become actively interested in his conversation; and, therefore, if the counselor expects frank responses to his queries, even though they may seem of an insignificant nature to him, he must provide assurance to the client that the interview is indeed on a one-to-one relationship, and that others are definitely precluded from overhearing or entering into the process.

It is also important for the counselor to recognize that, due to the disability, the blind individual referred to him may not find it possible to come to an office for discussion. In many instances, the interview may have to be held in the client's home or immediate neighborhood.

While this procedure is initiated for the convenience of the blind client, it may pose other interventions which would place severe restrictions on information gathered. For example, a client seldom feels free to discuss his problems in the presence of his family. We all recognize the importance of family support and participation in the rehabilitation process. But even in the interview situation, it is apparent that a well-intentioned but uninformed family can provide great blockage to the rehabilitation process.

In most instances it is comparatively easy for the counselor to make arrangements to interview the client privately at a local office in his community. This is certainly much easier than attempting to explain to a family why they should be excluded from a discussion that might have a vital impact on them. Other than following these few caveats, the initial counseling interview with a blind person follows the usual pattern of interviewing.

In preparing for the initial rehabilitation interview, one consideration is of extreme importance when dealing with any severely disabled person. It becomes vital when that person's disability is blindness. What with the pressures counselors are currently subjected to, a counselor may all too often resort to the technique of setting up the initial interview by correspondence. Anyone with experience in rehabilitation is familiar with the pitfalls that arise from this procedure, and with the number of cases that are closed from referral marked "not interested" or "uncooperative."

The problem is severely compounded when a written communication is sent to a blind or near-blind person. Even if the letter reaches him, he is unable to read it and may not have anyone available or interested enough to read it to him. The problem is further complicated if the blind person and his family have been made aware of social security or welfare benefits. In most instances, the tendency is to shy away from employment training that may be not only tenuous but also threaten the loss of cash benefit-payments. This aspect of the rehabilitation process must be carefully explained to both the individual involved and to the family constellation that will be affected.

In preparing for the initial interview with the client, whether at home or in an office situation, the counselor must be thoroughly familiar beforehand with the ophthalmological aspect of medical information. If sight restoration is possible through medical treatment or surgery, these facts must be brought to the immediate attention of the client and his family. If the condition is one that is causing deterioration of residual vision, treatment should be initiated as soon as possible. The benefits and risks must be clearly identified for the client and the family. The final decision regarding a plan of action, however, rests with the visually disabled person.

PSYCHOLOGICAL TESTING

A review of psychological testing of the visually disabled has been discussed by Raskin (1962) and need only be briefly updated here.

Administration of psychological tests to a blind individual does not differ markedly from test administration to sighted persons. The exception is that tests involving printed material must be read to the blind person and special allowances must be permitted for the time differential. Tests that are in widest use are verbal. In recent years, however, nonverbal tests have been developed and validated for the blind. The most noteworthy of these is the Haptic Intelligence Scale for the Blind developed by Harriet and Philip Shurrager (1964). For a complete review of tests now utilized by psychologists working with the blind, the reader is referred to Bauman's survey (1966–1967) and Bauman's manual of norms for the blind (1958).

A few projective tests have been adapted for the blind, for example, the Murray Thematic Apperception Test (Murray, 1943) and the sound recording projective technique developed by Tiffin and Teare (see Teare, 1966). A new test (as yet unpublished) for blind children has been developed by Davis.

At present, intelligence tests for both verbal and nonverbal factors, tests of interest, personality, performance skills, achievement, and vocational inventories, as well as tests for finger dexterity, hand coordination, and other manual skills, exist for the blind. There are also, as previously mentioned, a number of experimental projective techniques.

There is no reason to believe that the point has been reached at which all the diagnostic instruments necessary for psychological evaluation are available for the blind and visually handicapped client. However, considerable progress has been made during the past forty years in developing tests that will help in assessing the strengths and weaknesses of clients suffering this disability.

Perhaps the most important factors to be pointed out in any discussion of psychological diagnosis for the blind or visually impaired client is that the psychologist must have a thorough understanding of appropriate tests and their administration. He must also understand how to apply and relate his findings so that they are most useful to the counselor who is responsible for assisting the client to achieve his rehabilitation goals, whether vocational or nonvocational.

MULTIPLE HANDICAP

To serve the multiply handicapped individual who is also visually disabled, a great deal of effort must be expended to develop new techniques for overcoming the obstacles that are encountered when one or more disabling conditions are superimposed on blindness. It will be expensive, but there is every evidence that the challenge can be accepted to work toward solutions for the multiply handicapped blind child, the young adult, and the very large percentage of older blind persons in order to help them achieve a fuller life.

There are many who believe that so many learning and sensory aids have been made available to the normal blind child that this has become an area which need not be of great concern. There are braille, talking books, tape recordings, large print, optical-to-tactile systems which convert print into tactile stimuli, and a number of other devices which will be referred to later in the section on research. All of these are making the education of the blind or severely visually disabled child much less difficult. However, vast and complicated problems arise for the multiply handicapped blind child. We have only begun to scratch the surface.

As for the multiply handicapped visually disabled adult, one thing stands out. In spite of the thousands of jobs now practical for blind persons, a great deal of imagination must be employed if we are to make rehabilitation a practical goal for the multihandicapped blind. For example, it may be necessary to restudy the contributions that sheltered workshops can make for these persons. Sheltered workshops may prove to be one of the major avenues for training the multihandicapped blind for industrial and other semiskilled and skilled occupations. Such settings may also provide a very valuable long-term or terminal place of employment for those who cannot engage in outside competitive work.

A recent research project on employment for the multihandicapped (Hanger, 1968), conducted by National Industries for the Blind with the support of the Social and Rehabilitation Service, clearly indicated how certain packaging, assembling, and machine operations used in the production of articles purchased by the federal government could be re-engineered to make them practical for blind workers who had one or more other major disabling conditions. With proper re-engineering and training, such workers were not only able to earn substantial wages—many actually earning the minimum wage—but some earned in excess of this minimum in spite of the severity of their combined disabilities.

The author is not implying that there is a direct relationship between the severity of the multiply disabling conditions and the need for sheltered employment. There are many examples of individuals who qualify as multiply handicapped blind by any definition, but who nevertheless achieve a remarkable rehabilitation and compete in jobs requiring a high degree of physical and mental ability and skill.

Sheltered employment is, however, the answer for many whose combined mental and physical disabilities make outside competitive employment impractical in the foreseeable future. In addition, these workshops provide excellent long-term training facilities designed to prepare the multiply handicapped blind worker for ultimate competition with his sighted peers and in the interim provide productive employment. The sheltered workshop permits the individual to work toward independence and achieve a sense of dignity while so doing.

VOCATIONAL PLANNING AND PLACEMENT

In the three decades since the passage of P. L. 113 (Public Law 113, 78th Congress) in 1943, the vocational horizons for the blind and the visually handicapped client have been broadened considerably. There are now literally thousands of jobs that can be done without sight, and many times that number that can be done with limited vision. This, of course, lessens the importance of educational and work background history and heightens the emphasis on the vocational interests of the client.

The key to successful rehabilitation is the extent and quality of vocational training provided. A potential employer may be interested in hiring the disabled if it is feasible. He may also recognize the tangible values that can accrue from a highly motivated disabled worker and his effect on the morale of other individuals in the establishment. But the final decision will depend on whether the applicant can produce as much or more than his competitors. Training is a very strong determinant of this achievement.

Although counselors have been aware of the multiply handicapped blind person for more than a decade, until the passage of the rehabilitation amendments of 1968 (Vocational Rehabilitation Act Amendments, 90th Congress), all that could be done in evaluating the work potential of the multiply handicapped individual had to be accomplished in a few months. With the passage of these amendments, diagnostic evaluation was broadened in scope. For a number of disability groups, including the blind, an eighteen-month period of extended evaluation was permitted, with federal support. As these amendments are implemented throughout the country, the anticipated result will be the employment of thousands of multihandicapped blind and visually impaired workers in productive, competitive jobs for which they might previously have been considered completely unfeasible.

The responsibilities of the placement counselor have also undergone radical changes during the past quarter century. Less than two decades ago it was imperative for a counselor to "sell" the employer the advantages of employing a blind person, conduct a survey of the plant, demonstrate the capabilities of blind persons in certain job operations, and place and provide induction training for the client as well as follow-up supervision (MacFarland, 1954). While it is still necessary to some degree for the counselor to approach employers and to help blind clients in their approach to personnel departments and in their initial orientation on the job, emphasis in industrial placement is now on training provided a potential worker.

The simple, repetitive machine operations that were once the stock in trade of every effective counselor have been profoundly affected by automation. We no longer have simple repetitive single or multiple-spindled drill press operations. A drill press in many industrial plants today is an automated machine programmed and operated by tape, costing approximately $30,000, and requiring at least nine months' training before an individual is capable of coping with its intricacies.

Using this example alone, we can understand why the old concepts have undergone change. The change, fortunately, has been accompanied by more sophisticated training and increased federal and state funding for vocational rehabilitation programs. While other areas of employment for blind and visually handicapped persons never depended so heavily on the "placement" activities of the counselor, they have nevertheless been equally enhanced by training opportunities.

No one can deny that the era of automation came quickly, and, although we seem saturated with it at the moment, we can expect its effects to double in the 1970s. In spite of this rapid change from manpower to machine power, work opportunities for the blind and visually impaired in all areas of employment have increased many times over what they were in the early 1950s. And automation itself, as symbolized by the computer, has provided a new and lucrative opportunity for hundreds of blind workers, with ever-expanding horizons.

Follow-up supervision was always considered an integral part of the rehabilitation process for those who work with the blind or severely visually handicapped. It has not, however, always been accepted as a segment which could be supported by federal funds. This was rectified in the 1968 rehabilitation amendments. We have all come to agree that success can be maintained only if we are willing to review the strengths and weaknessess of the disabled person with the employer and the worker, and when he fails to measure up provide additional training, counseling, or other services in order to help him do so.

One final word on placement. It is the author's opinion that the "hard sell" approach to the employer is no longer necessary because of decades of educational information provided to the community at large and the employer in particular. Such information should be continually injected, through any media possible, into the mainstream of society. Although we can point with pride to thousands of success stories, those of us who are aware of the problems will freely admit that thus far we have barely begun to provide the total spectrum of social and rehabilitation services to the blind and visually impaired.

TRENDS, ISSUES, AND RESEARCH

A number of trends have evolved during the past three decades which seem to be the product of a natural evolution. A study of vocational rehabilitation for the blind and visually impaired immediately after the passage of the Barden-LaFollette Act (1943), would be the history of the struggle of counselors and other professional and subprofessional personnel to help the blind and visually impaired of the nation gain and maintain a foothold in competitive employment.

As the "success story" slowly unfolded, the imaginative thinkers and leaders of the field turned their attention to ways of utilizing the information gained through the provision of vocational rehabilitation services to other groups of disabled individuals. Older blind persons, for instance, could profit from all of the services that were developed and provided for vocational rehabilitation clients but which were not previously available to the elderly blind because the Vocational Rehabilitation Act specifically required that the provision of such services be contingent upon a vocational objective.

A second group, in which professional workers for the visually handicapped have developed a strong interest, is that of the multihandicapped blind. Until the Vocational Rehabilitation Act had been amended in order to include extended evaluation, services for multihandicapped blind persons were virtually nonexistent. For an individual who has one or more major disabling conditions in addition to blindness, thirty days, or even six months, of evaluation is not long enough to develop a training plan nor to set a vocational objective.

Interest in this group, as well as in the geriatric blind, has increased markedly during the past decade. However, services have been retarded because of the substantial financial support required and a shortage of key personnel. It is the author's opinion that services to both groups will be intensified in the 1970s, and that rehabilitation for independent living will be accepted as normal practice for all groups at the end of this decade.

There are a number of key issues which seem to be emerging and which will have a profound effect on services to the blind in the future. Perhaps the most crucial issue that will consume the attention of all workers in the field is the current trend to place a number of state agencies in one large administrative structure. The proponents of amalgamation maintain that such changes are inevitable and result in substantial savings in administrative costs. The effect on agencies providing services to the blind, however, can be disastrous. It is difficult to disperse or submerge a group of services and hope to maintain high standards or even viability. The many ramifications of this philosophical argument are discussed by Kohn (1969, 1970), Jernigan (1970), and Risley (1968).

One of the great leaps into the future that was taken in rehabilitation services for the blind and visually impaired came as a result of the addition of research and training funds to the Vocational Rehabilitation Act in 1954. As a result of this legislative change, it became possible to invest nearly 15 million dollars in research programs directly concerned with the blind and visually impaired. The research has been centered on the following areas: new teaching techniques, such as methods for instructing blind computer programmers (Sterling and Pollack, 1967), and resulting employment; psychological research, which has culminated in the development of some important diagnostic instruments, such as the Haptic Intelligence Scale (Shurrager, 1964); and longitudinal research designed to study social attitudes, evaluate rehabilitation, and pinpoint new areas of direction. One recent example is the research conducted by Scholl, Bauman, and Crissey (1969).

Most of the projects have been for the development of hardware such as the sight substitutes alluded to at the beginning of this chapter. A few examples of things which have been produced or are in the production stage are computer-to-braille transcription, print to tactile conversion (the Optacon), presentation on the skin of the back with neurosynaptic transmission to the brain for interpretation, a folding cane, a closed circuit television reading device, and many others (Switzer and Bledsoe, 1970).

Appropriations for the training program have made it possible to increase the number of professional personnel working in the field of service to blind and visually impaired. Examples include a graduate-training program in rehabilitation teaching at Western Michigan University, mobility instruction on the graduate level at the same school, and similar degree programs offered by Boston College and Los Angeles State College. In addition to support for long-term training in universities, training appropriations have provided the Office for the Blind and Visually Handicapped of the Rehabilitation Service Administration with valuable resources for developing short-term training programs in conjunction with public and private agencies. Through these grants the Office has been instrumental in expanding opportunities in professional, managerial, clerical, industrial, and recreational occupations.

In addition to planning and developing new delivery systems, as well as expanding those already in existence, P. L. 86-610, enacted in 1960, expressly states that rehabilitation research be included in the foreign aid program. Social and Rehabilitation Service is currently working with a number of developing nations in Southeast Asia and Africa as well as in Yugoslavia and Poland. The program can be expanded to other European countries and to South America. The primary thrust of this legislation was to support rehabilitation programs and practices in foreign countries, assisting some to adopt American techniques, and encouraging others to experiment with new techniques that could be beneficial to them as well as provide valuable resource information for agencies here in the United States. Specific information regarding SRS international programs for the blind is contained in *Blindness Annual,* (McCavitt, 1971) and in Lowenfeld (1966).

A fairly substantial part of the international program is concerned with research and demonstration projects designed to assist or to rehabilitate blind and visually handicapped persons. The projects range from the provision of mobile ophthalmological clinics in remote rural areas to training and placement programs in large industrial cities. That the philosophy of rehabilitation succeeds can scarcely be denied in light of what has taken place in some of the rehabilitation training and placement programs in India and Pakistan. India alone is said to have 30 million unemployed persons and 80 million underemployed. Yet, even with this discouraging backdrop, it is significant to note that several rehabilitation training programs for the blind have been established and are successfully training and placing blind persons for industrial work, thus proving the fundamental truth that successful rehabilitation can take place if the foundation for the program is based on adequate training.

APPENDIX

The American Foundation for the Blind (1969) published a list of all public and private agencies purporting to serve blind persons in the United States. Of the 800 agencies and organizations listed, the following are national in scope.

American Association of Workers for the Blind
1511 K Street, N.W.
Washington, D.C. 20005

American Foundation for the Blind
15 W. 16th Street
New York, New York 10011

American Foundation for Overseas Blind, Inc.
22 W. 17th Street
New York, New York 10011

American Council of the Blind, Inc.
539 New England Building
Topeka, Kansas 66603

American Printing House for the Blind
1839 Frankfort Avenue
Louisville, Kentucky 40206

Association for the Education of the Visually Handicapped
1604 Spruce Street
Philadelphia, Pennsylvania 19103

Library of Congress
Division for the Blind and Physically Handicapped

1291 Taylor Street, N. W.
Washington, D.C. 20542

National Center for Deaf-Blind Youths and Adults
105 Fifth Avenue
New Hyde Park, New York 11040

National Federation of the Blind
524 Fourth Street
Des Moines, Iowa 50309

Office of Education
Bureau for the Education of the Physically Handicapped
7th and D Streets, S.W., Room 2120
Washington, D.C. 20201

Blinded Veterans Association
2121 P Street, N. W.
Washington, D.C. 20037

National Society for the Prevention of Blindness, Inc.
79 Madison Avenue
New York, New York 10016

Recordings for the Blind, Inc.
215 East 58th Street
New York, New York 10022

Rehabilitation Services Administration
Office for the Blind and Visually Handicapped
330 Independence Avenue, S.W.
Washington, D.C. 20201

National Eye Institute
National Institutes of Health
Bethesda, Maryland 20014

Hadley Correspondence School for the Blind
700 Elm Street
Winnetka, Illinois 60093

National Braille Association
2060 Albion Street
Denver, Colorado 80207

National Accreditation Council
79 Madison Avenue, Room 1406
New York, New York 10016

National Council of State Agency Executives for the Blind
P.O. Box 12412
Austin, Texas 78711

REFERENCES

American Foundation for the Blind. 1969. Directory of agencies serving the blind and visually handicapped in the United States.

American Printing House for the Blind. January, 1970. Registration by school grades, and Braille and large type reading as registered under the federal act to promote the education of the blind. Louisville, Ky.

Barden-LaFollette Act. 1943. Public Law 113, 78th Cong.

Bauman, Mary K. Tests used in the psychological evaluation of blind and visually handicapped persons. American Association of Workers for the Blind. (The study on which this document is based was done in 1966–67.)

—— 1958. A manual of norms for tests used in counseling of blind persons; bound with tests used in the psychological evaluation of blind and visually handicapped persons. American Association of Workers for the Blind (published as a reprint, having been originally published by the American Foundation for the Blind).

Blasch, Bruce and Berdell Wurzburger. January, 1971. Mobility instruction: a professional challenge. The Long Cane News.

Carroll, Rev. Thomas J. 1961. Blindness, what it is, what it does, and how to live with it. Boston, Little Brown.

Cholden, Louis S. 1958. A psychiatrist works with blindness. New York, American Foundation for the Blind.

Dallenbach, K. M., M. Supa, and Cotzin. 1944. Facial vision: the perception of obstacles by the blind. American Journal of Psychology, Vol 57. See also review by Berthold Lowenfeld in Outlook for the Blind, December, 1944.

Davis, Carl J. Standardization of Perkins-Binet test. Watertown, Mass., Perkins School for the Blind, unpublished.

Duane, T. D. 1965. Ophthalmic research: U.S.A. New York, Research to Prevent Blindness.

—— 1967. The pros and cons of an eye institute. Blindness Annual.

Ebeling, Willi. 1950. The guide dog movement, in P. A. Zahl, ed., Blindness. Princeton, Princeton University Press.

Federal Register, Vol. 35, No. 230, November 26, 1970. Service programs for aged, blind and disabled, Title 45, Public Welfare. Chap. II, Pt. 222.

Finestone, Samuel. 1960. The demand for guide dogs and the travel adjustment of blind persons. Morristown, N.J., The Seeing Eye.

Goodman, Lawrence. 1967. A treatment program for multiply handicapped blind young adults. Blindness Annual.

Groth, Hilde. 1970. A manual for a motor skills training program for industrial placement of blind workers in Malaysia and an evaluation of the pre-industrial selection and training program for blind workers in Malaysia. American Foundation for Overseas Blind.

Hanger, J. W. 1968. Remunerative employment of multiply handicapped persons. New York, National Industries for the Blind.

Hoover, Richard. 1968. The Valley Forge story. Blindness Annual.

Howe, Samuel Gridley. 1865. The best of the past: Batavia address. Blindness Annual, 1965.

International Health Research Act. 1960. Public Law 86-110, 86th Cong.

Jernigan, Kenneth. July, 1970. The separate agency for the blind: why and where. Braille Monitor.

Kohn, Joseph. 1969. The future of services by state agencies for the blind. Proceedings of the National Rehabilitation Association. New York.

—— 1970. The challenge of the 70's. Contemporary Papers, Vol. VI.

—— Changing character of the responsibilities of state agencies. Contemporary Papers, Vol. VI.

Lesowitz, Nathan. 1970. Characteristics of clients rehabilitated in fiscal years 1965–69. Washington, D.C., Division of Statistics, Social and Rehabilitation Service.

Lowenfeld, Berthold. 1966. Vocational rehabilitation grant projects in Israel. Blindness Annual.

—— 1968. Multi-handicapped blind children in California. Sacramento, California State Department of Education, Division of Special Services.

MacFarland, D. C. March, 1954. Some guides to placement procedures. New Outlook for the Blind, Vol. 48.

—— 1968. Service needs of aged persons with severe visual impairments. Proceedings of the Research Conference on Geriatric Blindness and Severe Visual Impairment. Sept. 7–8, 1967. New York, American Foundation for the Blind.

Magers, George. 1966, 1971. Placement: key to employment. Blindness Annual. Also unpublished statistics from the Office of the Blind and Visually Handicapped.

—— 1969. State agencies serving the blind and visually handicapped. Blindness Annual.

McCavitt, Martin. 1971. Special foreign currency program of the social and rehabilitation service: international research and demonstrations. Blindness Annual.

Murray, Henry O. 1943. Thematic apperception test. Cambridge, Harvard University Press.

National Society for Prevention of Blindness. 1966, 1969. Updated Table I: Estimated statistics on blindness and vision problems.

Public Law 113. 1943. 78th Cong.

Raskin, S. J. 1962. Visual disability, pp. 341–75 in J. F. Garrett and E. S. Levine, eds., Psychological practices with the physically disabled. New York, Columbia University Press.

Risley, Bert L. 1968. The case for separate programs for the blind. Proceedings of the National Council of Citizens Advisory Councils. Washington, D.C.

Scholl, Geraldine, Mary K. Bauman, and Marie Skodak Crissey. 1969. A study of vocational success groups of the visually handicapped. Ann Arbor, University of Michigan.

Scott, Robert A. 1969. The making of a blind man. New York, Russell Sage Foundation.

Seward, Henry. 1968. History and development of workshops for the blind in the United States. Blindness Annual.

Shurrager, Harriet and Philip Shurrager. 1964. Haptic intelligence scale for the blind. Chicago, Illinois Institute of Technology Center.

Sterling, Theodore D. and Seymour Pollack. 1967. Training of the blind for professional computer work. Cincinnati, University of Cincinnati.

Switzer, Mary E. and C. Warren Bledsoe. 1967. Vocational rehabilitation training projects. Blindness Annual.

—— 1970. U. S. government sponsored research to study blindness; 1970 supplement prefaced by a composite listing of social and rehabilitation service research and demonstration projects 1954–70. Blindness Annual.

Teare, Robert. 1966. Test battery for use of the blind. Wichita, University of Wichita.

U.S. Congress. 1943. Barden-LaFollette Act. 78th Cong., Public Law No. 113. Washington, D.C., Government Printing Office.

—— 1960. International Health Research Act. 86th Cong., Public Law No. 86-110. Washington, D.C., Government Printing Office.

—— 1967. Social Security Act Amendments. 90th Cong., Public Law No. 248. Washington, D.C., Government Printing Office.

—— 1954. Vocational Rehabilitation Act Amendments. 83d Cong., 2d sess., S Doc No. 2759, Public Law No. 565. Washington, D.C., Government Printing Office.

—— 1965. Vocational Rehabilitation Act Amendments. 89th Cong., Public Law No. 333. Washington, D.C., Government Printing Office.

—— 1968. Vocational Rehabilitation Act Amendments. 90th Cong., Public Law No. 391. Washington, D.C., Government Printing Office.

U.S. Office of Education. 1967. Recommendations of ad hoc committee of advisers from the field on curriculum content and funding of orientation and mobility instructor training. Washington, D.C.

Vail, Derrick. 1959. The truth about your eyes. New York, Farrar, Straus.

Wagner, Elizabeth. April, 1967. Maternal rubella: a general reaction to the disease. New Outlook for the Blind.

Waterhouse, Edward J. 1967. Deaf-blind children: implications for education. Contemporary Papers, Vol. II.

Werntz, George. October, 1970. Letter to the editor. New Outlook for the Blind. See also C. Warren Bledsoe's Reflections on Dr. Robert Scott's Book. Blinded Veterans Association Bulletin, May–June 1970 and Reactions to Osti. Proceedings of the Pennsylvania-Delaware Chapter of the American Association of Workers for the Blind.

Wilson, Ronald. Characteristics of visually impaired persons in the United States, July 1963–64. National Center for Health Statistics, U. S. Public Health Series 10, Number 46. See also interpretation by Ronald Wilson in Blindness Annual, 1967, p. 144.

Worchel, Philip and Karl M. Dallenbach. 1947. Facial vision. American Journal of Psychology, Vol. 60.

EARLY PROFOUND DEAFNESS

DEAFNESS IS PROBABLY the least understood of all major disabilities. In contrast to such conditions as blindness, cerebral palsy, and amputation, profound hearing loss is invisible and rarely the subject of public notice or concern. Misconceptions about deafness abound, as indicated by the frequency with which deaf persons are asked if they use braille.

As invisible as deafness is on the surface, its manifestations are as drastic in the key adjustive areas that lie beneath the surface. Language development, communication, education, psychological maturation, and acculturation—all are aspects of the web of problems derived from early profound deafness. The emphasis of this chapter is upon persons with profound hearing losses as distinguished from those termed "the hard of hearing."

DEFINITIONS

There are many different ways to define the varying degrees and types of hearing loss. The definitions vary with their intended purposes. For example, the research audiologist might describe deafness as a total loss of hearing, which for him is a meaningful conceptualization but for the rehabilitation counselor is useless. The definitions that follow are the most functional available for those concerned with behavioral aspects of hearing loss.

MC CAY VERNON, Ph.D., is a Professor in the Department of Psychology, Western Maryland College, Westminster, Md.

Deafness: A hearing loss in the better ear severe enough to prevent the understanding of conversational speech whether or not a hearing aid is used.

Hard of Hearing: A hearing loss in the better ear severe enough to decrease the perception of conversational speech to some extent but involving sufficient hearing to permit understanding of speech under optimal conditions either with or without a hearing aid.

Hearing Impaired: Refers to all losses of hearing regardless of degree or type. This term is often used to describe deaf people and as such can be misleading and euphemistic.

The Prelingual Deaf: Deafness having its onset prior to the age at which the child has learned language (usually before three years of age).

These terms obviously do not represent airtight mutually exclusive categories. There is some overlap in that there are people who are on the borderline between being deaf or hard of hearing. By the same token there are precocious children who though "prelingually" deafened at three have well-developed language which is retained after loss of hearing.

Despite these problems these definitions are far more workable from a psychology of deafness viewpoint than definitions which are expressed in specific decibels of hearing loss. The main problem with these latter definitions, derived from the physics of sound, is that they lack isomorphism with behavior. In other words, people with identical hearing losses as measured audiometrically may vary greatly in the extent to which they can understand or interpret what they hear. For example, some persons who hear pure tones of low volume have such defective auditory mechanisms that speech sounds cannot be deciphered. They are perceived as just noise. Despite this, audiograms can be most helpful in interpreting hearing losses. Figure 1 gives some approximation of the relationships between various types of audiograms and functional hearing.

PREVALENCE

There are an estimated 8,500,000 Americans with significant hearing losses (Carhart, 1970). In fact, hearing loss is perhaps the most common health problem in the United States. Unfortunately, statistics of

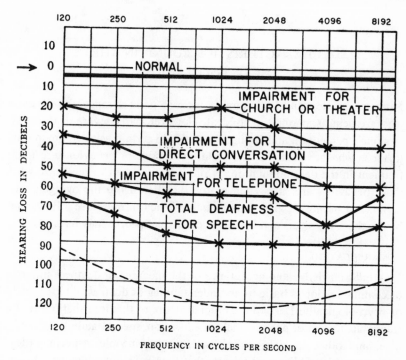

FIGURE 1. Audiograms and Functional Hearing Ability
(Courtesy of the American Hearing Society)

hearing disorders on a worldwide basis are vague and imprecise (de Reynier, 1970). This is a characteristic census problem of impaired hearing.

Among school-age children in this country, there are about 47,000 in
special schools for the deaf (Doctor, 1970). About 100,000 more require intensive management and approximately 250,000 others are au-
ditorially handicapped to an important degree in the regular school
environment. Overall, there are over 1 million children in the United
States who are hard of hearing (Berg and Fletcher, 1970).

Most estimates place the total number of deaf people in the United
States at about 250,000 to 300,000 (Switzer and Williams, 1967). This
is a tenuous estimate due to the lack of adequate census data on the
deaf. At present, a very extensive census is being conducted by the National Association of the Deaf which will result in valid prevalence figures.

CHARACTERISTICS FOUND IN THE
DEAF POPULATION

Human variation and individuality have as great a range among those who are deaf as among the nondeaf. However, early severe deafness alters one's perception and coping capacities in certain ways common only to those who are deaf. Hence, certain reactions or behaviors are more frequent in the deaf population. While it is important to recognize what these behaviors are, it is even more crucial to avoid the overgeneralization that because a given human being is deaf it therefore follows that he has the same assets and liabilities other deaf people may have.

COMMUNICATION

A full knowledge and acceptance of the meaning of deafness in terms of communication is basic to an understanding of deafness educationally or psychologically. Despite the crucial nature of this information, it is a tragic fact that most professionals in education, speech, audiology, medicine, and other specialties meet so few deaf people, especially deaf adults, outside of clinics or schools that they have only the vaguest concept of the true meaning of the communication implications of deafness, psychologically, socially, and vocationally. If deaf people spent their entire lives in clinics and schools instead of out in the world having to face the issues of economic and psychic survival, such gaps in professional knowledge would not be so destructive to them. However, deaf people do not desire a life of dependency, nor are clinics or schools at all anxious to assume lifelong responsibility for them. Consequently, the deaf person pays a very dear price for the failure of those whose professional responsibility it is to understand the essence of his disability—communication. For this reason, considerable time will be devoted to the problem here.

Most young people today who are termed deaf were born with their hearing loss or acquired it early in life before they were old enough to have learned to talk and to use language (Vernon, 1968). Under these circumstances, normal speech cannot be developed. Sometimes intelligible speech can be acquired, but in many cases the prelingually deafened client will not be able to talk in a way that is understandable to employers and the general public. If we will remember the trouble we may have had speaking a foreign language which we could hear, and if we will then imagine the difficulty we would experience in learning to articulate a foreign language if we could not hear our own voice, it is easy to understand why many capable deaf persons lack the ability to speak intelligibly.

Speechreading, commonly called lipreading, is another aspect of the communication problem faced by deaf persons. Only rarely do professional specialists in deafness fully understand the limitations of speechreading. Few recognize that 40 to 60 per cent of the sounds of the English language are homophenous, that is, they look just like some other sound on the lips (Lowell, 1959). Adding to this ambiguity inherent in the phonetics of the spoken language are factors, such as poor lighting, buck teeth, cigarettes in the mouth, mustaches, bad speech habits, small immobile mouths, head movements, and countless other interferences. These reduce the percentage of most speech that can be lipread to about 20 to 30 per cent at the most, provided the person is a good lipreader. Many deaf people are not.

Still another aspect of the communication problem is the fact that the person prelingually deafened does not have the chance to learn the vocabulary and syntax of language by hearing it. Consequently, he knows neither grammar nor word meaning until he goes to school. He does not know his name, the names of his parents, or the words for the food he eats and the clothes he wears. Because of this late start in learning language, coupled with the fact that his exposure to it is *through vision only,* the average deaf person does not develop a large vocabulary or a skill in the use of English syntax. His written language is generally poor and, in many cases, he is unable to clearly communicate complex ideas through writing.

In view of the communication problems deaf persons face with speech, lipreading, and writing, many find that they achieve greatest communication skill manually, that is, in the language of signs and fingerspelling (See Figure 2). Often deaf persons who lack any appreciable ability in oral or written communication can nevertheless express and receive complex ideas in the language of signs.

In years past most deaf youths attended state residential schools at

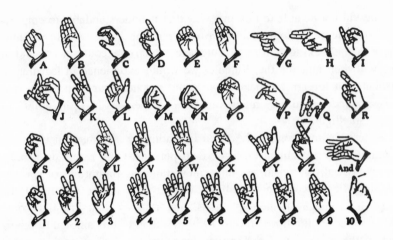

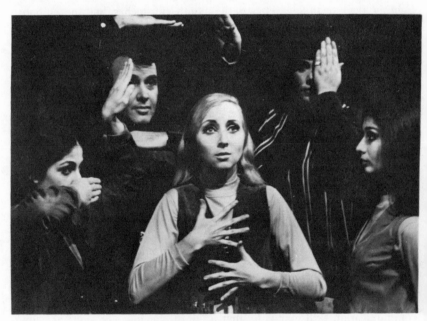

FIGURE 2. *Top*, Fingerspelling Alphabet (Courtesy of the
National Association of the Deaf);
Bottom, Sign for "Afraid" (Courtesy of the National
Theatre of the Deaf. Photo: Jay Aare)

least through their highschool age years. Manual communication was not customarily forbidden in most schools. Consequently, those who could not communicate orally were able to learn to communicate manually. This is no longer true. Today many deaf young people attend day classes or day-school programs with hearing students. This works out successfully for some. These few develop intelligible speech, can read and write, and are able to use lipreading for communication purposes. However, a large proportion of these youths do not learn to speak intelligibly, they cannot read and write enough to convey more than rudimentary daily needs, and they do not speechread successfully. Vocational counselors are facing more and more of these cases, especially in larger cities (Grinker, 1969).

INTELLIGENCE

Next to the auditory mechanism itself, undoubtedly the most-studied characteristic of deaf persons is their intelligence. Over fifty studies of IQ dating back to the early 1900s demonstrate rather conclusively that intelligence is distributed essentially the same in the deaf population as it is among the nondeaf (Vernon, 1968).

This fact is of major importance and must form a cornerstone of any judgment of appropriate achievement for deaf people. Corollary to these findings on intelligence, it has also been demonstrated that deaf persons have the same capacities for abstract thought as do the nondeaf (Furth, 1966; Vernon and Koh, 1970). This is most readily exemplified by the number of deaf professional mathematicians (Rose, 1967).

MOTOR SKILLS

Deaf persons are equal to the hearing in manual dexterity and most motor skills related to work (Boyd, 1967; Myklebust, 1960). Scores on motor subtest of the General Aptitude Test Battery are among the evidence of this (Kronenberg and Blake, 1966). More importantly, perhaps, competence in motor skills has been thoroughly demonstrated by studies of deaf persons in the world of work. Here it is found that 87.5 per cent are employed in manual occupations (Rainer, Altshuler, Kallmann, and Deming, 1963).

WORK HABITS AND VOCATIONAL ADJUSTMENT

Employers who give deaf persons an opportunity to prove themselves in work report them to be satisfactory (Furfey and Harte, 1964). The employment history of the deaf, until recent automation, has been one of high rates of employment and stable job tenure (Vernon and Koh, 1970).

However, despite having the same intelligence as hearing people, the deaf are frequently forced into manual labor of varying skill levels rather than having the opportunity to engage in professional employment. For example, five-sixths of the deaf are in some form of manual labor as contrasted to one-half of the general population (Boatner, Stuckless, and Moores, 1964; Kronenberg and Blake, 1966; Vernon and Koh, 1970). Only 17 per cent of deaf people do white-collar work, compared to 46 per cent of the general population. This is due primarily to a failure of the educational system to provide deaf persons with a chance to constructively utilize their potential.

EDUCATION

The education of deaf children poses unique problems. Imagine, for example, that you were faced with a child who spoke only Russian and that you were to teach this child through a glass, soundproof wall. Furthermore, you could not use the Russian language in any way. In a sense this fanciful situation represents the problem faced by the teacher and the deaf child as they embark upon the task of education. All of the communication problems and issues just discussed must be dealt with realistically and effectively if learning is to occur.

The results of the education of the deaf are discouraging, as the following information will show:

Boatner (1965) and McClure (1966). These two administrators of schools for the deaf did a study which included 93 per cent of all pupils enrolled in schools for the deaf in the United States who were sixteen years old or older and who were leaving school. Thirty per cent of these youth were functionally illiterate. Only 5 per cent achieved at a tenth-grade or better level. Of these youth, 60 per cent were at grade-level 5.3 or below.

Wrightstone, Aronow, and Muskowitz (1959). These investigators studied seventy-three school programs involving 53 per cent of all deaf school-age children. They found that from the age ten years to sixteen years the average gain in reading was less than one year. Furthermore, the average reading score for a sixteen-year-old deaf youth was at grade level 3.4.

Schein and Bushnaq (1962). These investigators found that admissions of deaf youth into college, including the special college for the deaf, were only one-eighth the per cent of admissions of normally hearing students into college. For example, if 40 per cent of the normally hearing get into college, then only 6 per cent of deaf get into college.

Babbidge Report (1964). The distinguished Babbidge Committee examined results from 269 schools and classes representing 23,330 deaf children, or 76 per cent of all deaf school-age children. Ninety per cent of public residential pupils were included. Day classes and schools were not represented. Results indicated that the median average on the Stanford Achievement Test for school leavers is 5.9.

A greatly increasing number of deaf youths now attend urban schools, a trend that will grow in the future. Research on the deaf of Chicago (Grinker, 1969) makes it clear that this aspect of an over-all weak educational system is by far the poorest. It is here that the dropout rate is highest and the waste and destruction of the potential of deaf youth is the most widespread (Grinker, 1969).

Changes in other aspects of the lives of deaf persons ultimately depend upon improvements in education. While rehabilitation has made efforts to compensate for educational retardation in its services to deaf adults, rarely is it possible for rehabilitation to overcome gross education retardation.

MARRIAGE PATTERN

Ninety-five per cent of deaf persons marry other deaf persons, the exceptions generally being those who are hard of hearing or those who become deaf later in life. This is understandable, and, in most cases, it represents a healthy adjustment to deafness. These marriages are basically stable; however, there is a slightly higher percentage of unmarried persons among the deaf, due in part to the somewhat higher ratio of men to women among the deaf (Rainer, Altshuler, Kallmann, and Demings, 1963).

SEXUAL ADJUSTMENT

There is little known about this area of the behavior of those who are deaf. One fact which stands out is that very few deaf adults obtained any sex education from their parents, schools, or any place else. In fact, few parents of deaf persons learn to fingerspell and to use the language of signs. Thus, most deaf children's only chance to learn from their parents about the complexities of sexual behavior and responsibility is through oral or written means. The children rarely possess the language comprehension required at the time sex information is essential. This unfortunate failure of parents to learn to communicate adequately with their children accounts, in part, for the somewhat higher prevalence of sexual adjustment difficulties among the deaf (Rainer, Altshuler, Kallmann, and Deming, 1963).

MULTIPLE HANDICAPS AND DEAF PERSONS

With both the deaf and the general population, IQ and a number of other traits are not distributed in a strictly normal curve. Instead there is a "bubble" at the lower end of the distribution (Jensen, 1969). This is due in the general population to genetic conditions such as mongolism and phenylketonuria and factors resulting from certain epidemics.

Within the deaf population this "bubble" is probably larger. It applies to the greater prevalence among the deaf of such conditions as cerebral palsy, aphasia, organically caused behavioral disorders, and visual problems. The reason for the somewhat elevated prevalence of these conditions among the deaf population is that the major causes of deafness (meningitis, prenatal rubella, complications of Rh factor, premature birth, and genetic factors) are also the leading etiologies of the conditions mentioned above (Vernon, 1969). Thus, they and deafness occur together more often than pure chance would decree. Undoubtedly this "bubble" accounts for some of the low achievement among deaf persons.

Multiple handicaps are not rare among deaf persons and they deserve the full attention of rehabilitation and education experts. However, an adequate discussion of this important problem is beyond the scope of this chapter other than making the often overlooked point that some of these multiply disabled persons have extensive potential, as exemplified by deaf cerebral-palsied college graduates (Vernon, 1969).

OTHER AREAS

Deficient education and underemployment have been documented earlier in the chapter. Obviously, a deaf person victimized by poor education and underemployment or unemployment will suffer in his social, psychological, family, and spiritual achievements and satisfactions. However, these spheres of life are hard to assess objectively.

A major effort in this direction, and one which can be generalized to other large urban areas, was the three-year study conducted at the Psychosomatic and Psychiatric Institute of Michael Reese Hospital in Chicago (Grinker, 1969). This extensive examination of the deaf and hard-of-hearing population of Chicago showed that a significant cause of low achievement begins early in the family life of the deaf child. At this time inappropriate counseling that encourages parents to limit themselves to *one* mode of communication, oral communication, and forbids them *total manual and oral communication* creates frustration and tensions in far too many families with deaf children. The deaf child, as a consequence of deficient communication, is denied full participation in family activities and their crucial psychological and educational benefits. The rather obvious fact is that if the deaf cannot hear spoken language, and that if it cannot be understood from the lips, the inevitable result is calamity. A major remediation in the opinion of many is total communication, that is, the use of manual and oral communication.

The naive assumption that this early deprivation in communication can be compensated for later in the life of the child is espoused by those who would withhold total communication until later years. Unfortunately, many adverse effects of early deprivation are irreversible.

Another finding of the Chicago study was that only a minority of deaf youth who attend urban public schools ever graduate (Grinker, 1969). The majority are forced out of the school system at ages fourteen to seventeen, functionally illiterate and unable to speak, lipread, or use the language of signs. Some of these remain socially isolated all their lives. Some live as dependent, frustrated burdens to themselves and their families. When their parents die, these dependent deaf persons are often institutionalized in state hospitals or other custodial facilities.

For most, the Division of Vocational Rehabilitation enters after the educational system has failed. It then attempts to pick up the pieces, give these youths a means of communication, and then provide vocational-technical education. Because many of these rehabilitation clients have average to high IQs despite their low communicative and academic achievements, it is possible to help them attain some form of vocational competence, learn to communicate with other deaf people, and to find some social satisfactions with deaf and hearing peers. The real point to be made is that the resultant achievement levels are totally unsatisfactory in terms of the potentials of the individuals.

KEY REHABILITATION NEEDS AND PROBLEMS

TOTAL COMMUNICATION

Research strongly indicates that "oral only" education has proved to be a failure (Vernon and Koh, 1970). Research has also indicated that total manual-oral communication can increase the present low levels of academic achievement (Vernon and Koh, 1970; see pp. 491–93 below). The Rehabilitation Services Administration has implemented these findings by: (1) emphasizing that its training programs in deafness teach prospective counselors fingerspelling and the language of signs; (2) establishing the Registry of Interpreters which provides interpreters for deaf people; (3) establishing communication skills programs which teach sign language; and (4) placing deaf persons in professional positions as counselors, teachers, and high-level policymaking federal administrators.

The author believes that were educators equally effective in implementing research and establishing total communication programs the present low academic achievement levels of deaf people could and would be significantly raised. Rehabilitation could then begin with clients who came to them with much higher educational levels. Until this comes to pass, if appropriate employment of the deaf is to be realistically possible, rehabilitative services must expand their efforts to provide deaf youths and adults with basic communication skills they should have been given in school. Along with this must be provided vocational-technical and remedial training and basic facts of psychosocial development.

To know the full ramifications of this issue of educational methodology, one has but to see the high priority it assumes in the deaf community. This is reflected in the policy of the National Association of the Deaf and in state associations of the deaf. Common sense, research findings of recent years, and experience cause defensive educators to try to evade the issue by saying, "It is an old argument," "It really doesn't matter," and "Hearing aids and preschool will solve the problem."

The issue of communication methodology is crucial. There is a growing belief that it must be met by total manual and oral technics from infancy through adulthood if achievement levels are to rise.

COUNSELING AND TRAINING

Deaf youth must be guided into and taught the vocational, technical, and professional skills of the future. If schools continue to direct young deaf persons into areas such as linotyping, shoe repair, and agriculture, which are diminishing in opportunity, they limit the development of these youths. Work-study programs in secondary schools, well-staffed vocational-technical education in topnotch existing facilities for the hearing, and upgrading of vocational teachers and rehabilitation counselors are some ways to assure that the guidance and training of deaf youth will lead to a marketable work skill with a future.

CLOSER RELATIONSHIPS BETWEEN SCHOOLS AND THE
DIVISION OF VOCATIONAL REHABILITATION

This has already begun in some residential schools and has proved tremendously successful. It is most badly needed in large urban programs where hundreds of bright deaf youths drop out every year, never even knowing about the opportunities open to them through vocational rehabilitation (Grinker, 1969).

CLOSING THE GAP BETWEEN NEED AND DEMAND

A major outgrowth of the three years of research on Chicago's deaf population was the discovery of a shocking gap between need for services and demand for them. This is a many-faceted, urgent problem.

For example, in Chicago alone were many times the number of multiply handicapped deaf than could be served by the only facility in the United States for such clients, the Arkansas Rehabilitation Center. Yet, these youths did not know of the Center's services nor did their families, their teachers, their ministers, or even their DVR counselors.

At the other end of the continuum were many bright deaf youths capable of college, junior college, or technical education who were oblivious to many outstanding new programs of the Rehabilitation Services Administration, as well as of such established facilities as Gallaudet College and the National Technical Institute for the Deaf.

The problem is one of communication. The establishment of a good program is but the first step in the delivery of services. Over the last ten years giant strides have been made in this initial step of starting facilities. But the task of informing and counseling those needing the services has only begun.

The eventual solution to this problem is a national, continually updated registry of deaf persons. Since at this time such a registry is not within the foreseeable future, other steps must be taken.

First, an annual listing of all postsecondary programs serving deaf clients should be sent to all counselors working with deaf clients, many general counselors, speech and hearing centers, and schools for deaf children. This listing should indicate what kind of training is offered and procedures for enrollment. In 1972 ASHA published an initial effort in this direction, which unfortunately is only a token of what is needed. Furthermore, this listing is not planned as an annual feature (Vernon and Snyder, 1972).

Second, special efforts must be made to locate and provide services to minority-group deaf persons. The Negro deaf are in great need of vocational-technical opportunities but are not well identified and often do not know about services available to them through rehabilitation (Bowe, 1971). In the Chicago project, mentioned previously, we were able to send to a college program serving the deaf, the National Technical Institute, several Negro deaf youths who had previously been totally unaware of such a possibility.

The gap between the need and the demand for rehabilitation is an important reason for the low achievement of the deaf population. While its remediation may lack the drama and appeal of other steps, the gap in "case finding" is a correctable problem and should be dealt with immediately.

RESEARCH ON URBAN EDUCATION

It is essential that the problem be researched and carefully described in order that operationally stated rehabilitative steps can be implemented. Many more residential training facilities will undoubtedly be a big part of the answer (Grinker, 1969).

MORE QUALIFIED DEAF PERSONS AT PROFESSIONAL LEVELS IN REHABILITATION

Perhaps the principal reason for the success of the Rehabilitation Services Administration (RSA) programs has been that the RSA has had deaf people in policymaking positions from the start. Its training programs have been open to and have encouraged qualified deaf applicants. Interpreters, instructors able to communicate manually, and other services have been provided to assure deaf students and staff equal opportunity. As a consequence, RSA and its programs have communication with the deaf community and an understanding of its needs. Clients who come to vocational rehabilitation counselors for services are increasingly seen by people who possess the skills needed to relate to the deaf. Instead of the routine referrals of the past for thirty lipreading and speech lessons for clients who have already studied these skills for twelve or more years, we are now getting meaningful programs based on counseling done by professionals able to communicate with deaf people.

There could be no stronger evidence for the employment and preparation of deaf persons at professional and policymaking levels than the success of RSA's using qualified deaf persons in key positions.

PLACEMENT EMPHASIS

Counselors and others who are out in the field meeting problems at the grassroots level recognize that placement service is the cornerstone of a successful rehabilitation program for deaf persons. Applying for positions is an Achilles' heel to most deaf persons, regardless of their vocational or professional competence. It is a somewhat frightening experience to hearing persons, but for the deaf applicant the reality of the situation puts him at a horrible disadvantage.

Employers, most of whom know nothing about deafness, have the idea that lipreading makes normal conversation possible and that the speech of persons born deaf should be understandable. In the job interview this generally proves not to be true. The embarrassment and discomfort that result jeopardize the chances of otherwise highly qualified applicants.

Deaf persons, knowing this, often take inferior positions or else remain for entire lifetimes in jobs far beneath their capacities due simply to the trauma and disadvantage they face in applying for a job. Often money spent in highly successful training programs goes down the drain, due to a failure at the placement stage of the over-all rehabilitative process.

Compounding the problem is the depreciation of the placement function by many counselors and college training programs. For deaf clients this has serious adverse effects in that they are not given the placement help they need. The problem must be corrected.

Meaningful rehabilitation for deaf clients must emphasize placement. RSA-sponsored college programs should be required to have a core course in placement for all counselors. Assessment of the work done by field counselors must have built into it a recognition and reinforcement of counselors who do effective placement.

PROGRAMS FOR MULTIPLY HANDICAPPED DEAF

Deaf persons with other disabilities pose a large and increasing challenge to rehabilitation (Sussman, 1970). Without specialized programs geared to their needs, multiply handicapped deaf persons have little or no chance in the world of work or in life in general. At present, educational programs are excluding many of these youths. With the huge influx to schools of post-rubella deaf children from the 1963–1965 epidemic, this problem can be expected to increase in the future.

In view of this and the demonstrated success of programs for the multiply handicapped, justification for the continuation and expansion of such programs is evident (Vernon and Snyder, 1972). This is especially true when one recognizes that without specialized training the multiply handicapped deaf person is relatively helpless to compete in today's job market. He is doomed to depreciating custodial care at state expense.

SUMMARY

Research findings indicate that deaf persons have essentially the same intelligence and manual dexterity that the hearing have. Their work habits are good and they are stable in job tenure, as shown in recent surveys. Yet, their achievement levels in education, technical and professional employment, and psychosocial areas are demonstrated to be unnecessarily low.

Evidence is given that demonstrates this low achievement to be primarily due to: (1) inappropriate educational methodology and inadequate educational programs; (2) lack of foresight in the directions of vocational-technical education and related counseling; (3) lack of closer working relationships between schools and rehabilitation; (4) a gap between needs of deaf people for services designed to prepare them for appropriate levels of work and the demand by deaf people for these opportunities; (5) inadequate preparation and use of deaf persons at professional decisionmaking levels; (6) a lack of understanding and research on the gross failure of schools to serve deaf youths adequately; (7) a lack of strong specialized job placement services for deaf clients; (8) a need for more counselors professionally prepared to serve deaf clients; (9) additional facilities qualified to give vocational-technical education to deaf youth, including those who are multiply handicapped; and (10) changes in education that will bring an end to presently ineffectual programs.

THE REHABILITATION PROCESS

COUNSELING

Granted there are certain differences which characterize most deaf clients, their job opportunities, and the nature of their communication. What then are modifications or requirements which help in providing good counseling with deaf clients?

Concrete vs. Abstract. There have been serious doubts raised about the value of abstract counseling and therapeutic approaches in work with the normal hearing client (Ullman and Krasner, 1965). With most deaf clients there is no real argument. Counseling must be concrete. Effort at the use of such techniques as classical psychoanalysis has failed, even in the hands of highly skilled therapists (Rainer, Altschuler, Kallmann, and Deming, 1963). Rogerians attempting to reflect affective overtones are responding with "hmmm's" which cannot be lipread and for which there is no sign. They soon see their technique as inappropriate with the average deaf client.

Successful counseling with most deaf persons and perhaps with people in general must be related in direct ways to the here and now. For example, this means the counselor goes with the client on a job interview instead of talking in his office in general terms about interview procedures. Counseling is best done on the job or in the job evaluation center, where actual behavior and specific incidents can be dealt with. It means environmental manipulation, talking to employers, getting the family to help, and giving support instead of abstractly discussing superego problems, displacement of unconscious drives, and other valid but intangible therapeutic concepts. The immaturity and the communication limitations of many deaf clients often make abstract procedures, when used, a useless tour de force.

Communication Modality. The few deaf persons who prefer speech and lipreading as the means of communication in counseling should have their wishes respected. The same is true for the overwhelming majority who prefer manual communication and those who want to write.

In the case of the counselor who cannot fingerspell or use the language of signs, an interpreter should be available to assist those clients needing this service. (Interpreters can be readily located by writing to the National Registry of Interpreters, 814 Thayer Street, Silver Spring, Maryland, 20910 or by contacting a local club for the deaf.)

It must be recognized that although the use of the language of signs can greatly facilitate communication, it is limited by the basic linguistic competence of the deaf client and the manual skills of the counselor or interpreter. Simply making a lot of signs does not insure communication, nor does it overcome the basic vocabulary problem of a semiliterate deaf client.

Job Placement. Good counseling deals realistically with the client's weaknesses as well as his strengths. As indicated earlier, locating a job and then applying for it often represents major, if not insurmountable, obstacles to many otherwise capable deaf persons. Counseling that ignores this or avoids it is oblivious to or unconcerned about the needs of a majority of deaf rehabilitation clients.

Unfortunately, some training centers are downgrading the placement function of counseling in their misguided efforts to elevate the status of counselors (Sussman and Stewart, 1971). This is a serious error in the case of programs preparing counselors to work with deaf clients. Job placement is an essential function of counseling the deaf. Furthermore, it should involve follow-up, wherein the counselor sees the employee and the supervisor to aid in working out possible difficulties. Good counselors have extensive contacts among employers, and they use these contacts as a service to both the employers and the clients.

General Information. Deaf clients often need guidance regarding the feasibility of their job desires, especially where levels of aspiration are not in keeping with abilities. Sometimes work evaluation programs are the best way to convey what is realistic in these cases. At other times, it is necessary to actually let the client try an inappropriate training program or job before it is possible to counsel in terms of more suitable goals.

Occasionally help in manners and appearance is necessary. For example, a deaf person may make offensive noises and not know it. Small things like this can mean the difference between success and failure in obtaining and keeping employment. Likewise, knowing how to dress for an interview or how to fill out the forms is important.

Counseling vs. Psychotherapy. Professional journals and meetings are replete with articles and papers on the differences between counseling and psychotherapy. However, the distinctions made are artificial, as Dr. Roy R. Grinker, Sr., has indicated (Grinker, MacGregor, Selan, Klein, and Kohrman, 1961). Counselors must, therefore, be prepared to meet the responsibilities of the therapeutic relationship with a recognition that certain cases will need to be referred for more intensive care than the rehabilitation counselor is able to provide.

Training Opportunities. The training needs of some deaf persons can be met by the use of available local facilities established for the hearing. Coordinating these services into a rehabilitation program is an important function of counseling. However, many deaf people require highly specialized training staffs if they are to be properly prepared for work. In recognition of this, the Vocational Rehabilitation Administration in conjunction with state governments initiated a number of such programs. These have been increased by the Social and Rehabilitation Service. Gallaudet College, the National Technical Institute, and the Riverside City College Program are examples of postsecondary opportunities especially designed to serve the deaf. The Hot Springs Rehabilitation Center is an example of a training facility for vocational and/or social adjustment skills. Any counselor serving deaf clients should be aware of all of these programs as well as of community resources. He should not only know what the programs offer but also how a deaf person goes about enrolling for them. Unfortunately, some of the special programs for the deaf do not adequately inform vocational counselors about their services and these programs, and consequently have vacancies that could meet the needs of some deaf people. This tragic failure is inexcusable. It must be corrected if rehabilitation is to be efficient and effective.

Oral Training and Hearing Aids. The naive counselor often sees the hearing aid and a few lessons in oral communication as the answer to the problems of the deaf client. As indicated earlier, too often otologists and other specialists are subject to the same fantasy. For many deaf people this sort of treatment is all they ever get. The real problem of deafness is ignored. Instead, worthless prostheses and lessons continue to be prescribed. Individuals who have gone through six to twelve years of oral training (as have most deaf persons) and have not developed speech and speechreading are not likely to do so as adults. Additional time and money spent for these services are frequently wasted. Hearing aids can be of value if the impairment is not too severe, but in losses averaging 70 decibels or greater in the speech range, they are rarely helpful to adults who have never used them. Even in milder losses they do not always help. It is important that counseling about this be based on the client's wish and advice from a specialist who knows deafness, and not just those from audiology or otology who know the ear.

Theoretical Consideration. The orientation of this chapter has been essentially descriptive and pragmatic. Theoretical considerations of the effects of deafness on basic personality dynamics and the relationship of these effects to psychotherapeutic interaction and counseling have been avoided. One reason for this is that the present state of "the psychology of deafness" has not yet yielded extensive verified information of this depth. Certain facts have been established or at least some basic questions have been asked.

It is known that organic brain damage is disproportionately prevalent among the deaf and may account in part for the number of impulse disorders reported among the deaf. Vernon (1969) studied major etiologies of deafness which are also associated with brain damage and has reported on the behavioral correlates of these disease conditions. While interesting relative to the relationships between brain lesions and behavior, this work is difficult to apply directly in counseling.

Myklebust (1960) and Vernon and Rothstein (1967) have speculated on the effects of auditory deprivation on nerve tissue and on conceptual organization, but no conclusive body of research data has evolved. Work with the deaf mentally ill in New York City (Rainer, Altshuler, Kallmann, and Deming, 1963) has provided useful descriptive and demographic findings but has not dealt extensively with the theoretical aspects of the deafness variable in human behavior.

SUMMARY

Federal and state programs are rapidly making adequate counseling services for deaf persons a reality. In order that it be effective, the counseling process as it relates to deaf clients must be better understood in terms of the counselor, the counselee, and the interaction between them.

The major characteristic of a deaf counselee requiring adaptations of the counseling process is the communication difficulty associated with early profound hearing loss. This in turn manifests itself in low academic achievement despite a normally distributed intelligence. Vocational patterns and goals are subject to the double effect of both limited educational levels and varying degrees of communication difficulty. Despite these difficulties, the income of deaf workers approaches national norms, and the deaf as a group demonstrate stability of job tenure and satisfactory work habits. While most deaf people are employed with hearing people, they generally prefer to spend their social life with other deaf individuals.

Standards and requirements of counselors desiring to work with the deaf are rising, but the most important criterion of all remains the proficient use of the language of signs. Without this, there can be no counseling with the majority of deaf rehabilitation clients.

In the counseling process itself certain things should be emphasized. Among them are the need to be concrete and specific in communicating, the role of job placement, and the responsibility of the counselor to know about available special vocational-technical training facilities. Care must be taken to appraise realistically the advantages of oral training and hearing aids for adult clients with no history of success in speech or the use of amplification.

EVALUATION

Medical. The leading etiologies of deafness frequently leave the client with other disabilities in addition to the hearing loss. Conditions such as prenatal rubella, meningitis, complications of Rh factor, and prematurity, which account for from one third to one half of all deafness of early onset, are also known to be associated with brain damage, learning disabilities, aphasia, mental illness, and other disorders (Vernon, 1969). In the case of the deaf client the very presence of the hearing loss is already evidence of major neurological damage, evidence which increases the probability of other pathology within the nervous system.

The medical examination of impaired hearing assumes primary importance. First, it must assess the nature and degree of the hearing loss with particular attention to whether or not the loss is surgically correctable or whether referral for hearing aid evaluation is in order. Second, it is important to determine if there are other disabilities present, particularly visual ones. Where so crucial a sensory modality as hearing is defective, special care must be taken to protect those remaining.

Psychological. The deaf person who is characterized by the kinds of problems which most rehabilitation services are designed to handle requires special psychological procedures for psychodiagnostics and interviewing (Levine, 1971, 1960). It is the purpose of this section to summarize cautions and techniques that will lead to more effective psychological evaluations.

The communication difficulties caused by deafness were discussed earlier. It is these problems that make the proper psychological evaluation of deaf persons a difficult and specialized procedure. When it is realized that conventional psychological evaluation consists of interviewing or the use of psychometric instruments involving sophisticated levels of language development, it becomes readily apparent that the deaf client's language deficiency and his limitation in oral communication make these conventional approaches inappropriate for and unjust to the deaf client. Instead of measuring his intelligence, personality, and vocational aptitudes, most traditional tests reflect his communication disability. There is ample proof of this evaluation injustice in the cases of mentally normal deaf individuals hospitalized as mental defectives on the basis of IQ tests involving language. Later, in nonlanguage IQ tests, these same individuals are found to be average or even above average in intelligence and to have the ability to function adequately in a public-school program for the deaf.

Interviewing. If interviewing is to be a part of psychological screening, it is essential that the deaf client be provided with the opportunity to have his interview conducted through fingerspelling and the language of signs if he feels this would be helpful. Either an examiner known to be qualified in manual communication should be used or else a person certified by the National Registry of Interpreters should be engaged to interpret the interview.

Psychological Testing. Tests are often used by psychologists or by employers to provide information concerning areas such as intelligence, personality structure, educational achievement, and vocational aptitudes. Where clients with average hearing are to be evaluated in these areas, then the same process should be followed for the applicant with profound hearing loss. However, specific tests used, their administration, and their interpretation must be adapted to the communication problems of deaf persons. A clear understanding of the factors that follow should precede any efforts to test or interpret test findings with deaf clients.

In intelligence testing:

1) To be useful as a measure of the intelligence of a person with a severe hearing loss of early onset, an intelligence test must in most cases be a nonlanguage performance instrument. Verbal-intelligence tests are almost always inappropriate because they measure language deficiency due to deafness rather than intelligence.

It should be noted that not all nonverbal tests are appropriate. One reason is that while many nonverbal tests have performance items, their administration may nevertheless require verbal directions. Hard-of-hearing persons may give the impression of being able to understand verbal tests, but this is often misleading. In testing such a client it is essential to begin with a performance measure and then, if desired, to try a verbal instrument. In cases where the score yielded by the former is appreciably higher, the probability is that it is the more valid measure. The lower score on the test involving language may be entirely due to the subject's hearing impairment.

2) There is far more danger that a low IQ score is wrong than that a high one is inaccurate. This is due to the many factors, such as illness, motivation, etc., that can lead to an individual's not performing to capacity. In contrast, only remarkable luck in guessing, cribbing, or practice on the test can lead to spuriously high scores.

3) Tests given to deaf persons by psychologists not experienced with the hearing impaired are subject to appreciably greater error than is the case when the service is rendered by one familiar with deaf persons. The faulty responses of deaf clients to testing are felt to be one of the outcomes of this. For example, deaf youths sometimes think it very important to finish quickly and will therefore answer randomly. A tester experienced with the deaf can pick this up far more readily than one who does not "know" the deaf.

4) It must be noted that the performance part of some conventional intelligence tests is only half or less of the test. Therefore, to approach the validity of a full IQ test with a deaf person, it may be necessary to use nonlanguage portions of a variety of tests.

5) Group testing of deaf and hard-of-hearing-youths is a dubious procedure that, at best, is of use only as a gross screening device.

In personality testing:

1) Personality evaluation is a far more complex task than is IQ testing, especially with deaf persons. Because of this, test findings should be carefully interpreted in light of case history data and/or personal experience with the individual.

2) Because of communication problems inherent with a severe hearing loss, personality tests are more difficult to use with deaf subjects than with the general population. Not only do these tests depend on ex-

tensive verbal interchange or reading skill, but they also presuppose a rapport on the part of the subject that is difficult to achieve when the person examined cannot understand what is being said or written. The need for fluency in manual communication by the examiner is especially evident in the area of projective testing. The use of an interpreter for personality testing is a questionable procedure because it would require that the interpreter be not only fluent in manual communication but also adept in psychology and testing. Obviously such an individual would be doing the examining himself and not interpreting for another. In view of the lack of available personality tests and the total absence of norms for deaf populations, it is necessary in personality evaluation to look very carefully at full and accurate case history data (Levine, 1960).

In testing educational achievement:

Most clients who have attended an educational program for the deaf or hard of hearing have already taken educational achievement tests. This experience is helpful and makes such testing easier. However, here again it is important that the person doing the educational achievement evaluation be an experienced teacher or psychologist with the deaf.

In vocational aptitude testing:

It is not feasible to recommend specific tests of vocational aptitude which should be used, because their selection is a highly individual matter depending on the person being evaluated and the available vocational offerings. In general, however, nonverbal tests should be used, qualified examiners experienced with hearing-impaired youth should administer them, and interpreters should be used in giving directions and answering questions if the examiners are not fluent in manual communication. The kinds of tests commonly used with the deaf can be found in reviews by Levine (1960, 1971) and Vernon (1964).

TRENDS AND ISSUES

Rehabilitation in the near future will be determined by several major issues in addition to those described earlier. In brief these are as follows:

1) The degree of involvement of the deaf community in policymaking and leadership roles.

2) The extent to which services, training, and research in deafness change from "soft money" short-term grants and demonstration projects into permanently legislated and funded programs.

3) The exceptions to governmental policy generalizations on defederalization which will permit certain primary policy decisions to remain centralized federally.

4) The extent to which those with little knowledge of or contact with the adult deaf community cease to be in decisionmaking roles in rehabilitation and education.

5) The power of the deaf community and professionals in deafness to exercise effectively their political rights and influence in the interests of deaf youths and adults.

PSYCHOLOGICAL COUNSELING:
AN ILLUSTRATIVE CASE

We conclude this chapter with one of the few, if not the only, published verbatim account of a counseling session between a deaf counselee and a deaf professional psychological counselor (Sussman, 1970). It is illustrative not only of some of the problems of deaf persons stemming from communication tensions, and this despite good communications skills, but also of the rapport possible when a qualified psychological counselor who is himself deaf deals with a deaf patient. We quote as follows:

Mary was a 27-year-old woman born with a severe hearing loss. When she was four years old her parents, noting that she did not respond to sounds other than loud noises, had her examined by an audiologist. The audiologist diagnosed the problem as one of serious loss of hearing, but told her parents that if she wore a hearing aid and attended public school, Mary would be "just like any other child." The parents were told that under no circumstances was Mary to be allowed to use sign language, for its use would destroy her chances for leading a normal life. The parents, being from an ethnic group that gave unswerving loyalty to the voice of authority (in this case, the audiologist), vowed to themselves that they would do everything in their power to see that their daughter grew up like "everybody else." To this end they had Mary fitted with a hearing aid, sent her to a preschool class for hearing-impaired children, talked to her constantly without using sign language, and forbade her to have friends who used sign language. She soon

enrolled in public school and, assimilating her parents' negative evaluation
of deafness, tried every way within her power to appear as a "hearing person." In school she would sit in the front row and strain unceasingly to follow her teacher's speech through lipreading and what little residual hearing
remained. In order to avoid the uncertainty and anxiety of having to communicate normally in a group of her peers, Mary would go home after
school rather than join groups of her schoolmates in the school snackbar, at
school activities, and the like. She went through junior and senior high
school in this manner, barely managing to pass her courses and becoming
something of a "loner." Following graduation from high school Mary went
into her parents' business, helping out in a role that brought her into contact with people with whom she found it difficult to communicate. Many
embarrassing situations developed from her misunderstanding of comments
and requests made by customers. Yet she continued at her parents' insis-
tence. Later her mother died and her father, deeply affected by his wife's
death, grew listless and despondent and gave the burden of the family business to Mary. Mary, struggling to keep the business going, made mistake
after mistake with customers because of deafness. Finally, out of frustration,
she and her father sold the business and her father retired. Mary, then 22
years old, met and became friends with an audiologist who encouraged her
to study toward her bachelor's degree in the education of the deaf. Encouraged by the first person who accepted her for what she was, she enrolled at
a large state university and finally reached her senior year there. It was at
this time that Mary came for counseling. She had struggled her way through
semester after semester of courses having large groups of students and little
close contact with the instructors. She finally entered the practicum courses
in the teacher preparation program, and had to do practice teaching in public school with normally hearing children. By this time, however, Mary had
developed a severe anxiety reaction. She was extremely nervous when talking to others. Her voice, soft and clearly understandable when she was with
friends, would become harsh and strident when she was with people she did
not know well or when she felt she was under pressure. She was also given
to frequent periods of sleeplessness and despondence. Her college faculty adviser, who had a master's degree in education of the deaf, scolded her often
for not trying to lipread better and for ostensibly using her deafness as a
crutch. The audiologist who had advised Mary to attend college noted her
tense state and suggested she seek counseling and tutoring in sign language.
Interestingly, Mary made no progress in the manual communication class,
and her teacher reported that she was not capable of learning the language.
When Mary came for her first counseling session she appeared extremely
tense and ill at ease. She began speaking to the counselor, who explained
that he could not hear and that she would have to speak slowly and fingerspell and sign for him. Following is an excerpt from the first session:

Counselor: Mary, I cannot hear so you will have to speak slowly for me, or if you can sign that will help. We can also write if we find it necessary.

Mary: (Stuttering and having difficulty speaking) . . . I . . . I cannot sign. Maybe, may—be my teach—er told you I can't . . . learn to sign? (Smiles apologetically, swallowing with difficulty, and averts her head in painful self-consciousness.)

Counselor: We won't worry about that right now. Let's just get to know each other a little better. I understand that you wanted to see me because you were having difficulty learning to use sign language. Can you explain a little about why you want to learn signs and just what problems you are having in learning? (Note: The counselor spoke and used sign language simultaneously. Mary could understand him quite well through lipreading, but he intentionally used sign language to help her become accustomed to it.)

Mary: (Looking away, then returning her gaze to the counselor, painfully) . . . I . . . I don't know why . . . I can't learn. I am so nervous . . . (Looks distressed) . . . I am trying to learn because my speech teacher . . . thinks it will help my speech. But (hopelessly shaking her head) . . . I just can't seem to learn. My sign language teacher has spent a lot of time with me and says . . . she says I just can't learn to fingerspell. (Note: Mary was speaking slowly and haltingly, obviously very anxious, but she would occasionally spell a word for the counselor in surprisingly good fingerspelling.)

Counselor: One of the best ways to learn to use sign language is to practice with deaf people. Do you have any deaf friends or acquaintances, or do you ever practice in the classroom?

Mary: Oh, no! I do not know any deaf people. My parents did not want me to learn signs and would not let me bring home any deaf people who signed, so I have no one to practice with. (Here Mary had forgotten herself and was speaking and signing without hesitation.)

Counselor: That must have been hard on you. Do you communicate well with people who do not use sign language?

Mary: I can read lips quite well, and I can hear some. I do okay when a person is speaking directly to me, but in class and in groups I get lost.

The first session continued mostly in this manner. As it turned out, Mary could sign quite well when she relaxed, but she seldom relaxed with people who did not understand her hearing loss. Over the course of the next few sessions this was discussed with Mary, who admitted that her problem was that she would become nervous and panic-stricken in her sign language classes as well as in many other situations. Thus, what appeared as an inability to sign was actually acute anxiety and inability to function. Subsequent sessions revealed that Mary had an extremely negative self concept.

She perceived deafness and anything associated with it (e.g., sign language) as undesirable, yet she was acutely conscious of the fact that she was deaf. She had spent years denying her deafness and putting on a false facade, as shown in the following exchange:

Counselor: You have difficulty following what is being said in a group, and yet you refuse to tell others you have a hearing loss. Why do you think you do like that?

Mary: (Shaking her head slowly) I . . . I . . . I just can't do it. With you I can be myself because I don't have to hide anything. You understand my problem, and you accept me as I am. I can't be this way with other people. It makes me so ashamed for others to know I am different.

Counselor: I am not sure I understand just what you mean, Mary. What I see in what you are saying is that I know what you are, and I accept you as you are, and your being what you are is still good. On the other hand, it seems you think if others knew what you are—deaf—they would see you as unworthy and would not accept you. This you could not stand. Is this true?

Mary: (Thinking for a few moments) . . . I think that is it. I know my deafness means nothing to you, but with others I feel it means everything. I just can't stand for others to know. I know, really, that deafness is not that bad, but I can't help feeling this way. I have thought and thought about it and I know I am being silly, but that doesn't change how I feel.

Counselor: I believe I can understand how you feel, Mary. Your feelings about your deafness are a part of you, and although you know consciously that your deafness is something that is not your fault, you can't help being ashamed. (Pause) . . . Can you tell me whether the rejection —or negative feelings—you perceive in others could possibly be your own feelings toward yourself, rather than real feelings people have toward your deafness?

Mary: (Appearing shocked) You mean other people don't see me as bad, that the feelings I see in others are really my own feelings? (Becoming angry now.)

Counselor: I see this idea is upsetting you. Can you help me understand why it bothers you?

Mary: (With some hostility) . . . Yes! It does bother me! I am not imagining things. You make me feel like you don't believe me! You make me feel like it is all my fault, like my adviser said.

Counselor: I can see that this really bothers you, so there must be something important in what we are saying. But, I did not say that it was your fault. I said only that perhaps the bad feelings you have about having others know about your deafness actually reflect some of your own attitudes to-

ward deafness. In other words, you see deafness making you unworthy
. . . inferior . . . and you think others feel the same way.
Mary: (Looking shaken) . . . I . . . I can . . . hardly believe what you are
saying. But it hurts . . . you are right . . . I hate myself (begins to cry
brokenly).

This was the turning point for Mary, who had absorbed her parents' deval-
uation of her deafness and who had for years carried the heavy burden imposed upon those who try to be what they are not. In subsequent interviews
Mary became more and more aware of her own attitudes toward deafness
with her entire being, and of rejecting herself as a person just as she rejected
her deafness. With this realization and through social interaction with other
deaf adults, Mary was slowly able to work through the negative feelings she
had accumulated toward herself and her hearing loss. At the termination of
counseling, Mary had learned to use manual communication very well, was
more relaxed with others, readily mentioned her hearing loss when she
could not understand someone, was going steady with a deaf man, and had
obtained a job as a teacher of young children in a school for the deaf.
Everything was not rosy, however; Mary still experienced periods of anxiety
and self-doubt. The roots of self-rejection, planted in childhood, are not so
easily uprooted. Perhaps this is a lesson for those who would deny a deaf
child any method of communication, or not permit him to make effective
adjustments in life as a *deaf* person rather than as a poor facsimile of a
hearing person (Sussman, 1970).

MAJOR NATIONAL ORGANIZATIONS

There are organizations of adult deaf people, rehabilitation agencies,
special education facilities, parent of deaf children associations, speech
and hearing associations, and almost countless other programs which
have some relationship to services for the deaf. These are listed annually in the *Directory* issue of the *American Annals of the Deaf,*
available at many libraries or from the business office at 5034 Wisconsin Avenue, Northwest, Washington, D.C. 20006.

Investigator	Sample	Results
Meadow (1968)	56 deaf children of deaf parents (manual group)	1) Manual group better in reading (2.1 yrs.) 2) Manual group better in math (1.25 yrs.)
	56 matched deaf children of hearing parents (oral group)	3) Manual group better in overall education achievement (1.28 yrs.) 4) Manual group better in social adjustment 5) No differences in speech and lip-reading 6) Manual group better in written language
Stuckless and Birch (1966)	105 deaf children of deaf parents (manual group)	1) No difference in speech 2) Early manual group better in speech-reading
	337 matched deaf children of hearing parents (oral group)	3) Early manual group better in reading 4) Early manual group better in writing 5) Early manual group possibly better in psycho-social adjustment
Montgomery (1966) *	59 Scottish children	1) Exposure to, use of, and preference for manual communication did not negatively affect speech or speech-reading skills
Stevenson (1964)	134 deaf children of deaf parents (manual group)	1) 90 percent of manual group did better than matched oral students
	134 deaf children of hearing parents (oral group)	2) 38 percent of manual group went to college versus nine percent of oral group

RESULTS OF EARLY MANUAL COMMUNICATION (*continued*)

Investigator	Sample	Results
Quigley and Frisina (1961)	Sixteen non-residential deaf children of deaf parents (manual group). Sixteen non-residential deaf children of hearing parents (oral group)	1) Manual group better in vocabulary, speechreading and better in educational achievement. Oral group better in speech.
Hester (1963)	Deaf children in New Mexico School for Deaf. One group had finger-spelling beginning at school age, one group taught orally.	1) Fingerspelling group superior on standardized achievement tests.
Quigley (1969) †	Sixteen orally educated deaf children matched with sixteen combined orally and manually educated deaf children.	1) Combined manual oral children did better in language, speechreading, and general academic achievement.
Denton (1965)	The academic top ten percent of deaf children ages twelve, fifteen, and eighteen from 26 schools for deaf. Manual group had deaf parents, oral group hearing parents.	1) Mean achievement test score of manual group 8.2, of oral group 7.7.

* The Montgomery study did not involve preschool manual communication specifically.

† Quigley, S. P.: The influence of fingerspelling and the development of language, communication, and educational achievement in deaf children. Mimeographed report. Department of Special Education, University of Illinois, Champaign, Illinois, 1969.

COMPARISON OF EARLY MANUAL AND EARLY ORAL PRESCHOOL AND EARLY ORAL DEAF CHILDREN WITHOUT PRESCHOOL EDUCATION [1]

Variables	Children with Early Manual Communication and No Preschool [2]	Children with Three Years of Tracy Clinic Oral Preschool Education	Children with No Preschool, but an Early Oral Environment	Tests for significance of Difference
Matching Variables				
Age	18.2 years	18.5 years	18.7 years	$F_{(2,66)} = .29 \, p > .05$
IQ	116	114	114	$F_{(2,66)} = .29 \, p > .05$
Stanford Achievement				
Test Scores				
Paragraph meaning	7.6	6.1	6.2	$F_{(2,66)} = 3.60 \, p < .05$
Word meaning	7.0	5.9	5.8	$F_{(2,66)} = 2.50 \, p > .05$
Reading Average	7.3	6.0	6.0	$F_{(2,66)} = 3.51 \, p < .05$
Total Stanford Average	8.9	7.9	7.8	$F_{(2,66)} = 1.39 \, p > .05$

[1] Table based on original research by Vernon, M., and Koh, S., Michael Reese Hospital, 1969; sample: 23 matched pairs.
[2] Had deaf parents.

REFERENCES

Babbidge, H. D. 1964. Education of the deaf: a report to the Secretary of Health, Education and Welfare by his Advisory Committee on the Education of the Deaf. U.S. Department of Health, Education and Welfare. Washington, D.C.

Berg, F. S. and S. G. Fletcher. 1970. The hard of hearing child. New York, Grune and Stratton.

Boatner, E. B. November 6, 1965. The need of a realistic approach to the education of the deaf. Paper presented at the joint convention, Calif. Assn. Teachers of the Deaf and Hard of Hearing, and the Calif. Assn. of the Deaf.

Boatner, E. B., E. R. Stuckless, and D. F. Moores. 1964. Occupational status of the young adult deaf of New England and demand for a regional technical-vocational training center. West Hartford, Conn., American School for the Deaf.

Bowe, F. G. 1971. About Black and Puerto Rican deaf people. Deaf American 24:16.

Boyd, J. 1967. Comparisons of motor behavior in deaf and hearing boys. Amer. Annals of the Deaf 112:598–605.

Carhart, R. 1970. Human communication and its disorders: an overview. Bethesda, Md., National Institute of Neurological Diseases and Stroke, Monograph No. 10, p. 10.

Doctor, P. V. 1970. Summary statement of pupils and teachers in the U.S. Directory Issue, Amer. Annals of the Deaf 115:405.

Furfey, P. H., and T. J. Harte. 1964. Interaction of deaf and hearing in Frederick County, Maryland. Washington, D.C., Catholic University.

Furth, H. G. 1966. Thinking without language. New York, Free Press.

Grinker, R. G., H. MacGregor, K. Selan, A. Klein, and J. Kohrman. 1961. Psychiatric social work: a transactional casebook. New York, Basic Books.

Grinker, R. G., ed. 1969. Psychiatric diagnosis, therapy, and research on the psychotic deaf. Final Report Grant # RD-2407-S, Social Rehabilitation Service, Department of Health, Education and Welfare (available from Dr. Grinker, Michael Reese Hospital, 2959 S. Ellis, Chicago, Ill.

Jensen, A. R. 1969. How much can we boost IQ and scholastic achievement? Harvard Educational Rev. 39:1–123.

Kronenberg, H. H. and G. D. Blake. 1966. Young deaf adults: an occupational survey. Department of Health, Education and Welfare, Vocational Rehabilitation Administration. Washington, D. C.

Levine, E. S. 1971. Mental assessment of the deaf child. Volta Review 73:80–105.

—— 1960. The psychology of deafness. New York, Columbia University Press.

Lowell, E. L. 1959. Research in speechreading: some relationships to language development and implications for the classroom teacher. Report of the Proceedings of the 39th Meeting of the Convention of American Instructors of the Deaf, pp. 68–73.

McClure, W. J. 1966. Current problems and trends in the education of the deaf. Deaf American 18:8–14.

Myklebust, H. 1960. The psychology of deafness. New York, Grune and Stratton.

Patterson, C. H. and L. G. Stewart. 1971. Principles of counseling with deaf people, in A. E. Sussman and L. G. Stewart, eds., Counseling with deaf people. New York, New York University Deafness Research and Training Center, pp. 43–86.

Rainer, J. D., K. Z. Altshuler, F. J. Kallmann, and W. E. Deming, eds. 1963. Family and mental health problems in a deaf population. New York. New York State Psychiatric Institute.

de Reynier, J. P. 1970. Deafness in the world today. WHO Chronicle 24:1.

Rose, E. F. Civil Service. Paper given at the Institute for Advanced Study, De Paul University, Chicago, July, 1967.

Schein, J. D. and S. Bushnaq. 1962. Higher education for the deaf in the United States—a retrospective investigation. Amer. Annals of the Deaf 107:416–20.

Sussman, A. E. 1970. The comprehensive counseling needs of deaf persons. Hearing and Speech News 38:12–13, 22, 24.

Sussman, A. E. and L. G. Stewart, eds. 1971. Counseling with deaf people. New York, New York University Deafness Research and Training Center.

Switzer, Mary E. and B. R. Williams. 1967. Life problems of deaf people. Arch. Envir. Health 15:249–56.

Ullman, L. T., and L. Krasner. 1965. Case studies in behavioral modification. New York, Holt, Rinehart, and Winston.

Vernon, M. 1970. Potential, achievement, and rehabilitation in the deaf population. Rehabilitation Literature 31:258–67.

—— 1968. Fifty years of research on the intelligence of deaf and hard of hearing children: a review of literature and discussion of implications. J. Rehabilitation of the Deaf 1:1–12(b).

—— 1968. Current etiological factors in deafness. Amer. Annals of the Deaf 113:1–12(a).

—— 1969. Multiply handicapped deaf children: medical, educational, and psychological aspects. Washington, D.C., Council of Exceptional Children.

Vernon, M. and D. W. Brown. 1964. A guide to psychological tests and testing procedures in the evaluation of deaf and hard of hearing children. Journal of Speech and Hearing Disorders 29:4:414–23.

Vernon, M. and S. D. Koh. 1970. Early manual communication and deaf children's achievement. Amer. Annals of the Deaf 115:527–36.

Vernon, M. and D. A. Rothstein. 1967. Prelingual deafness: an experiment of nature. Archives of General Psychiatry 16:325–33.

Vernon, M. and J. Snyder. 1972. Post-secondary programs for deaf people. ASHA.

Wrightstone, J. W., M. S. Aronow, and S. Muskowitz. 1963. Developing reading test norms for deaf children. Amer. Annals of the Deaf 108:311–16.

HARRY J. SPAR

THE DEAF-BLIND

FEELINGS OF REVULSION during early contacts with obvious and seri-ously handicapping disabilities are quite common and are probably in-stinctive. The wolf pack, for example, or the chicken flock are known to ostracize and sometimes to attack any of their members who become disabled. Man, who is a social animal, undoubtedly retains vestiges of some of the same drive for preserving the natural strength of the social group of which he is a part that motivates more primitive social animals to reject any of their group who exhibit weaknesses that threaten group security.

These feelings of revulsion and a sense of guilt for experiencing them tend to create avoidance of seriously handicapped individuals by most people who have not had much contact with them. Coping with this avoidance is a major problem of deaf-blind persons. It is made particu-larly difficult by the special limitations in their ability to communicate.

Action research in methods of reducing the barriers between the community and its deaf-blind members corroborates the observations of many workers with the deaf-blind that contact with such persons gener-ally dissipates the barriers (Rusalem, 1964, 1967). Information about the nature and implications of deaf-blindness and about the achieve-ments of deaf-blind individuals can develop an acceptance of deaf-blind persons on an intellectual level which is usually accompanied by dimin-ished or suppressed feelings toward their disability. Personal contacts with deaf-blind persons generally result in genuine acceptance and fre-

HARRY J. SPAR is Associate Director, National Center for Deaf-Blind Youths and Adults, New Hyde Park, N.Y.

quently lead to convictions and enthusiasm about them as human beings that have important and extensive spill-over effects.

Wide dissemination of information through public education media may help to create a favorable atmosphere in the community toward deaf-blind persons, but it is difficult to assess the quality or the durability of this atmosphere. The public cannot be expected to devote the time nor to possess the capacity necessary to acquire a sound and lasting understanding of the special problems of all the numerous small subgroups in the community. To improve understanding and acceptance of deaf-blind persons therefore requires a selective concentration of effort on individuals and segments of a community who are in the best position to improve social, vocational, and economic opportunities for deaf-blind persons. These efforts, it seems clear, can best be served by helping to bring the deaf-blind into direct contact with appropriate individuals and groups so that deaf-blind persons themselves can exercise their influence on the feelings and attitudes of those in the community who are important to their welfare.

PROBLEM OF DEFINITION

A major problem in the effort to identify the deaf-blind population lies in the fact that there is not as yet any common accord as to what constitutes deaf-blindness.

In an agreement between the United States Department of Health, Education and Welfare and The Industrial Home for the Blind in connection with the operation of the National Center for Deaf-Blind Youths and Adults, "Deaf-Blind" and "Deaf and Blind" persons are designated as those "who have substantial visual and hearing losses such that the combination of the two causes extreme difficulty in learning." This designation encompasses a fairly broad group of visually and auditorily impaired individuals. The size of the group can be significantly affected by subjective interpretation of "extreme difficulty in learning" as well as by the influence of mental ability, motivation, and other factors which are extraneous to the degrees of visual and auditory losses involved. However, the designation provides practical parameters in which to develop a simple, objective, and restrictive definition of deaf-blind, with room for exceptions to the restrictions where clearly warranted in individual cases and with a basis for giving priority attention to those most severely handicapped by visual and auditory losses who are least likely to receive any services from local resources.

The National Center currently employs a restrictive definition of "deaf-blindness":

Blindness is defined as central visual acuity of 20/200 or less in the better eye with correcting glasses, or central visual acuity of more than 20/200 if there is a field defect such that the peripheral field has been contracted to an extent that the widest diameter of visual field subtends an angular distance no greater than 20 degrees and deafness is defined as a chronic impairment of hearing so severe that most speech cannot be understood, even with optimum amplification.

In recent years, the increased incidence of brain damage accompanying deaf-blindness has pointed up the need for adding a specified decibel loss within the speech range to the definition of deafness to help assure that the inability to understand most speech results primarily from a major hearing loss rather than from major mental deficiency. Particular care must be taken to avoid dissipating resources being developed for the rehabilitation of deaf-blind persons through misapplication to persons with communication difficulties who are not deaf and who might be more effectively served in programs specifically designed to meet the problems related to their particular handicaps.

The blind have enjoyed a widely accepted definition of "blind" for over thirty years. It grew out of a definition of "economic blindness" developed by a Committee of the Section on Ophthalmology of the American Medical Association in 1932 (*Journal of the American Medical Association,* 1934). With minor modifications, it was incorporated into many federal and local laws and regulations, and made it possible for the blind to be among the first handicapped group to enjoy several special benefits and services such as exemptions on earnings of recipients of public assistance, special tax exemptions, etc.

The advantages of being able to identify a handicapped group by definition lie, first, in the ability of any legislative body to obtain a reasonably accurate estimate of the dimensions of any special service or benefit which it is asked to provide for the particular group; and, second, in the ability of any specialized agency or program established for the group to use its resources for the purpose for which they are provided rather than diverting them to more easily attainable purposes.

In recent years, unfortunately, many agencies for the blind have been enticed into changing their designations from "for the blind" to "for the visually handicapped" by the fact that their work could be made easier by broadening their clientele to include less severely disabled individuals. Generally, they have rationalized this action by pointing out that it enabled them to serve more people, and in so doing to receive more substantial support for their work and in the case of sheltered workshops to produce a wider variety of goods and services. They have maintained that these advantages would accrue to the benefit of the blind members of their clientele. However, experience is demonstrating that services for these blind members are being significantly replaced by services for an increasing proportion of their clientele who are not sufficiently visually handicapped to be classified as "blind." For example, under regulations issued pursuant to the Wagner-O'Day Act, where 75 per cent of the direct labor is required to be "blind labor" in order for a workshop to receive priority in the opportunity to manufacture goods for the federal government, a number of workshops for the visually handicapped have so reduced the number of their blind clientele that they can no longer qualify for government work.

On the basis of experience with the blind, it seems clear that more deaf-blind persons will receive more of the specialized services required in their rehabilitation if a fairly restrictive and clear definition of deaf-blindness can be developed and widely applied. Some controversy exists as to whether the definition should be liberal or restrictive. Unquestionably, many individuals with moderate impairments of vision and hearing could benefit from specialized services designed to meet the problems related to such impairment. But these individuals may generally expect to receive some meaningful services from generic agencies and programs in the community. Those with severe impairments of vision and hearing will rarely receive any meaningful rehabilitation services from generic agencies and community programs. Because of the severity of their disabilities, failure to serve these individuals will have far more damaging consequences for them, their families, and their communities than failure to provide specialized services for those with moderately impaired vision and hearing. This particular controversy will probably be best resolved by establishing a fairly liberal definition of deaf-blindness for determining eligibility for specialized services when these can be offered without denying them to those persons who might be given a first priority in their use on the basis of satisfying the conditions of a more restrictive definition of deaf-blindness.

PROBLEM OF CENSUS

Problems of definition inevitably create problems of enumeration. Testifying before a select Committee of the House of Representatives on July 18, 1967, Peter J. Salmon, Administrative Vice President of The Industrial Home for the Blind and Director of the National Center for Deaf-Blind Youths and Adults, summed up the situation as follows:

We do not know how many deaf-blind people there are in the United States, and we never will know until service is available to them. Estimates of the numbers seem to center around 4,000 or 5,000; but we dare say that there may be twice as many as this.

One of the problems of recent origin which will have a marked effect on the deaf-blind population in the immediate future is the impact of the considerable number of infants who are deaf-blind as a result of the epidemic of German measles of 1964 and 1965. This brings a factor into the picture which is completely new, and one which has given great concern to those interested in the education of deaf-blind children. Those of us who are primarily concerned with rehabilitation aspects will need to plan for the rehabilitation of these children in the immediate years ahead.

Dr. Salmon's statement realistically presents the problem of identifying the deaf-blind population in the United States, or, for that matter, in any sizeable geographic or political area.

To take a reliable census of any severely handicapped population is difficult because members of such populations are reluctant to call attention to themselves and often are skeptical about the benefits which might result from their doing so. Families and friends seem to share this skepticism. In some cultural settings, families feel guilty about the very existence of their handicapped members and try to mitigate their feelings of guilt by sheltering them from the embarrassment of public sympathy and protecting them from physical needs and the anguish of aspirations which they are assumed to be incapable of satisfying.

In the case of those who cannot be reached by either the printed or spoken word of the news media, the protective isolation imposed by families and friends becomes almost impregnable. Ordinarily, when services for the severely handicapped prove beneficial, word of such achievement will reach a great many who were previously undiscovered by those in a position to serve their needs; and they will apply for or at least inquire about such services.

However, where the deaf-blind are concerned, motivation to apply for or inquire about services must be initiated by individuals who generally have little or no confidence in the value which outside service may hold or in their ability to make use of such service. The families and friends of uninspired and untrained deaf-blind individuals find a palliative for the concern and guilt they feel in the care which they themselves provide. Rarely do they appreciate the inadequacy of such care. Rarely are they aware of the extreme frustration and the painful loneliness of an overprotected and under-challenged deaf-blind individual. They fail to realize that such an individual would often grasp at even a dubious opportunity to enter the mainstream of life if only he had the information and help he needs to make the effort and to act on his decision.

Efforts over many years to develop a register of deaf-blind persons in the United States on the basis of referrals of individuals thought to be deaf-blind have proved to be highly unsatisfactory (Zumalt and Silver, 1971). Many years will be required before services for the deaf-blind can be sufficiently developed to reach a substantial portion of such persons directly. But only in this way will it be possible to verify the deafness and the blindness of these persons and make projections that will provide a basis for a reliable estimate of the number of deaf-blind persons in the United States.

THE DEAF-BLIND POPULATION

The individual who was born deaf and later becomes blind experiences challenges in learning, in thinking, and in general functioning that are quite different from those experienced by the individual who was born blind and later becomes deaf. Similarly, but to a lesser extent, the age of onset of deafness, the age of onset of blindness, the degree of residual hearing, and the degree of residual vision all influence the way an individual perceives, the way he conceptualizes, and the way he functions. This makes for considerable diversity in the deaf-blind population.

Despite the diversity, the deaf-blind population does not appear to contain any specific subgroups which are clearly defined in terms of practical implications for the organization and content of rehabilitation services. In order to constitute a subgroup within the deaf-blind population, there must be a number of deaf-blind individuals with closely similar histories and similar current degrees of residual vision and hearing within a fairly small geographical area. Fortunately, even with a very liberal definition of deaf-blindness, there are not likely to be enough deaf-blind persons in a given area to constitute subgroups within the deaf-blind population. Some rehabilitative activities may be effectively administered on a group basis even if the groups are not highly homogeneous; but these do not predominate. In the rehabilitation of individuals with handicaps as severe as deafness plus blindness, effective rehabilitation services are best administered on an individual basis.

An analysis of the characteristics at the time of intake of 171 deaf-blind adults who were served from 1962 to 1969 by The Industrial Home for the Blind (under a regional research and demonstration project partially supported by the United States Rehabilitation Service Administration) revealed findings that are fairly consistent with the findings obtained on other and smaller groups. According to information supplied by the group members, 47.9 per cent became blind as a result of retinitis pigmentosa; 44.4 per cent were congenitally deaf; and 24.5 per cent of the adventitiously deaf became deaf prior to the age of six years. In addition to deafness and blindness, there were other handicapping conditions present which were considered to have rehabilitation significance. These included: physical conditions, 22.8 per cent; emotional conditions, 11.1 per cent; physical and emotional conditions, 5.9 per cent; intellectual conditions, 4.1 per cent; emotional and intellectual conditions, 1.8 per cent; physical, emotional, and intellectual conditions, 2.3 per cent. Fifty-two per cent were considered to have no significant handicap in addition to deafness and blindness (Salmon, 1970).

Actual characteristics of deaf-blind persons, including children and the aged, could be expected to show that a higher proportion of the deaf-blind population than indicated in the above figures suffer from significant handicaps in addition to deafness and blindness. There is strong evidence of the need for rehabilitation services for the multihandicapped deaf-blind, particularly for those who lack the capability of achieving vocational rehabilitation objectives. Some of these people may be capable of advancing from institutions providing complete custodial care to relative independence in such protective settings as homes for the aged, boarding homes, or family residences. However, many will require permanent rehabilitation maintenance in institutions for the deafblind if their initial rehabilitation is to result in more humane ways of living and in less costly support by their communities.

The periodic upsurge of rubella (German measles), with a concomitant high incidence in the late 1940s and early 1950s of retrolentalfibroplasia and other conditions affecting the central nervous system, has resulted in fairly substantial numbers of multihandicapped deaf-blind persons. The 1964–1965 epidemic of rubella alone is estimated to have resulted in approximately 1,000 severely damaged deaf-blind children.

While it may be expected that many of these children will require total and lifetime custodial care, some will have enough vision and/or hearing to be capable of benefiting from specialized programs for the blind, the deaf, the mentally retarded, etc.; and others—a substantial number—will undoubtedly require very closely supervised sheltered employment and residence. Within the next eight to ten years, if not earlier, it will become necessary to provide special programs of rehabilitation and rehabilitation maintenance for these severely damaged deafblind persons that will need to be different in many important ways from the rehabilitation programs now being developed for deaf-blind youths and adults who have good potential for vocational rehabilitation.

HISTORICAL BACKGROUND OF SERVICES
FOR THE DEAF-BLIND

The education of deaf-blind children is generally considered the beginning point of organized services for the deaf-blind. In 1837 Laura Bridgman, a seven-year-old deaf-blind child, was admitted to the Perkins School for the Blind, then known as the Perkins Institution for the Blind, in Watertown, Massachusetts. The fact that this child, who was totally deaf and practically blind since shortly after the age of two years, was able to learn to read, to communicate—though she never acquired the ability to speak—and to develop intellectually created a great deal of interest among educators and writers.

About half a century later, the remarkable Helen Keller was admitted to Perkins at the age of eight years after her mother had read about the work with Laura Bridgman in *American Notes* by Charles Dickens. Helen, who had become totally deaf and blind as a result of an illness contracted at eighteen months of age, had been trained and tutored for some years prior to her admission to Perkins by Anne Sullivan, a former student at Perkins who had had a major visual handicap all her life.

The lectures and writings of Helen Keller brought her to the attention of persons of influence throughout the world. Other deaf-blind persons, not as well known as Laura Bridgman and Helen Keller, were also demonstrating that deafness and blindness need not constitute a barrier to useful and productive living.

Several schools for the blind in the United States opened special departments for deaf-blind children. But until recent years, the education of deaf-blind children in these educational institutions tended to be reserved for the most promising and to focus on the development of scholastic attainments rather than on the practical skills of self-care, social intercourse, and vocational preparation.

However, with the development of rehabilitation services for deaf-blind persons, the educators came to recognize that successful living as a deaf-blind person does not necessarily correlate with academic achievement and need not be limited to the intellectually gifted. Even if a deaf-blind person is not able to read, to write, to compute, or to perform any academic activity above a very basic level, he can still be a helping member of his family, engage in remunerative employment, and accomplish many of the objectives of his nonhandicapped peers if he is able to care for himself, relate to others, perform manual work tasks, and maintain acceptable work discipline. With this realization came the recognition that many more deaf-blind children than had been supposed could benefit from properly designed and properly administered educational programs. Recognition of this fact was strengthened by the increase in the number of multihandicapped deaf-blind children that resulted primarily from the 1964–1965 rubella epidemic. Responding to the need for expanded educational services for such children, Title VI of the Elementary and Secondary Education Act was amended by Public Law 90-247, Part C, on January 2, 1968 to establish model centers for deaf-blind children by the Division of Educational Services in the Bureau of Education for the Handicapped of the United States Office of Education. In April 1970, this Law became Part C (Sec. 622) of Public Law 91-230, Title VI, the "Education of the Handicapped Act."

In regard to deaf-blind adults, over the years there have been numbers of small islands of services for such persons throughout the United States. Usually, the services were motivated and sustained by a desire to serve a few deaf-blind individuals in the sheltered workshops of particular agencies for the blind. When the deaf-blind clients would retire or for some other reason withdraw from the labor market, the services that had been built around them were generally discontinued.

An outstanding exception is The Industrial Home for the Blind, which has provided specialized continuous services for deaf-blind adults for over fifty years. In 1945 these services were organized into a formal rehabilitation program for the deaf-blind, and in 1962, as a result of the regional research and demonstration project referred to earlier in this chapter, they were greatly intensified and expanded to reach deaf-blind persons mainly within the fifteen northeastern and central eastern states. Prior to 1962, the specialized services for deaf-blind adults offered at The Industrial Home for the Blind were designed to enable the deaf-blind clients of the agency to make maximum use of the services that the agency provided for its hearing-blind clientele.

With few exceptions, it was found to be impracticable to serve deaf-blind children or deaf-blind adults through services for the deaf. Understandably, workers with the deaf center their efforts in education, rehabilitation, and employment on the sense of sight. This being the case, a person who is blind as well as deaf can seldom be satisfactorily served in settings designed for deaf persons who can see.

The experience of The Industrial Home for the Blind has demonstrated that certain deaf-blind persons can make good use of many of the services designed for hearing-blind persons. Examples are training in suitable methods of communication and special instruction in physical orientation and independent mobility. However, integration of the deaf-blind with the hearing-blind could not be easily accomplished, and often was, in fact, virtually impossible to achieve. With reluctance, it was concluded that separate residential accommodations, separate recreational programs, and a number of separate rehabilitation evaluation and training services were required to achieve maximum rehabilitation for most deaf-blind persons. For some few who were free from any major handicap other than deafness and blindness, and who possessed good mental capacity and high motivation, integration with their hearing-blind peers was possible, and in some cases integration with their nonhandicapped peers as well.

As a result of the work of the regional research and demonstration project, a number of deaf-blind persons were successfully placed in fully competitive employment. Agencies for the blind cooperating with the project began to appreciate the rehabilitation potential of their deaf-blind clients, and a number of them instituted small but durable and effective programs of specialized service for their deaf-blind clients.

CURRENT NATIONAL CENTER REHABILITATION SERVICES FOR THE DEAF-BLIND

The 1967 amendments to the Vocational Rehabilitation Act authorized the establishment and operation of the National Center for Deaf-Blind Youths and Adults. Based on proposals submitted by organizations interested in operating the Center, the Social and Rehabilitation Service selected The Industrial Home for the Blind to operate the National Center under an agreement with the United States Department of Health, Education and Welfare.

The proposal of The Industrial Home for the Blind for operating the Center outlined a comprehensive program of rehabilitation services, including rehabilitation evaluation and training, training of professional personnel, and research. The program was initiated at the Center's temporary headquarters and through three field offices in the first three years of its operation. The program is to be implemented by permanent facilities, additional field offices, and trained staff.

The service components of the program are offered by the National Center when necessary, and through or in conjunction with cooperating agencies where possible. The services include:

DIRECT SERVICES

1) Services in the clients' home communities for the initial assessment of their physical and psychosocial functioning in order to determine the feasibility of planning extensive rehabilitation for them, either at the National Center or in their home communities.

2) Services in the home communities of clients preparing to enter the National Center designed to ready them for the comprehensive diagnostic and intensive training services of the Center.

3) Multidisciplinary evaluative services to determine the rehabilitation potential of each deaf-blind client at the National Center.

4) Medical, surgical, psychiatric, corrective, and other treatment services and special devices at the National Center or, where feasible, in the clients' home communities to enhance rehabilitation potentialities.

5) Social casework; rehabilitation counseling; low-vision rehabilitation; training in independent travel, physical fitness, communication skills, including speech therapy and language development, skills of daily living, skills of social interaction, homemaking, industrial arts, and recreation at the National Center or, where feasible, in the clients' home communities to help achieve the most appropriate rehabilitation objective for each client.

6) Residence at the National Center and transportation for clients where required for their rehabilitation.

7) Transportation and short-term residence at the National Center for family members or close friends of clients when dictated by the rehabilitation needs of clients.

8) Direct placement and placement consultation services to obtain suitable employment for deaf-blind individuals in their home communities when practicable or elsewhere when necessary.

9) Referral, when feasible, for suitable educational or vocational placement.

10) Recreational and social activities for clients at the National Center and consultation on the development and maintenance of such activities for deaf-blind individuals in their home communities.

11) Referral to rehabilitation centers prepared to offer any appropri-

ate rehabilitation services to deaf-blind persons and consultation to help assure success of such services.

12) Referral, consultation, and long-term follow-up services to assist in the resettlement of deaf-blind persons in their home communities, or, when necessary, in other communities on the completion of rehabilitation training.

13) Distribution to clients in the National Center and to interested deaf-blind individuals throughout the country of publications in both Braille and large type to provide them with a means of keeping up with current events and of receiving other new information on as nearly a current basis as possible.

TRAINING FOR PROFESSIONAL WORKERS
AND VOLUNTEERS

1) Liaison with programs of education for deaf-blind children throughout the country and consultation service for schools serving the blind, schools serving the deaf, and other educational programs in which deaf-blind children may be enrolled.

2) Residencies, offered in conjunction with approved institutions of higher education, for graduates of professional training programs in the disciplines which comprise professional services for deaf-blind persons.

3) Short-term, intensive training programs for professional and paraprofessional personnel engaged in or planning to enter programs of services for deaf-blind persons.

4) Orientation and training programs for volunteers.

5) Consultation on the recruiting and training of volunteers.

6) Information service to provide appropriate material for inclusion in the curricula of schools offering programs of training in the helping professions.

7) Field training for students enrolled in professional or technical training in schools affiliated with the National Center.

8) Fellowship and scholarship assistance for the training of prospective workers with deaf-blind persons, where such assistance is not otherwise available.

9) Residence and/or part-time employment for students preparing for service to the deaf-blind or for a field of work in which deaf-blind persons are likely to be served.

RESEARCH

1) Conducting a continuous program of case finding through reviews of the registers of clients of agencies for the blind and agencies for the deaf, through surveys of institutions for mentally retarded, mentally ill, aging, and indigent persons, through encouraging routine vision tests of clients of agencies for the deaf and hearing tests for clients of agencies for the blind, and through other means of identifying deaf-blind persons to whom the National Center might be of service.

2) Maintaining a register of deaf-blind persons within the jurisdiction of the United States for rehabilitation and research purposes.

3) Conducting programs of research to expand and improve methods of case finding.

4) Encouraging the initiation of and cooperating in programs of research into the causes of deaf-blindness, and into methods of reducing or eliminating these causes by the National Institutes of Health and other medically oriented agencies or individuals.

5) Conducting studies of the problems of deaf-blind youths and adults and conducting related research to develop and improve methods of meeting these problems.

6) Encouraging and, to the extent feasible, cooperating in any research conducted anywhere in the world which promises to contribute to the rehabilitation of deaf-blind persons.

7) Conducting studies, including follow-up studies of clients, to evaluate and to improve the services offered by the National Center.

8) Encouraging and, to the extent feasible, cooperating in research in any area of service that may contribute to the rehabilitation of deaf-blind persons—such as language development, learning, vocational adjustment, and re-entry into the community.

9) Conducting research and development studies in cooperation with appropriate research organizations to develop and improve mechanical and electronic devices that might contribute to the rehabilitation of deaf-blind persons.

10) Maintaining affiliations with one or more departments of research in universities or other appropriate organizations in order to have available to the National Center the skills, knowledge, and resources essential to purposeful, diversified research of a high standard.

11) Conducting studies to develop and evaluate methods of recruiting, training, and using volunteers.

PUBLIC EDUCATION

1) Publicizing the work of the National Center through newspapers, magazines, radio, and television.

2) Developing special programs of community education and information to increase understanding and acceptance of deaf-blind persons by the general and professional public.

3) Developing special programs of public education designed to stimulate interest in serving as volunteers at the National Center and in other communities where volunteer services might be helpful to deaf-blind persons.

4) Disseminating the findings of research conducted at the National Center and, where indicated, helping to disseminate the findings of other research pertinent to the rehabilitation of deaf-blind persons.

5) Writing, editing, and publishing pamphlets, books, and other literature on the subject of deaf-blindness.

6) Preparing and making available tapes and films describing and portraying the work of the National Center and of competent deaf-blind persons for use by interested agencies and individuals.

7) Preparing exhibits concerned with the rehabilitation of deaf-blind persons and displaying the exhibits at appropriate conferences, conventions, and other gatherings.

8) Maintaining communication between the National Center and all programs known to serve deaf-blind persons, with a view to facilitating the exchange of information that might contribute to the improvement and expansion of services for the deaf-blind.

TYPES OF PERSONNEL REQUIRED

The implementation of the foregoing program requires far more and better-trained and experienced personnel than has been produced by the various programs of service for deaf-blind persons which preceded the inauguration of the National Center for Deaf-Blind Youths and Adults. Expanded service suggests very strongly a need for specially trained *professional generalists.* The special focus of the social worker, the re-habilitation counselor, the travel instructor, the communication instruc-tor, etc. cannot be economically nor effectively utilized in many situa-tions in which deaf-blind persons are found.

While social work and rehabilitation counseling can be helpful in working with the more sophisticated deaf-blind individual and with some families and close friends of deaf-blind persons, a great many deaf-blind persons, because of severe educational and cultural depriva-tion or mental deficiency, cannot comprehend the abstract concepts that are entailed in the supportive function of social work or the guidance function of rehabilitation counseling. Limited education and/or strong skepticism concerning the potentialities of deaf-blind persons frequently place the families and friends of these persons beyond the influence of the social worker and the rehabilitation counselor. A great many deaf-blind persons, members of their families, and others interested in them require concrete services to develop confidence in the possibilities that rehabilitation might hold. Help to improve a deaf-blind person's ability to move about, even in a protected environment, help to improve his ability to communicate, or any service which he can identify and evalu-ate, will often do far more to inspire hope and motivation for rehabili-tation than any amount of social work or rehabilitation counseling. Fur-ther, the level of learning and the initial goals that may be achieved by many deaf-blind persons do not require highly specialized instructors. The wide disbursement of the small deaf-blind population makes it very costly to serve deaf-blind individuals in their home communities with teams of highly specialized personnel. The cost of such a practice is sel-dom justifiable in view of the fact that a single worker, properly trained and adequately experienced, can often effectively meet a variety of instruc-tional needs and other services of a deaf-blind person.

In addition, recent experience with providing comprehensive evaluation and training services to deaf-blind persons at the National Center—particularly, in providing these services to multihandicapped deaf-blind persons—has pointed up the desirability of using carefully selected and trained aides to substantially supplement the work of pro-fessionally trained personnel. Much of the training of deaf-blind persons requires repetitive attention to the problem of conveying simple infor-mation and developing basic skills. When a deaf-blind trainee does not have sufficient language to be useful in introducing him to new concepts, as is often the case, the connection between a word and the object it symbolizes can often be established for him only through painstaking trial and error. There must be careful exploration of the knowledge that the deaf-blind trainee possesses and the ways in which his curiosity and interest can be stimulated and exploited in the process of broadening and strengthening the relationship between what he knows and the related concepts he is acquiring in order to significantly improve his understanding of his environment.

The effort to develop information and skill in a deaf-blind individual who does not yet have sufficient meaningful vocabulary to be substantially useful depends upon a worker's sensitivity to his responses, ingenuity in motivating and encouraging him, and in the capacity to establish the kind of rapport with the individual that will show respect for his efforts and minimize feelings of embarrassment or tendencies to cling to childish behavior to conceal or excuse his limited development.

Properly selected aides trained through carefully designed short courses and on-the-job experience can effectively provide many of the services required by deaf-blind trainees. The use of such aides proves far more economical than the excessive use of professionally trained personnel and, very often, the aides feel better rewarded for their efforts and apply themselves more consistently to their work than do professional personnel employed in work which they may feel does not make adequate use of their professional preparation. However, planning, directing, and coordinating approaches and techniques employed by aides in serving deaf-blind persons must remain the responsibility of professionally trained and experienced personnel if the best results are to be realized from the combined efforts of professional and paraprofessional workers.

Another important advantage of employing aides to supplement the work of professional personnel is that it makes possible an increase in the number of people with whom the deaf-blind trainees can establish meaningful contacts.

A deaf-blind individual receives a large part of his knowledge of the environment and of the thinking and attitudes of others through the relatively few persons who communicate with him. The knowledge he receives in this way is inevitably filtered and modified by the attitudes and views of those who transmit it. Because of this, every effort should be made to have as many persons as possible communicate with each deaf-blind individual in order that he may have the benefit of a diversity of attitudes and views with which to develop the broadest possible understanding of his environment and of the thinking of others.

THE REHABILITATION PROCESS:
SPECIAL CONSIDERATIONS

The rehabilitation process for deaf-blind individuals, in its broad outline, is not essentially different from that employed for individuals with other types of handicaps. However, a number of special considerations, special emphases, and various adaptations are particularly important to rehabilitation of the deaf-blind. While it is convenient to think of individuals with problems in common as constituting special groups which are defined by these common problems, it is nevertheless important not to lose sight of the fact that individuals in any group are far more different than they are alike, and that rehabilitation is therefore an individualized process.

Unfortunately, there is a persistent tendency among rehabilitation workers to try to fashion those whom they serve after their own image; to try to impose the worker's standards of appropriate behavior and proper attitudes upon the client. Because of problems of communication, this kind of well-meaning indoctrination is particularly difficult for a deaf-blind person to fend off. Not infrequently, the "rehabilitated" deaf-blind person suffers a suppression of his social and cultural differences, which serves to further alienate him from his family and his home community while equipping him with a shallowness of affect that prevents him from giving adequate expression to his own personality and deriving adequate satisfaction from the role he is trying to fill.

Lack of sight and hearing does not diminish an individual's rights as a member of a democratic society. In providing rehabilitation services for the deaf and blind person, particular care must be taken to safeguard his right to freedom from needless dependency; his right to personal identity, including the retention of idiosyncrasies, uncommon attitudes, and unpopular views when these do not infringe on the rights of others; his right to an opportunity to contribute to his community and to the welfare of those for whom he has a personal responsibility; and his right to respect for the dignity of his individuality and the worth of his contribution. Following are some special considerations in the rehabilitation of deaf-blind persons.

HEALTH STATUS

Before entering a program of rehabilitation evaluation and rehabilitation training, a comprehensive health-status report, based on recent examinations, should be obtained to determine: (a) the possibility of restoration so as not to needlessly train around a remediable disability; (b) the possible need for precautions to conserve any residual capacity that might be endangered by improper activities during rehabilitation and subsequent endeavors; and (c) whether the individual entering the program is apt to provide a hazard for others in the program.

After entry into the program, the deaf-blind rehabilitant should receive comprehensive medical and medically related re-examinations by physicians and other specialists involved who are experienced in serving deaf-blind persons. Too often, examinations of deaf-blind persons are found to be superficial and incomplete because of problems related to communication. Also, physicians and other specialists who are not accustomed to serve individuals who have major sensory deficits are apt to discount the value of partial restoration of such deficits. The correction of any eye condition, for example, which might restore only 5 per cent of vision may not seem worthwhile in a patient who has nearly normal vision, and the ophthalmologist who is oriented to this kind of situation may not appreciate the enormous value of restoring 5 per cent of vision to a patient who has little or no vision. Similarly, the gains which may be realized by improving the usefulness of residual vision or residual hearing through the fitting of low-vision aids or the fitting of high-powered hearing aids may not be appreciated by optometrists or audiologists who measure such improvements against full capacity instead of against minimal residual capacity.

COMMUNICATION

Communication is an ability which not only requires major emphasis in the rehabilitation program of a deaf-blind person but which also has a pervading influence on the counseling and training services he receives. A first and major step in the rehabilitation process of a deaf-blind person is the determination of which method of communication can best be employed and how much knowledge and understanding the deaf-blind person has been able to achieve through his communication ability. Occasionally, deaf-blind persons appear to have no communication ability because of their having depended on an improvised method of communication which may not be detectable except by trial and error unless the deaf-blind person is accompanied by someone who can explain the special method of communication he has employed in the past. Printing on the thigh, writing in Braille, and using a foreign language are among the avenues of communication that have had to be discovered through trial and error or through devious surmises and deductions by rehabilitation workers. Counseling with a deaf-blind rehabilitant requires, at a minimum, a preliminary assessment of the extent and quality of the communications ability and knowledge of the rehabilitant. If these are substantial and sound, counseling may proceed on the basis of commonly recognized principles of counseling. However, the principle of self-determination, for example, may have to be abandoned, at least temporarily, if the deaf-blind rehabilitant has not had sufficient experience to provide him with a frame of reference in which to select the types of training and the training objectives from among the alternatives available to him. In such a case, it becomes initially necessary to make decisions for him. If he has never traveled alone, for instance, his ignorance and his fear of such an activity may cause him to reject out of hand all methods of independent travel. It may be necessary, nonetheless, to attempt to train him in a particular method, despite his initial resistance to the training, until he has had sufficient experience with the training and has acquired sufficient related knowledge to enable him to make a valid judgment as to the appropriateness of it for him.

A selection of a primary method of communication for a deaf-blind person (Dinsmore, 1959) is crucial in determining the quality of his intellectual development. Whether he has useful residual vision, useful residual hearing, whether he reads with some regularity, and whether he has a capacity for and a need for precise communication are among the factors that should influence his selection of a primary method of communication. The use of signs if he has sufficient vision to see them under selected conditions, or the reading of lips by touch (the Tadoma Method) if he has been able to acquire this skill, provide relatively rapid means of communication. However, as the use of such methods depends on inferring conceptually a good deal of what is being communicated, they do not help to develop or to preserve precise understanding of vocabulary. This fact may not present a problem for those deaf-blind persons who read with some regularity; but it does tend to make it very difficult to retain the kind of understanding of vocabulary and sentence structure which is essential to clear, incisive thinking. Therefore, the one-hand manual alphabet (fingerspelling), requiring word-by-word communication, has been found to be the fastest and otherwise most satisfactory method of communication for most deaf-blind persons who are capable of learning it.

ORIENTATION AND MOBILITY

Physical orientation and independent mobility, perhaps, next to communication, present the greatest challenge to those deaf-blind persons who do not have sufficient sight or hearing to be helpful in the exercise of these abilities. Such persons experience difficulty in maintaining their equilibrium because they can neither see the surface on which they are walking so as to maintain a perpendicular position in relation to it, nor hear the sounds refracted by the surface and by large solid objects. Hearing blind persons depend upon these sensory cues to maintain their equilibrium. Many deaf-blind persons will be observed to veer from one side to the other because they are not aware of their departure from a perpendicular position until the departure is so great as to result in a significant shift in their weight and stimulate protective muscle reaction. In an effort to anticipate a tilting to one side or to the other, many deaf-blind persons walk with their toes turned out in an effort to maintain an awareness of the relationship of their bodies to the floor or the ground on each side of them as well as in front and in back of them.

Methods of independent travel developed for hearing blind persons have been adapted for use by the deaf-blind. Through the use of a button that identifies them as deaf and blind, which can be displayed when required, of a card that explains how a stranger may communicate with them, and through the use of a series of cards with carefully planned questions, such as "Will you please help me board the Seventh Avenue bus?" ". . . let me know when we stop at Tenth Street," ". . . help me across the street," etc., many deaf-blind persons are able to meet their important travel needs without having to depend on a regular guide.

To detect obstacles and descents in the path of travel, a long cane is employed. The cane is held where the shaft meets the crook with the forefinger extended along the shaft. The cane is moved from side to side in an arc, an inch or two high and slightly longer than the width of the body. The movement of the cane is synchronized with the movement of the feet so that it touches the ground in front of the foot that is to the rear. This provides warning of an obstacle or a descent two full steps before the obstacle or the descent is encountered. The use of the cane in this way has a unique value for the deaf-blind traveler. It provides three almost simultaneous contacts with the surface on which he is walking, repeated with sufficient frequency and regularity in a triangular rela- tionship, so that he obtains the information he needs in order to main- tain his equilibrium, and to minimize, almost to the vanishing point, the troublesome tendency to veer (Anne Sullivan Macy Service, 1966).

INDUSTRIAL ARTS

Industrial arts fill an important role in the rehabilitation evaluation and training of deaf-blind persons, both for those who are preparing to enter industrial employment as well as for those who do not have such employment as an objective. The most commonly understood purpose for which industrial arts are used is to familiarize trainees preparing for industrial employment with both hand tools and motive power ma- chinery, to familiarize them with their components and their uses, to enable them to overcome fear of using them, and to instruct them in tool and machine skills in which they might find employment.

In addition to the commonly understood use of industrial arts in re- habilitation, industrial arts can be effectively coordinated with voca- tional aptitude testing and corrective physical therapy. Work-perfor- mance tests and tests of basic, transferable abilities can be devised through the use of selected hand tools, machines, and specially designed work projects—as, for example, a kick press to test hand-foot coordina- tion or a tactile inspection project to test tactual perception. Employing such tests in combination with conventional aptitude testing, it is possible to obtain a broader base for evaluating transferable abilities than through the use of vocational aptitude testing alone.

While some deaf-blind trainees feel comfortable in the structured, controlled setting of a formal testing situation, others, especially those who have had little formal education, often show best performance in the work-like setting of work performance tests. Further, vocational aptitude tests are frequently misleading when applied to deaf-blind persons because, often, they do not test the same ability in a deaf-blind person as they do in persons who can see.

Vocational aptitude tests are ordinarily designed on the assumption that the individuals to whom they are administered use their vision to control the movements of their hands. A deaf-blind person must depend upon kinesthetic memory to control the movements of his hands. As a vocational aptitude test does not have sufficient duration to permit kinesthetic learning to take place, a deaf-blind person may not be able to demonstrate his true ability in his performance on vocational aptitude tests. When work performance tests are employed, several hours or longer can be used to allow kinesthetic learning to take place, and thereby to provide a fair measure of a deaf-blind person's use of his kinesthetic memory in combination with whatever physical ability may be in the process of being tested. Thus, hand-foot coordination, bimanual coordination, finger dexterity, tactual perception, ability to cope with boredom and frustration, and a wide variety of other components of a deaf-blind person's functioning ability can best be tested through the use of work performance tests in conjunction with vocational aptitude tests.

Industrial arts are coordinated with corrective physical therapy in the rehabilitation of deaf-blind persons by the use of work exercises to complement corrective physical therapy exercises. Work exercises are work tasks selected to strengthen or improve particular work abilities as, for example, an operation involving extensive use of a hammer to strengthen finger and wrist muscles or a fine assembly operation to improve finger dexterity. Corrective physical therapy can provide exercises which are purer and more intensive than work exercises, but, because of their intensiveness and nonproductive nature, they induce fatigue and monotony which limit their use to only short periods of time. Work exercises entail the production of things, the disassembly of things, or some other type of measurable results of effort expended. Although the results of the exercises may be incidental to the purpose of the effort when the purpose is simply exercise, they nevertheless provide a means by which the trainee can measure the outcome of his effort and thereby be motivated to sustain maximum effort for an extended period of time. Thus, by combining work exercises with corrective physical therapy exercises, the advantage of both intensity and sustained effort can be combined to achieve a broad attack on the problem of developing physical functioning ability.

SKILLS OF SELF-CARE

Training in skills of self-care—such as applying makeup, shaving, marketing clothes for their selection to avoid incongruous color combinations, and other skills of personal grooming; training in using eating utensils properly, reaching for food and water containers gracefully, and other skills of acceptable table conduct—helps the deaf-blind person to develop confidence in his personal appearance and his ability to cope with many of the challenges of social intercourse.

HOMEMAKING

Training in homemaking—housecleaning, preparation of food, mending, etc.—is provided for deaf-blind women on as extensive and sophisticated a level as their needs and abilities dictate. It is also provided to deaf-blind men, at least on a rudimentary level, both as a type of contingency survival training and as a means of helping them to appreciate what homemaking entails.

HOME REPAIR AND AUTOMOTIVE REPAIR
AND MAINTENANCE

Training in home repair and in simple automotive repair and maintenance provides obvious economic advantages, especially for deaf-blind men. However, such training offers two other important advantages. It provides content for interesting conversation in many social circles and, for the man particularly, it often provides an opportunity to acquire or regain status as the head of the household who can be looked to for the fixing of things and the solving of related problems.

RESEARCH NEEDS

Research in the rehabilitation of deaf-blind persons has been most productive and most promising in the development of mechanical and electronic devices to meet some of the problems of communication. Research into methods of reducing some of the social barriers between deaf-blind persons and their communities has been limited thus far, but has produced worthwhile and encouraging preliminary results. However, research into the methods of perception available to deaf-blind individuals and the potentialities of these methods has been extremely meager and, generally, has been marked by a lack of imagination, poor insight, and a failure to draw upon the unique contribution which intelligent deaf-blind individuals themselves can make to this kind of research.

There are a number of popular assumptions which have never been adequately investigated and that serve to preclude for many deaf-blind persons opportunities for education and rehabilitation. It is commonly assumed that if blindness or deafness sets in before the age of about five or six years, the visual or auditory images gained prior to the onset of blindness or deafness cannot contribute significantly to the orientation and conceptualization of the affected individual. It is assumed that a lag of five or six years between the level of functioning of a child and his chronological age will result in such damage to his potential for learning as to be virtually irremediable. It is assumed that the possession of sight or hearing which is so slight as to have no overt usefulness, no "economic" value, may be totally discounted. Ophthalmological and optometric reports, or otological and audiological reports, will frequently indicate the total absence of sight or hearing in an individual who possesses sufficient sight or hearing to hold important psychological value for him.

It is difficult to refute the kind of assumptions cited above because they apply to so few individuals and because these individuals are generally so victimized by them as to be denied the opportunity for the type of education and the kind of rehabilitation that could render them capable of contradicting the assumptions. Assumptions that are positive in their forecasts can lead to important new knowledge, even if that knowledge serves to refute. However, assumptions that are negative in their forecast are totally indefensible because they are both harmful and self-perpetuating. Extreme care must be taken to guard against false professional pride, defensiveness, or any motivation that can serve to foreclose opportunities for the growth and development of any human being.

There is some evidence to suggest that the ability to see no more than very gross forms and very strongly contrasting degrees of brightness, even after this ability is lost, can result in the ability to visualize. There is some evidence to suggest, too, that information acquired through senses other than the sense of sight can serve to enhance a visual image.

We know very little about the functioning of the kinesthetic sense, the precise interrelationship between the senses, and the ways in which perception might be enhanced through adjusting and developing this interrelationship. So little practical research has been done in this area that we lack adequate vocabulary to facilitate such research. There is no adequate parallel, for example, to the word "visualize" for referring to the production of images by the other senses. We do not speak of "tactilizing," "kinestheticizing," or "auditorizing," etc.; and yet, the exploration of the ways in which the senses function could be greatly facilitated by the existence of a commonly accepted vocabulary. Discussions with sensorially deprived individuals are made slow and difficult because of the absence of adequate vocabulary. Nonetheless, such discussions sometimes produce highly pregnant information and raise very provocative questions.

Research into the methods of perception of sensorially deprived individuals will necessarily have to be cautious, slow, and sometimes unorthodox. It will not submit to rigid timetables nor lend itself to early publication; and it will not respect professional authority. Much of the findings such research may hold will necessarily depend upon the insight and the perceptiveness of its subjects, and upon the ability of the investigators and the subjects to probe together on the basis of mutual respect with no hierarchy of authority. Only after many impressions are gleaned from such exploration will it be possible to apply techniques of statistical analysis to separate the valid from the invalid findings. Such findings as may in time be found to be valid will need to be transferred into terms that will render them useful to the instructor, the counselor, and other professional practitioners in rehabilitation. If this is done, it will not only greatly benefit the deaf-blind, the deaf, and the blind, but it may very well hold important implications for all education and training.

REFERENCES

Anne Sullivan Macy Service. 1966. Instruction in physical orientation and foot travel for deaf-blind persons. New York, The Industrial Home for the Blind.

Dinsmore, Annette B. 1959. Methods of communicating with deaf-blind people. Rev. ed. New York, American Foundation for the Blind.

Journal of the American Medical Association. 1934. Definition of blindness 102:205.

Rusalem, Herbert. 1964. The diffusion effect of an orientation program on deaf-blindness. The New Outlook for the Blind. 58:2:44–46.

—— 1967. Engineering changes in public attitudes toward a severely disabled group. Journal of Rehabilitation 33:3:26–27.

Salmon, Peter J. 1970. Out of the shadows, final report of the Anne Sullivan Macy Service for deaf-blind persons. New Hyde Park, N.Y., National Center for Deaf-Blind Youths and Adults.

—— 1971. A report of progress, March 24, 1970–March 23, 1971, p. 18. National Center for Deaf-Blind Youths and Adults.

Zumalt, L. E. and S. Silver. 1971. Report of a content analysis performed on the register of deaf-blind persons (unpublished paper). New Hyde Park, N.Y., National Center for Deaf-Blind Youths and Adults.

SUGGESTED READINGS

GENERAL

Deaf/blind persons—world-wide round-up of services following Council Meeting in New Delhi, India. October, 1969. Watertown, Mass., Perkins School for the Blind; Brooklyn, The Industrial Home for the Blind.

Industrial Home for the Blind and U.S. Office of Vocational Rehabilitation. 1958. Rehabilitation of deaf-blind persons. I. A manual for professional workers (out of print); II. Communication—a key to service for deaf-blind men and women; III. Report of medical studies on deaf-blind persons; IV. A report of psychological studies with deaf-blind persons; V. Studies in the vocational adjustment of deaf-blind adults; VI. Recreation services for deaf-blind persons; VII. Survey of selected characteristics of deaf-blind adults in New York State, fall, 1957. Brooklyn.

Lawson, Lawrence J., Jr. and Helmer R. Myklebust. September, 1970. Ophthalmological deficiencies in deaf children. Exceptional Children.

Meshcheryakov, A. I. March, 1968. Initial teaching and development of the deaf and blind and mute child. Southern Regional Association for the Blind. London Review.

Peare, Catherine Owens. 1959. The Helen Keller story. New York, Thomas Y. Crowell.

Rothschild, Jacob. 1962. Deaf-blindness, in James F. Garrett and Edna S. Levine, eds. Psychological practices with the physically disabled. New York, Columbia University Press, pp. 376–409.

Sculthorpe, Arthur. October, 1966. The adjustment to deaf-blindness in adult life. New Beacon.

Smithdas, Robert J. 1958. Life at my fingertips. Garden City, Doubleday.

Waterhouse, Dr. Edward J. December, 1967. Rubella: implications for education, in Contemporary Papers. Washington, D.C., American Association of Workers for the Blind, II, 18–25 (reprinted from The New Outlook for the Blind, April 1967).

RESEARCH

Dinsmore, Annette B. June 1967. Field testing the tactile speech indicator. The New Outlook for the Blind, pp. 192–93.

Frank, W. E. 1955. Instrumentation requirements in sensory aids. New York Academy of Science Annals 60:869–876.

Holbert, N. 1969–70. Development of person perception in the pre-school deaf, partially sighted, non-verbal child. Perkins School-Boston College Teacher Training Class, 17 pages.

Myklebust, H. R., and M. Brutten. 1953. A study of visual perception of deaf-blind children. Acta Oto-Laryngologica. Lund, Sweden.

Rusalem, H. March 1965. A study of college students' beliefs about deaf-blindness. The New Outlook for the Blind.

Waterhouse, E. J. 1956. Socialization problems of deaf-blind children. The Lantern 25:3.

Zumalt, L. E., S. Silver, and L. C. Kramer. January, 1972. Evaluation of a communication device for deaf-blind persons. The New Outlook for the Blind.

THE INTERNATIONAL SCENE

HOWARD A. RUSK, MARY E. SWITZER,
AND EUGENE J. TAYLOR

INTERNATIONAL PROGRAMS IN
REHABILITATION

BEFORE THE EIGHTEENTH CENTURY, educational and health services were primarily concerns of the individual and his family, with the Church in some instances giving aid to the indigent. Slow but steady scientific and social progress, rising nationalism, and the Industrial Revolution contributed to a growing interest in cooperative provision of medical services which were beyond the means of most families. These were usually provided to some degree by religious and voluntary societies and, to a very limited degree, by governments.

Throughout the world, the first rehabilitation services to emerge have traditionally been those for the blind and the deaf. Most of the original institutions for the blind in the "developed" nations in Europe and North America were established in the nineteenth century. The first public effort to benefit the blind, however, was a hospital for 300 blind

DR. RUSK is President, the late MARY SWITZER was Vice President, and EUGENE J. TAYLOR is Secretary-Treasurer of the World Rehabilitation Fund, Inc. Dr. Rusk is also Professor and Chairman of the Department of Rehabilitation Medicine, New York University School of Medicine; Past President of the International Society for Rehabilitation of the Disabled; and Chairman of the Board, American-Korean Foundation. Miss Switzer was former Commissioner, United States Social and Rehabilitation Service, and a member of the Council of the International Society for Rehabilitation of the Disabled. Mr. Taylor is Adjunct Professor of Rehabilitation Medicine, New York University School of Medicine and former President of the American–Korean Foundation.

persons founded in Paris in the year 1260 by Louis IX. It was over five hundred years, however, until the first school for the blind was founded in Paris in 1784 by Valentin Haüy, a pioneer in education of the blind. France also established the first institution in Europe for the deaf, a school for deaf-mutes which was opened by the Abbé Michel de l'Épée in 1760 in Paris on the Rue des Moulins. In 1791 this school was designated as a national institution, and then in 1794 it moved to 254 Rue St. Jacques, where it is still in operation.

This pattern of services for the blind and the deaf preceding services for persons with other disabilities undoubtedly resulted from the compassion resulting both from the severity of the disabilities of blindness and deafness and their obviousness to persons coming in direct contact with persons having these disabilities. A secondary factor is that although techniques and skills in education of the training of the blind and the deaf were quite rudimentary, there was nevertheless a certain body of knowledge and techniques for providing services to such persons. However, in the case of persons with orthopedic and neuromuscular disabilities, medical science had not progressed to the stage that definitive measures were available to alleviate these conditions except for the provision of very crude prosthetic and orthotic devices and means of transportation, usually sedan chairs for the wealthy.

Modern rehabilitation had its genesis in World War I with the establishment of the specialty of orthopedic surgery and the development of the then new disciplines of physical and occupational therapy. Some key institutions for the treatment of the war-disabled were developed in those nations engaged in World War II. Among such institutions in the United States were the Institute for the Crippled and Disabled, New York City, the Cleveland Rehabilitation Center and the Milwaukee Curative Workshop. The modern concept of rehabilitation as a service to meet the physical, emotional, social, and vocational needs of the disabled individual developed during World War II. This was based on the premise of treating the "whole man" and not his physical disability alone, a concept developed first in Great Britain by the Royal Air Force and then in the United States by the Army Air Forces.

Writing in *The New York Times Magazine* in 1953, the British social philosopher, Arnold Toynbee, said, "the twentieth century will be chiefly remembered . . . as an age in which human society dared to think of the welfare of the whole human race as a practical objective."

One, and perhaps the most significant, feature of social development which gives hope for Mr. Toynbee's objective becoming reality is the increasing recognition throughout the world that the security and welfare of the human race are interdependent within each geographic area of the world, and that the security and welfare of each geographic area is dependent upon the security and welfare of the world as a whole.

This growing recognition of interdependence has not resulted solely from practical necessity. We believe that it also represents man's ability, as society matures, to give fuller expression to a feeling that is as old as humankind itself: the desire to share with and help one's neighbor.

This concept has long been practiced by religious groups, but it is only since World War II that technical assistance programs, both governmental and voluntary, have become significant. The first global recognition of this multilateral responsibility came with the establishment of the United Nations and its Specialized Agencies. This was closely followed by bilateral governmental technical assistance programs and then by multilateral and bilateral voluntary assistance programs.

Rehabilitation of the handicapped has a unique role to play in the development of the international understanding that must form the foundation of any lasting peace. Most individuals regard technological improvement in agriculture, industry, and utilities as somewhat removed from their immediate personal problems. Rehabilitation, however, has highly tangible and visible results. It epitomizes the prime democratic concept of equal opportunity for all.

In the United States and other developed parts of the world, we have seen a remarkable growth of interest in rehabilitation during the past three decades. This interest has not been prompted by humanitarian motives alone. It has resulted from the growing incidence of the physically handicapped resulting from spectacular lifesaving advances in medicine, surgery, and public health, and a prolongation of the life span, which has in turn increased public assistance costs dramatically. The result has been that the developed nations of the world can no longer afford not to provide rehabilitation services for their disabled. The pressing problems of public assistance costs do not exist in the developing nations of the world, where the disabled individual remains a responsibility of his family rather than of society. Nor is there a need for manpower. The undeveloped nations have far more manpower than they can profitably utilize in their present stage of industrial development.

The real reason seems to be that many of these nations, particularly those of the African and Asian areas, have, after long years of colonization, received their long-sought dreams of political independence. Now they are searching for ways for proving to the world and, more importantly, to themselves, that they have the political and social maturity to justify their political independence. In these countries, which are faced by mass problems of public health, unemployment, and underemployment, rehabilitation is not an economic necessity but rather an expression of humanitarianism, human rights, and the dignity of the individual.

The major contributing factor to the tremendous growth of interest in international activities in rehabilitation is the internationalism which grew out of World War II and which was epitomized by the establishment of the United Nations. This spirit of international cooperation and technical assistance was to be found immediately after World War II not only in the United Nations and its Specialized Agencies, but also in the rapid growth of international and national concern, both governmental and voluntary, in the establishment, extension, and improvement of rehabilitation services globally.

THE UNITED NATIONS AND ITS
SPECIALIZED AGENCIES

THE UNITED NATIONS

On July 13, 1950, the United Nations Economic Council adopted a proposal recommending the establishment of a coordinated program for the social rehabilitation of the physically disabled. Five months later, in December 1950, this proposal was approved by the General Assembly of the United Nations and became the basis for all subsequent UN programs for rehabilitation of the disabled.

The resolution requested the Secretary General "to plan jointly with the specialized agencies and in consultation with the interested nongovernmental organizations a well-coordinated international program for rehabilitation of physically handicapped persons. . . ." Member governments were also requested to take the lead in studying and solving the problems confronting physically and visually handicapped persons and to affect appropriate measures for this purpose, including necessary legislation.

A request to include funds for employing a staff to initiate such a United Nations program in the UN budget estimates for 1951 led to what is now the Rehabilitation Unit for the Disabled within the United Nations Social Development Division. This unit has been responsible not only for initiating, but also for implementing the UN program for rehabilitation of the disabled. As a first step to implement the Economic and Social Council resolution, an Ad Hoc Technical Working Party was created, consisting of representatives of the UN, including United Nations Children's Fund (UNICEF), UN Educational, Scientific, and Cultural Organization (UNESCO), the International Labour Organisation (ILO), the World Health Organization (WHO), and the International Refugee Organization (IRO). Three Working Party meetings held during 1950 and 1951 served to coordinate international activities and recommended future programs. Also, in October 1951, a conference was called for nongovernmental organizations interested in the handicapped and cooperating with the United Nations. This resulted in the formation of The Council of World Organizations Interested in the Handicapped (CWOIH) in 1953. The Council, represented by nongovernmental organizations, both professional and voluntary, interested in all areas of physical disability including blindness and deafness, has continued to function.

Programs of conferences prepared by the Working Party stressed the human rights of the handicapped by emphasizing the responsibility of governments to prevent the occurrence of disabling conditions and also to provide all appropriate means for assisting, educating, and rehabilitating their disabled citizens. The roles to be played in rehabilitation programs by the UN, the Specialized Agencies, and the nongovernmental organizations were set down in detail.

The ECOSOC resolution also opened the way for the inclusion of rehabilitation projects in the regular UN program for technical assistance. The first UN Advisory Mission in the field of rehabilitation was undertaken by Dr. Henry H. Kessler of the United States, who went to

Yugoslavia in 1950. Since that time, UN experts have been sent to advise governments throughout the world on the establishment and development of rehabilitation services. The experts have covered a variety of specialities within the field of rehabilitation, such as the manufacture of braille machines for the blind, equipment for the deaf, services for the mentally retarded, problems in physical therapy, occupational therapy, prosthetics, special education, and administration. Experts are sent as individuals, or in some instances as members of teams. Usually teams of experts are sponsored by the United Nations and one or more of its Specialized Agencies, such as the World Health Organization and the International Labour Organisation. In some instances, teams have also included representatives of voluntary agencies.

Specialized information is provided in United Nations Publications dealing with various aspects of rehabilitation, and a "Summary of Information on Projects and Activities in the Field of Rehabilitation of the Disabled" is published annually. This summary provides comprehensive information on activities in all fields of rehabilitation in different countries by the nongovernmental organizations, the UN, and the Specialized Agencies.

An interesting development can be noticed in the ECOSOC resolutions on rehabilitation. While the title of the first resolution in 1950 was "Social Rehabilitation of the Physically Handicapped," the one adopted in 1955 is simply "Rehabilitation of the Disabled." Thus, the scope of the United Nations Role in the field of rehabilitation was broadened and, particularly, the door was opened for the United Nations to deal with the problems of mentally handicapped persons. A more definite step in this direction was made by the Commission for Social Development when, at its twenty-first session in March 1970, it decided that "appropriate work on the problem of mentally retarded persons should be included in the program of the Commission."

A recent development involving rehabilitation in the United Nations and its Specialized Agencies was the creation in 1970 of a new Rehabilitation Liaison Program which is concerned with ways in which the United Nations and its Specialized Agencies may work in closer cooperation among themselves and with the World Rehabilitation Fund in improving and expanding rehabilitation services for the handicapped throughout the world. The Rehabilitation Liaison Program was estab-

lished when the Directors General of the United Nations and its Specialized Agencies, or their representatives, and officers of the World Rehabilitation Fund met in New York City in October 1970 and agreed that the objectives of the Rehabilitation Liaison Program should be:
1) To improve the efficiency of the rehabilitation services provided by the United Nations and its Specialized Agencies and the World Rehabilitation Fund through increased cooperation and particularly information-sharing and joint planning.
2) To increase the amount of funds available for such rehabilitation services from the World Rehabilitation Fund through its solicitation of financial contributions for this purpose from private sources.
3) To attempt to increase the amount of funds available for such rehabilitation services from the United Nations Development Programme.
4) To induce national governments in their planning and establishment of national goals to recognize the importance of rehabilitation services for the handicapped as part of the process of economic development.

Under this new program the rehabilitation officers of the United Nations and its Specialized Agencies and the officials of the World Rehabilitation Fund meet annually, in New York in the fall and in Geneva in the spring, for discussions and decisions on methods of implementation of the objectives of the program.

One objective which has been achieved has been the recognition by the United Nations Development Programme that rehabilitation services for the handicapped are an integral part of economic development.

Currently it is estimated there are one billion persons in the developing parts of the world who are, or should be, in the labor force. Of these, there are 300 million who are unemployed or underemployed to the extent that they can also be considered unemployed for practical purposes and for planning. In addition, there are another 300 million persons in this population with physical, mental, and emotional disabilities who could become employable or self-employed if they had adequate rehabilitation services. Based on United Nations population growth estimates, it can be anticipated that the total number of disabled in the developing parts of the world will reach 400 million by 1980.

One fundamental objective for the second decade of the United Nations Development Programme is full employment throughout the world. This objective recognizes that the developing nations must have a national strategy for the training of skills for which employment can be found within the developing national economy. The strategy is based on training for all who can benefit from such training, including the disabled. It recognizes that the only difference between the general unemployed and underemployed and the disabled is that the disabled person requires certain basic medical rehabilitation services and, in some instances, a different type of training than the unemployed and underemployed, who are simply without job skills.

As a result of the recognition by the United Nations Development Programme of the economic validity of the contribution of rehabilitation services, the United Nations Development Programme, as a policy, is approving the use of United Nations Development Programme funds to support rehabilitation services when national governments include such projects within their national plans for economic development, and request financial support for specific projects.

WORLD HEALTH ORGANIZATION (WHO)

The World Health Organization has a technical assistance program similar to that of the United Nations involving surveys, services of expert consultants, and equipment and fellowships which are available to the governments of nations requesting such services through the regional offices of WHO. The program is coordinated through the Headquarters of the World Health Organization in Geneva, Switzerland. Programs of technical assistance in rehabilitation are related to the medical aspects of rehabilitation with particular emphasis upon training and the development of training resources in the specialty of rehabilitation medicine and allied health professions such as physical therapy and occupational therapy. WHO has an expert committee on rehabilitation.

INTERNATIONAL LABOUR ORGANIZATION (ILO)

The International Labour Organization operates a technical assistance program in rehabilitation similar to that of the United Nations and WHO but with emphasis on vocational rehabilitation. It, too, provides technical assistance upon the requests of the governments of nations for surveys, consultations, expert consultants, fellowships, and equipment. The primary emphasis has been on assisting in the development of vocational rehabilitation and sheltered workshop facilities. The program is administered directly from ILO Headquarters in Geneva, but in contrast to the United Nations and WHO, the International Labour Organization has a number of permanent regional consultants whose services are available to nations within the particular geographical area of the world in which the consultant is stationed.

UNITED NATIONS EDUCATIONAL, SCIENTIFIC AND
CULTURAL ORGANIZATION (UNESCO)

UNESCO operates a technical assistance program in special education of the handicapped similar in purpose and methodology to the technical assistance programs in rehabilitation of the UN, WHO and the ILO. The program is relatively new and an expert in special education of the handicapped to coordinate the program was appointed to the staff of UNESCO only in 1969.

UNITED NATIONS CHILDREN'S FUND (UNICEF)

The United Nations Children's Fund has provided technical assistance to governments of nations requesting such aid primarily in medical rehabilitation services designed to serve children. Technical assistance has consisted primarily of equipment and supplies but has included other types of aid, including fellowships.

PAN AMERICAN HEALTH ORGANIZATION (PAHO)

The Pan American Health Organization, the regional office of WHO for the Americas, has conducted technical assistance programs in rehabilitation in the Americas similar to those conducted by WHO in other parts of the world. The volume and range of technical assistance provided by PAHO in the Americas has been somewhat larger than similar assistance programs sponsored by WHO in other parts of the world. PAHO has a full-time physician on its staff whose activities are devoted to direction and coordination of the program. It also has a full-time expert consultant in prosthetics and orthotics who is assigned primarily to long-term training programs but who also serves as a short-term consultant.

OTHER ORGANIZATIONS

Some technical assistance in rehabilitation has also been provided under regional organizations, such as the Organization of American States, to nations in Central and South America and through the Colombo Plan to nations in Southeast Asia. The Organization's programs have included the provision of expert consultants and fellowships. A notable project under this program was the assistance provided by Australia in establishing modern prosthetic and orthotic services in the National Orthopedic Hospital in Manila in the early 1960s.

BILATERAL TECHNICAL ASSISTANCE PROGRAMS

The volume of bilateral technical assistance from one nation to another in rehabilitation is fairly limited when compared to the size and scope of the multilateral programs of the UN and its Specialized Agencies. The United States Agency for International Development (AID) and its predecessor agencies have supported some such activities, primarily consultation services and fellowship training. The major emphasis in this program was in the 1950s, when the AID Public Health Mission in Mexico had a United States expert on rehabilitation on its staff to serve as a consultant to the government of Mexico and to provide short-term consultation services and fellowships to the Central American republics and the republics on the west coast of South America. Most of the fellowships were of a "third country" nature, in which the recipients of the fellowships received professional and technical training at resources in Mexico under joint funding of AID, the government of Mexico, and the recipient republic.

AID has also provided substantial support to the development and expansion of rehabilitation services within the Republic of Vietnam through contracts with the World Rehabilitation Fund involving medical rehabilitation aid to the National Rehabilitation Institute in Saigon and its branches in Cantho and Danang, and vocational rehabilitation aid to the government of South Vietnam.

Outside the framework of the traditional bilateral technical assistance programs, the United States Social and Rehabilitation Service of the

Department of Health, Education and Welfare began conducting a special international program of research and demonstration grants in 1959 utilizing "counterpart" funds. These are funds which the UN owns in national currencies which have resulted from the sale of excess agricultural commodities. The basic objective of the program is to complement, supplement, and strengthen the domestic research programs of the Social and Rehabilitation Service. Projects are selected to test and evaluate new rehabilitation techniques and develop innovative approaches in promoting effective programs for the handicapped. Frequently it is feasible to conduct research in a more natural setting, in countries other than the United States. Often unusual research talents in the form of a single individual or institution in other countries can conduct certain research more effectively than could be done in the United States.

For example, in such a project at the Konstantin Rehabilitation Center near Warsaw, Polish scientist Dr. Marian Weiss did the basic research which has led to new concepts and techniques in the immediate and early fitting of prostheses after surgery. These techniques are now widely utilized not only in the United States but also throughout the world. The Social and Rehabilitation Service has a small supplementary dollar appropriation which is used primarily to pay maintenance costs of scientists from other countries who are in the United States for specialized research training or international research conferences.

In the period between 1961 and 1971, a total of 291 different projects, costing national currencies equal to 27,162,000 United States dollars, were conducted in Brazil, Burma, Ceylon, India, Israel, Morocco, Pakistan, Poland, Syria, Tunisia, the United Arab Republic (Egypt), and Yugoslavia. During the same period, 336 American experts visited projects in these countries and 307 foreign nationals were brought to the United States for short periods of research training or to attend international conferences. As of 1971 the program was operative in India, Israel, Morocco, Pakistan, Poland, Tunisia, the United Arab Republic (Egypt), and Yugoslavia.

The United States Social and Rehabilitation Service in 1971 sponsored an international seminar on the utilization of research results in vocational rehabilitation under a grant to the International Association of Rehabilitation Facilities, which is primarily a United States organization. Scientists were brought to the United States for the seminar, not only from the nations in which the SRS sponsors research and demonstration grants, but also from leading institutions throughout the world. The same year it also sponsored, in association with the American Association for Mental Deficiency, a similar three week seminar on the utilization of research findings in the vocational rehabilitation of the mentally retarded. Later in 1971, a Pan-Pacific Conference on mental retardation, to which leaders in this field from the Asian nations were invited, was held in Hawaii under the auspices of the President's Committee on Mental Retardation.

The external Aid Office of Canada has also assisted the National Rehabilitation Institute in Vietnam through the construction, equipping, and providing expert consultants and other aid for a branch of the National Rehabilitation Institute in Qui Nhon. The construction and equipping of the Center was provided by the World Rehabilitation Fund under a contract with the External Aid Office of Canada; the provision of expert consultants and other assistance is provided by the Rehabilitation Institute of Montreal under a similar contract with the External Aid Office of Canada. Under this contract, the Rehabilitation Institute of Montreal is also assisting in the establishment of a school of physical therapy in Vietnam, with a three-year curriculum designed to meet the standards of the World Confederation for Physical Therapy. The External Aid Office of Canada is also providing technical assistance in medical rehabilitation in Cameroon in association with Cardinal Leger and his endeavors.

Leaders in technical assistance in rehabilitation in Europe have been the Scandinavian countries, particularly Denmark. The government of Denmark has regularly given substantial contributions to the United Nations over and above its assessment, particularly for bringing personnel from undeveloped nations to Denmark for long- and short-term training in various aspects of rehabilitation services. Postgraduate training of physicians in Denmark under this program, which has included observation visits to rehabilitation facilities in Norway, Sweden, and Finland, has been conducted in cooperation with the World Health Organization. Similar long-term training and particularly short-term courses and conferences in prosthetics and orthotics in Denmark, have been cooperative projects with the United Nations.

Bilateral technical assistance in rehabilitation provided by other nations of Western Europe has been relatively limited but has grown in recent years, particularly in aiding rehabilitation services in the developing nations of Africa. Israel has supported projects in Africa, and Japan and Taiwan have conducted technical assistance projects in rehabilitation in Vietnam.

INTERNATIONAL VOLUNTARY AGENCIES

INTERNATIONAL SOCIETY FOR REHABILITATION
OF THE DISABLED (ISRD)

The International Society for Rehabilitation of the Disabled was organized in 1922 when the Ontario (Canada) Society for Crippled Children asked to become affiliated with the National Society for Crippled Children (United States), which had been formed in 1921 by state societies for crippled children in Michigan, New York, Illinois, and Ohio. The program was later expanded to include other states in the United States and other provinces in Canada. In 1927 the Rotary International arranged to have Paul H. King of the United States be Chairman of a conference on the problems of crippled children, which was held at the Rotary International's annual meeting in Ostend, Belgium. Two years later the World Federation of Educational Associations, met in Geneva with 100 delegates from twelve countries. The International Society was asked to join in the planning of educational programs for handicapped children. This first World Congress ended with the appointment of a Committee of International Development headed by Mr. King, with representatives of the twelve countries attending the meeting.

The second World Congress was held at The Hague in 1931, with 170 delegates from 23 nations. The third World Congress convened in Budapest in 1936, and plans were made to organize a national society for crippled children and adults to function in the United States and for the International Society (then known as the International Society for the Welfare of Cripples) to become a truly international organization, with headquarters in Cleveland. The reorganization took place in 1939.

The new organization held a fourth World Congress in London in 1939. Delegates from thirty nations attended this Congress, at which tentative plans were made to hold another World Congress in two years, in Norway or Palestine. The war in Europe had started before the delegates reached their homes. Primarily through the efforts of Belle Greve, who served as the voluntary Secretary-General of the International Society, contacts were maintained with the European members during the war, and new contacts were developed in Mexico and Latin America. In 1949 the International Society established its first Secretariat, with paid staff, in New York City, and Donald V. Wilson as Secretary-General. Since then, the International Society has constantly increased its membership and services, and in 1971 it had 87 organizations in 62 nations as its members. It also has four international associations as its affiliates—International Cerebral Palsy Society, with headquarters in London; World Federation of Hemophilia, with headquarters in Montreal; International Bureau for Epilepsy, with headquarters in London, and Cardinal Leger and his Endeavors, with headquarters in West Montreal. The organization is the only world-wide nongovernmental federation devoted solely to work for the prevention of all types of disability and for the rehabilitation of disabled persons.

Since World War II, world congresses on rehabilitation sponsored by the International Society have been held in Stockholm in 1951, The Hague in 1954, London in 1957, New York City in 1960, Copenhagen in 1963, Wiesbaden in 1966, Dublin in 1969, and Sydney in 1972. At the eighth World Congress, held in New York City in 1960, the name of the Society was officially changed from the International Society of the Welfare of Cripples to the International Society for Rehabilitation of the Disabled. At the World Congress in Wiesbaden in 1966, Mr. Wilson resigned as Secretary-General and was succeeded by Mr. Norman Acton, a member of the International Society's staff in the early 1950s.

The International Society has also sponsored five Pan Pacific Congresses on Rehabilitation—in Australia in 1958, the Philippines in 1962, Tokyo in 1965, Hongkong in 1968, and the fifth Pan Pacific Congress in Australia in 1972, in conjunction with the twelfth World Congress.

The Society sponsored sessions or working groups at many other international professional meetings, such as the meetings of the International Conference of Social Work. It has also cosponsored many regional and national meetings devoted to regional problems, and programs of rehabilitation on specific aspects of rehabilitation, such as legislation, employment, vocational rehabilitation, and public relations.

In 1970 the International Society adopted a new working name, "Rehabilitation International." At its Council meeting in Rome in 1971 the International Society voted to change its national affiliate, which had been the National Easter Seal Society for Crippled Children and Adults, to a newly incorporated body, "Rehabilitation International, U.S.A." As the principal international spokesman for its field, Rehabilitation International maintains official status with the United Nations Economic and Social Council, the World Health Organization, the International Labour Office, the United Nations Educational, Scientific and Cultural Organization (UNESCO), UNICEF, and several regional bodies. It provides the Secretariat for the Council of World Organizations Interested in the Handicapped, a coordinating body of all major international nongovernmental organizations active in rehabilitation and working with the agencies in the United Nations family.

The program of Rehabilitation International is planned and carried out with the assistance of four standing Commissions dealing respectively with the educational, medical, social, and vocational aspects of rehabilitation. Among the principal activities are the preparation and distribution of information needed for professional training and public education, the organization of World Congresses and of more specialized technical meetings, the provision of expert guidance to those who are developing programs, the collection and dissemination of data about relevant research projects, and the granting of technical assistance to the developing countries.

INTERNATIONAL PROFESSIONAL ORGANIZATIONS

Working in close cooperation with the United Nations and its Specialized Agencies are a number of international professional organizations concerned with various aspects of rehabilitation. Among them is the International Federation of Physical Medicine, with its Headquarters in the Netherlands; The World Confederation of Physical Therapists, with its Headquarters in London; The World Federation of Occupational Therapists, which currently has its Headquarters in Canada; the International Society of Prosthetists and Orthotists, which has its Headquarters in Denmark; the International Association of Technicians in Orthotics and Prosthetics, which has its Headquarters in New York; and the World Council for the Welfare of the Blind, which has its Headquarters in Paris.

UNITED STATES VOLUNTARY AGENCIES

WORLD REHABILITATION FUND

The World Rehabilitation Fund was founded in 1955 to assist in developing, extending, and improving rehabilitation services throughout the world. Its primary emphasis has been on the training of rehabilitation personnel. During its first fifteen years the World Rehabilitation Fund has provided postgraduate training in rehabilitation medicine on a long-term basis (one to three years) for over 500 physicians from 57 nations. It has also assisted over 1,000 physicians, therapists, and other rehabilitation personnel from other countries to participate in short-term training programs and observation periods in the United States.

Since 1960 the World Rehabilitation Fund, in cooperation with many other agencies, has conducted a series of four- to six-month training programs in prosthetics and orthotics in underdeveloped countries. Approximately 350 technicians have received training in these programs. It has also provided technical consultation in prosthetics and orthotics in most of the underdeveloped nations in Latin America, the Near East, and Africa. Under a contract from the United States Department of State, the World Rehabilitation Fund constructed and equipped the John F. Kennedy Memorial Center for Spastic Children and the World Rehabilitation Fund Day Centre in Hong Kong, and then supplied trained personnel. Since October 1965 the World Rehabilitation Fund, under a contract with the United States Agency for International Development, has been assisting the National Rehabilitation Institute in Saigon and its branch centers in Cantho, Danang, and Qui Nhon in strengthening and expanding its services. The Qui Nhon Center was constructed by the World Rehabilitation Fund under a contract with the External Aid Office of Canada.

In March 1971 the World Rehabilitation Fund began a new contract with AID to provide for a team of United States experts in vocational rehabilitation, special education, and sheltered workshops to advise the

Republic of Vietnam in establishing vocational rehabilitation facilities and training programs. Its activities have included providing operational funds for the San Pablo Rehabilitation Center in a rural area of the Philippines; the collection and overseas shipment of used but serviceable artificial limbs and braces; and provision of such professional literature as audio tapes, films, books, and periodicals. The principal officers of the World Rehabilitation Fund are Howard A. Rusk, David A. Morse, and Eugene J. Taylor. The late Mary E. Switzer was also a principal officer of this Fund.

COMMITTEE ON THE HANDICAPPED, PEOPLE TO PEOPLE PROGRAM

The Committee on the Handicapped disseminates information on rehabilitation and employment of the handicapped internationally, aids rehabilitation specialists from other countries visiting the United States in planning their itineraries, assists Americans interested in rehabilitation in planning itineraries for visitations to rehabilitation facilities in other nations, and solicits and ships rehabilitation equipment and supplies to rehabilitation programs in other countries.

GOODWILL INDUSTRIES OF AMERICA

The Goodwill Industries of America has been active for more than twenty years in a growing program of providing technical guidance to voluntary groups in other countries wishing to establish vocational rehabilitation facilities or sheltered workshops patterned after the programs of the Goodwill Industries. Its major activities have been in, but not limited to, the Caribbean and Central and South America.

AMERICAN FOUNDATION FOR THE OVERSEAS BLIND

The American Foundation for the Overseas Blind operates a network of services for the blind in seventy countries. Included are education, rehabilitation, professional preparation, and braille publishing facilities. Major projects in Europe, Asia, Latin America, and the Middle East include teacher-training programs, prevention of blindness, rehabilitation centers, international conferences, and development of specialized techniques for multihandicapped blind children. The Foundation maintains offices in Asia, Europe, and Latin America.

THE AMERICAN-KOREAN FOUNDATION

As a part of its program of technical assistance to Korea, the American-Korean Foundation has provided fellowships for Koreans for training in rehabilitation in the United States as well as assisting a number of rehabilitation projects in Korea.

THE PRESIDENT'S COMMITTEE ON THE
EMPLOYMENT OF THE HANDICAPPED

Although its program is directed primarily toward public and employer education on the values of employing the handicapped, the President's Committee for many years has had international participation in its annual meeting, and in 1970 established a Subcommittee on International Affairs.

CARE

As a part of its worldwide program, CARE has from time to time provided equipment and other support for rehabilitation projects in other countries. It also provides overseas shipping of used but serviceable artificial limbs collected in the United States by the World Rehabilitation Fund.

AMERICAN NATIONAL RED CROSS

American National Red Cross has assisted from time to time in the recruitment and provision of personnel in other countries, particularly in the Caribbean, which have suffered such disasters as major polio epidemics. It has also participated in such disaster programs involving rehabilitation sponsored by the International League of Red Cross Societies. Major among these was the large-scale rehabilitation project in Morocco in 1959 in which 10,000 Moroccans became paralyzed as a result of using adulterated cooking oil.

RELIGIOUS ORGANIZATIONS

CHURCH WORLD SERVICES

Church World Services has sponsored a number of rehabilitation activities in other countries, such as the Church World Service amputee project in Korea, which provided equipment, prosthetic, and orthotic equipment; the Fund for the Disabled in Ethiopia; and the provision of the services of American physical therapists in Korea and Vietnam.

CATHOLIC RELIEF SERVICES

Catholic Relief Services, as a part of its worldwide program, has assisted in some overseas rehabilitation activities. It also provides overseas shipping for used but artificial limbs and for braces collected by the World Rehabilitation Fund.

THE SALVATION ARMY

Some rehabilitation services have been included in the overseas medical missionary work of the Salvation Army, particularly in India.

THE AMERICAN FRIENDS SERVICE COMMITTEE

The American Friends Service Committee has assisted in overseas rehabilitation projects, a major one being the sponsorship of a large medical rehabilitation center in Quang Ngai province, Vietnam.

A number of other religious organizations, such as the Central Mennonite Committee, have assisted in various rehabilitation projects in other countries. Since this book is primarily for American readers, no attempt has been made to list or describe the bilateral international assistance activities of many of the national voluntary agencies in other countries.

In conclusion, the underlying theme of all current international effort on behalf of the disabled has been set by the United Nations as follows:

First, that the handicapped person is an individual with full human rights, which he shares in common with the able-bodied. He is entitled to receive from his country every possible measure of protection, assistance, and opportunity for rehabilitation.

Second, by the very nature of his physical handicap he is exposed to the danger of emotional and psychological disturbance, resulting from a deep sense of deprivation and frustration, and therefore has a special claim on society for sympathy and constructive help.

Third, he is capable of developing his residual resources to an unexpected degree, if given the right opportunities of so doing, and of becoming in most instances an economic asset to the country instead of being a burden on himself, on his family, and on the state.

Fourth, handicapped persons have a responsibility to the community to contribute their services to the economic welfare of the nation in any way that becomes possible after rehabilitation and training.

Fifth, the chief longing of the physically handicapped person is to achieve independence within a normal community, instead of spending the rest of his life in a segregated institution, or within an environment of disability.

Sixth, the rehabilitation of the physically handicapped can be accomplished successfully only by a combination of medical, educational, social, and vocational services, working together as a team.

The first task, which confronts all international agencies, is that of using all possible means to secure general acceptance throughout the world of this new conception of physical disability (United Nations, 1963).

REFERENCES AND RESOURCES

Proceedings of the World Congresses of the International Society for Rehabilitation of the Disabled: Stockholm 1951; The Hague 1954; London 1957; New York 1960; Copenhagen 1963; Wiesbaden 1966; Dublin 1969. New York, International Society for Rehabilitation of the Disabled.

Rehabilitation of the Disabled in 51 countries. December, 1964. Washington, D.C., United States Department of Health, Education and Welfare, Superintendent of Documents, United States Government Printing Office.

Rehabilitation: New talent for the community. 1969. Proceedings of the 4th Pan Pacific Rehabilitation Conference, September 1st–7th, 1968. Hong Kong; Joint Council for the Physically and Mentally Disabled.

Taylor, Wallace W. and Isabelle W. Taylor. 1967. Services for handicapped children in England and Wales. New York, International Society for Rehabilitation of the Disabled.

——1970. Services for the handicapped in India. New York, International Society for Rehabilitation of the Disabled.

United Nations. 1963. Rehabilitation of the Handicapped.

United Nations Secretariat. Summary of Information on Projects and Activities in the Field of Rehabilitation of the Disabled. Annual Reports.

Sources of information concerning international rehabilitation activities include the following organizations:

Committee for the Handicapped
People-to-People Program
1146 16th Street, N.W.
Washington, D.C. 20036

Community Health Services
World Health Organization (WHO)
1211 Geneva 27, Switzerland

Division of Equality to Access to Education
United Nations Educational, Scientific and Cultural Organization (UNESCO)
B. P. 3.07
Place de Fontenoy
75 Paris-7^e, France

Division of International Activities
Social and Rehabilitation Service
Department of Health, Education and Welfare
Washington, D.C. 20201

Human Resources Development Department
International Labour Organization (ILO)
CH 1211 Geneva 22, Switzerland

International Society for Rehabilitation of the Disabled
219 West 44th Street
New York, New York 10017

Pan American Health Organization (PAHO)
525 23rd Street, N.W.
Washington, D.C. 20037

Rehabilitation Unit for the Handicapped
United Nations, New York 10017

United Nations Children's Fund (UNICEF)
United Nations, New York 10017

World Rehabilitation Fund, Inc.
400 East 34th Street
New York, New York 10016

INDEX

Abercrombie, M. L. J. and others, cited, 244

Abilities, Incorporated, 103

Abrams, R. D. and J. R. Finesinger, 178

Acton, Norman, 540

Adams, G. F. and S. B. McComb, cited, 322

Addiction in cancer therapy, 159

Adler, Alfred, cited, 180

Adler, E., cited, 295, 315, 316

Africa: rehabilitation activities in, 530, 537, 538, 539, 542, 543, 544, 545

Aged: homebound, services for, 81, 109; cancer patients, 161; heart patients, 231; osteoarthritis, 367, 381; amputees, 398, 400, 402 (chart); blind, 434, 442, 448, 453

Agency, rehabilitation, defined, 14

Age of occurrence of disability: chronic illness, 121; cerebral palsy, 249, 299; hemiplegia, 294, 295, 299-300, 315; stroke, 331; arthritis, 364, 367, 368, 369, 370, 371; amputation, 399-400, 402 (chart), 403; blind, 434-35; deaf-blind, 503

Agnosia, 338-39

Agrammatism, 341

Alexander, F., cited, 379, 381

Alexander, Franz, 178; cited, 180

Allen, R., cited, 301

Ambulatory programs: heart disease, 212-13; hemiplegia, 310-11

American Academy for Cerebral Palsy, 281

American Academy of Physical Medicine and Rehabilitation, 310

American Association on Mental Deficiency, 263

American Cancer Society, 196; cited, 151, 153, 157, 163, 168; Reach to Recovery Program, 166

American Congress of Rehabilitation Medicine, 310

American Foundation for the Blind, 455; *Directory of Agencies Serving the Blind and Visually Handicapped in the United States,* 438, 455-56

American Foundation for the Overseas Blind, 543

American Friends Service Committee, 545

American Heart Association, cited, 210, 295, 308

American-Korean Foundation, 544

American National Red Cross, 544

American Printing House for the Blind, 455; cited, 434

American Rheumatism Association, 365; cited, 366, 380

Amputation, 144; cancer patients, 156, 164-66, 190, 192; causes, 399, 402 (chart); incidence, 399-400, 402 (chart); age of occurrence, 399-400, 402 (chart), 403; types, 400-3, 407-8